DEMON DOCTORS

Physicians as Serial Killers

DEMON DOCTORS

Physicians as Serial Killers

Kenneth V. Iserson, M.D.

GALEN PRESS, LTD. • TUCSON, ARIZONA

Galen Press, Ltd.
P.O. Box 64400
Tucson, AZ 85728-4400
Phone: (520) 577-8363   Fax: (520) 529-6459
Orders: (800) 442-5369 (U.S./Canada)

www.galenpress.com

ISBN: 1-883620-29-5

Cover photos: Dr. Marcel Petiot (large), who was guillotined in Paris in 1946; Dr. Thomas Neill Cream (top small), who was hanged in 1892; Linda Burfield Hazzard, D.O. (bottom small), who starved her patients to death.

Library of Congress Cataloging-in-Publication Data

Iserson, Kenneth V.
    Demon doctors : physicians as serial killers / Kenneth V. Iserson.
       p. ; cm.
    Includes bibliographical references and index.
    ISBN 1-883620-29-5 (pbk.)
       1. Physicians. 2. Serial murderers. 3. Serial murders. 4. Physicians—
    Miscellanea. I. Title.

R706 .I83 2002
610—dc21   2002068426

Printed in The United States of America

10   9   8   7   6   5   4   3   2   1

Table of Contents

Preface

The Hippocratic Oath reads, in part:

> I swear by Apollo Physician and Asclepias and Hygeia and Panacea . . .
> that I will keep the sick from harm and injustice. I will neither give a
> deadly drug to anybody, even if asked for it . . . Whatever houses I may
> visit, I will come for the benefit of the sick, remaining free of all inten-
> tional injustice, of all mischief . . . If I fulfill this oath and do not violate
> it, may it be granted to me to enjoy life and art, being honored with
> fame among all men for all time to come; if I transgress it and swear
> falsely, may the opposite be my lot.

The physicians whose stories are related in this book all subscribed to this or a
similar covenant. Clearly, "the opposite" was their "lot."

For more than thirty years, I have studied, practiced, taught, and written about
medicine. My medical practice has been that of an emergency physician at
major medical centers. Before that, in the early (pre-paramedic) days, I drove
an ambulance. I love the profession to which I have devoted my life. So, imagine my shock when, while doing research for another book (*Death to Dust:
What Happens to Dead Bodies?*, Galen Press, Ltd., 2001), I stumbled upon a list
of physician-killers. I take seriously the Hippocratic injunction "to do good,
but at least do no harm." Therefore, I was appalled to find that, over the years,
some of my colleagues had not only killed but also become infamous.

vii

Endeavoring to learn more about medicine's dark underbelly, I plunged into the obscure and nearly forgotten world of "old medicine," including the strange practices that were once the norm. I initially believed that few physician-killers would be of the type described in this book: serial killers, mass murderers, and the notorious killers detailed in Chapter 8, *The Minor Players*. I was wrong. The more I researched this bizarre topic, the more physician-killers I discovered. So many, in fact, that several will be the subjects of a second book called *Demonic Doctors: More Physician-Killers*.

This book describes some of those physicians who, either as individuals or as part of a group, have intentionally killed. Given their power, their prestige, the pressures they are under, and the knowledge that they possess or can easily obtain, it is surprising that so few physicians have strayed this badly— *or, at least, that so few have been caught.*

How could it happen that physicians continue to engage in murderous careers, some spanning decades, without the medical establishment intervening? In some cases, colleagues remain silent; in others, they tacitly abet the killer. Nurses may point out problems, but no one wants to listen. And those charged with overseeing the profession are too often engaged in damage control—or simply not paying attention. We are lucky that few physicians are bent on murder; it seems to be easy for them to get away with it.

These stories of medical murderers also offer a look at societies and medical practices during the past two centuries. It's an apt method for presenting medical history, for, as Ralph Waldo Emerson said, "There is properly no history; only biography." More specifically, as Richard Cobb noted in his book, *A Second Identity*, "Murder trials light up the years and give a more precise sense of period than the reigns of monarchs or the terms of office of presidents."

To add some flavor of the events and to introduce each villain or group of villains, every chapter (except for *The Minor Players*) begins with a *fictionalized account in italics*, characterizing the events about to be described. While this book is a non-fiction account of what transpired, I have taken some liberties in these italicized sections. To the best of my knowledge, they represent what probably occurred—although there generally were few, or no, surviving witnesses. To ensure accuracy and to provide a sense of the times, I have used direct quotations from contemporary periodicals and records of official proceedings wherever possible. Finally, each chapter (except *The Minor Players*) has an addendum that illuminates unusual or historical aspects of the story or of society at that time.

Acknowledgements

Only one name appears as the author of this book. Any project of this magnitude, however, requires the assistance and support of multiple individuals. I am grateful for their help.

At every stage of production, my wife, Mary Lou Iserson, contributed enormously. She acted as in-house editor (sometimes offering cruel and unusual suggestions), reference checker, and a source for new ideas. Without her assistance, this book would not have been published.

She was ably assisted by the excellent editorial work of my friend and editor, Jennifer Gilbert, who carefully emended the manuscript while teaching me the rules of English usage I consistently tried to ignore. Lisa Bowden produced the book's eerie cover and Anne Olson designed the interior, making reading it more enjoyable.

Three individuals suffered through the gestational pains of birthing this book, reading early drafts of each chapter and giving me excellent advice on ways to clarify the text. Despite their own busy schedules—only busy people could have provided this type of feedback—they offered me useful and unique comments. I owe a great debt to Don Witzke, Ph.D. of the University of Kentucky Medical School at Lexington (as a psychologist who works with the school's pathology department, Don was not overly disturbed by the content); Steve Nash, J.D., executive director of the Pima County, Arizona, Medical Society (who liked the book "just a little too much"); and Alan Reeter, M.S.E.E., president of Medfilms Inc. in Tucson, Arizona (whose nurse-wife said that the subject was too horrible to read about).

Hannah Fisher, R.N., M.LS., AHIP, Associate Librarian, is an unbelievably knowledgeable reference librarian at the University of Arizona Health Sciences Library. She continues to be a valuable resource in locating and verifying many of the bizarre and obscure citations.

An extraordinary detective has helped me at every step in preparing this text. Nga T. Nguyen, B.A., B.S., Senior Library Specialist, is able to locate sources and information when everyone else has declared the search "impossible." Similarly, Robert Fisher, M.LS., who can only be described as a walking encyclopedia and a genuinely nice guy, has continued his noble efforts as my research assistant.

Throughout the book's preparation, the entire University of Arizona Health Sciences Library Information Services Section helped beyond measure. Of special note are Mary L. Riordan, M.LS., Associate Librarian; Fred Heidenreich, M.LS., Librarian; and the interlibrary loan staff.

A number of very special people reviewed the book in part or in its entirety. While any errors or misstatements are mine alone, these individuals helped reduce their numbers. Professor Sheldon Harris, of California State University at Northridge and the author of *Factories of Death: Japanese Biological Warfare, 1932–45, and the American Cover-Up*, reviewed the chapter on Japan's biowarfare experiments. Brian Whittle, editor of Cavendish Press in Manchester, England, and co-author of *Prescription for Murder: The True Story of Mass Murderer Dr. Harold Frederick Shipman*, reviewed that infamous killer's chapter. My longtime friend, Kris Foti, Ph.D., a clinical psychologist with First Correctional Medical, and my new friend, Ronald Holmes, Ph.D., a professor at the University of Louisville, co-author of *Profiling Violent Crimes: An Investigative Tool, 2nd ed.*, and an expert on serial killers, reviewed the Introduction to correct both psychological and historical inaccuracies. Some of my relatives were also kind enough to offer their comments, including my brother, Lawrence S. Iserson of Lakewood, New Jersey, and my nephew, David Iserson (a talented budding TV-comedy writer and screenwriter; does anyone have a job opening?), who lives, naturally, in Hollywood, California.

When I needed additional information, clarification, and translation of source materials, some wonderful people came to my assistance. Professor David Soren, a true Renaissance educator and archeologist from the University of Arizona, sat with me for many hours while we extracted information on the terrifying French psychopath, Dr. Marcel Petiot. Adaline Klemmedson, vice president of Administrative & Corporate Relations at University Medical

Center in Tucson, Arizona, and her family, helped with the Russian for the chapter about Stalin's "Doctors' Plots." Jennifer Uno, a friend from the emergency department, reviewed the Japanese proper names with her mother. When I needed someone to review the infectious disease material related to biowarfare, I turned to Rod Adams, M.D., an infectious diseases specialist at the University of Arizona College of Medicine. Likewise, when I needed technical information about toxins, my source was Stacy L. Haber, Pharm.D., a clinical assistant professor at the University of Arizona College of Pharmacy.

W. Seth Carus, Ph.D., author of *Bioterrorism and Biocrimes: The Illicit Use of Biological Agents Since 1900* and a senior research professor at National Defense University, not only provided great source material from his book but also kindly provided me with (non-classified) information and sources to flesh out the information about the various Japanese killers. One of those sources was Mr. Masaaki Sugishima at Asahi University Law School in Gifu, Japan.

Several individuals helped track down pictures for the book, among them are: Bob Schuler in Special Collections at the Tacoma (Washington) Public Library; Daniel Coleman, Special Collections, Kansas City, Missouri Public Library; Marilyn Rader with A/P Wide World Photos; and Sharon Wells of PictureQuest.

Finally, thanks go to the wonderful professionals at Galen Press, Ltd., who believed in the importance of *Demon Doctors*, and without whom this book would not have been possible. If I have inadvertently omitted anyone, I truly regret it. The list above, however, attests to the wonderful cooperation I received while compiling this book. For the help these people provided to me, I owe a great debt of thanks.

It is now time for careful readers to detect any other errors I may have made. Enjoy!

Kenneth V. Iserson, M.D.
Tucson, Arizona

Introduction

Physicians as Multiple Murderers

The subject of real-life murder is morbid and sordid, a far remove from the neatly arranged fictional treatment of the crime. Yet both factual and fictional murder is one of the most popular subjects in literature.

— Orlo Miller, *Twenty Mortal Murders:*
Bizarre Murder Cases from Canada's Past

Murder has always fascinated us. The Old Testament, for example, first grabs the reader with the temptations and excesses in the Garden of Eden and, soon afterwards, with Cain's murder of his brother. As Henry Thomas Buckle noted in his nineteenth-century book, *The History of Civilization in England*:

> Of all offences, it might well be supposed that the crime of murder is one of the most arbitrary and irregular . . . the fact is that murder is committed with as much regularity, and bears as uniform a relation to certain known circumstances, as do the movements of the tides, and the rotation of the seasons.

Today, the media has made murder seem routine. At least one killing is almost obligatory in most novels, television programs, and movies. Newspapers, news magazines, and news programs routinely try to outdo themselves in following the editor's traditional injunction: If it bleeds, it leads.

One reason for our fascination is that we see ourselves as potential victims. It is not just that John F. Kennedy and John Lennon were murdered—the next life taken could be our own or that of a loved one. In reality, killers and their victims are most often friends or family, making murder the most personal of crimes. While murder might seem beyond the capability of the people we know, a national survey in the United States found that 67 percent of men and 57 percent of women believe that anyone is capable of committing murder if pushed far enough by rage or passion.

Although we may identify with the victims, we continue to believe that we share nothing in common with their killers. Alexander Solzhenitsyn noted:

> If only it were all so simple! If only there were evil people somewhere committing evil deeds, and it were necessary only to separate them from the rest of us and destroy them. But the line dividing good and evil cuts through the heart of every human being. And who is willing to destroy a piece of his own heart?

Theodore Reik agreed in *The Unknown Murderer*:

> Middle-class society likes to represent the gulf between itself and the law breakers as unbridgeable, and is frightened to find that even mass-murderers are made of the same stuff and behave in all walks of life like the rest of us—your very neighbor might be a murderer.

Ordinary murders do not capture our imagination. Rather, we remember those that have no discernible motive, a horrible method, or a large number of victims. That rarest of breeds, the doctor-killer, has always exerted a hold on the public's imagination, and any such case becomes a "cause célèbre." We are horrified that a doctor who is supposed to save lives would deliberately take them. But at the same time, we are fascinated because this symbol of middle-class success and respectability, with intimate access to the victims, has broken society's rules.

Although isolated murders have become commonplace, repeated or serial killing is a heinous deviation. John Douglas, the famous Federal Bureau of Investigation (FBI) profiler, wrote in *The Anatomy of Motive*, "As decent, sensitive human beings, anytime we see someone capable of multiple murders, we are instantly repulsed. The circumstances hardly matter." The continuing production of serial killer-based books and movies attests to our enduring fascination with individuals who consciously decide to kill. While serial killers are not common and the chance of encountering one is less than that of being struck by lightening, their dark and foreboding image, like the shark from *Jaws*, has become a permanent resident of the modern psyche.

What is the difference between mass murderers, serial killers, spree killers, and assassins?

Different types of individuals with unique motivations commit multiple murders, which some have described as "multicide." Although multiple murderers, by definition, kill many people, FBI profilers have divided them into three basic categories based on the killer's behavior: mass murderers, serial killers, and spree killers or assassins.

Mass Murderers

Mass murder is defined as killing four or more victims in a single episode at one location. The killings are all part of the same emotional experience, although the incident may occur within a few minutes or over a period of hours. White males in their mid- to late forties generally commit these crimes, although adolescents have recently begun committing mass murder.

Mass murderers are considered "mission oriented." When they kill, it is usually in a location with which they are familiar—their school, work site, or home—where they open fire (most use firearms) and kill indiscriminately. Their goal is to make a statement and, usually, to either kill themselves or commit "suicide by cop," dying in what they would term a "blaze of glory."

Typically, these killers are asocial loners who rarely blend into the community. In most cases, acute stress precipitates the act. Before the murders, these killers seethe with anger and frustration; they are often described as "pressure cookers waiting to explode." Mass murderers are generally much more comfortable with the written word, and may write letters to newspapers and government officials or vent their frustrations, hate, and anger in a diary. Eventually, they exact revenge on those who they feel ignored them. These depressed, paranoid individuals may see themselves as heroic agents of good or of retribution, but those who survive find that the experience increases their mental anguish.

Of the physician-killers in this book, only the Japanese doctors in Chapter 8 fall into this category. They repeatedly committed mass murder for nationalistic and scientific purposes. FBI profilers did not have that type of organized group killing in mind when they devised their categories. The motives and attitudes of these Japanese doctors were distinctly different from the norm. So was the outcome: These physician-killers not only escaped, but also prospered.

Serial Killers

Serial murder is defined as killing people in three or more separate events (although the range experts use is from two to four) with an emotional cooling-off period between the murders. Most other physicians in this book, with the exception of the Russians in Chapter 5 and the "Minor Players" in Chapter 7, are serial killers. Usually serial murders occur at separate locations, but not always. (Drs. Holmes and Petiot constructed specially designed killing structures, and did not need to change locations.) These episodes are emotionally distinct and separate, and demonstrate deliberate premeditation. In rare cases, serial killers work in pairs, as did Henry Lee Lucas and Ottis Toole, who both had the same psychopathology.

Serial killers carefully select their victims to fulfill their fantasies, which may include hunting humans for the sexual thrill. They meticulously plan their killings, and strike only when the time is right, carefully managing their activities to avoid detection. They almost uniformly believe that they can outwit the police and will stop killing temporarily if they feel that they may be caught. Thus, the period between their killings can be days, weeks, or even months.

Unlike mass murderers, serial killers most often project a completely normal persona. As Douglas & Olshaker noted:

> Often, when a serial killer in the United States is apprehended, neighbors, acquaintances, or coworkers will express shock, saying that he was the last person in the world they would have suspected of being a vicious murderer. He seemed so charming, or he seemed so ordinary. He seemed to get on so well with his wife or girlfriend.

So thoroughly do they conceal their psychopathology and killings that only in rare cases are the killer's intimates aware of their activities.

In reality, these individuals are obsessive, hyper-narcissistic ritualistic killers. Fantasies of their victims and killings preoccupy them. Often, they keep souvenirs, such as those found in Jeffrey Dahmer's refrigerator; some even keep detailed records. The pain these deviants cause originates from a pathological desire for complete mastery over their victims: they want to engulf and to annihilate them. The serial-killing cannibals, such as Dahmer or the semi-fictional Dr. Hannibal "the Cannibal" Lector, go even further and actually consume their victims.

Spree Killers and Assassins

Two other groups warrant mentioning, although they are not represented among the physician-killers in this book. Spree killers murder many victims at different locations within hours or days of each other. Bonnie and Clyde may be the best-known U.S. spree killers. Unlike serial killers, they remain on an emotional high and have no cooling-off period between killings. The authorities must recognize a pattern to identify serial killers: police generally know who spree killers are, but must determine *where* they will strike next.

Assassins act like stalkers. Before the killing, they shadow the intended victim, who may be a famous person, criminal, or simply the object of their obsession. Assassins are sometimes professionals (or think that they are). It is often difficult to identify and locate assassins, especially if they have no direct connection with the victim.

Some murderers do not fit neatly into any one category. As Douglas & Olshaker wrote:

> We sometimes see these designations of killers combined. The most common of these would be the serial killer who degenerates into a spree killer, as Ted Bundy did at the end. As he worked himself up into more and more of a frenzy, his cooling-off period grew shorter and shorter until it essentially went away. At that point, the stresses grew; he became more intense, sloppier; he exercised poorer judgment in terms of being able to get away. And we're always looking for that phase with a guy who's on the loose and active.

Most multiple murders are sociopaths, but the psychological terminology can be confusing. The characteristics that are central to this psychopathology include a lack of interpersonal affect, lack of concern with conventional morality, lack of gross psychopathology, and low ideological commitments. In addition, these killers often rape their victims, not solely for sexual gratification, but as an expression of power and anger. Nancy H. Allen noted that the presence of certain elements results in a higher likelihood of an individual becoming a multiple murderer. These factors are listed in the box on page 6.

See Chapter 10, *Serial Killers: Psychology and Behavior* for more detailed information about serial killers.

How were the killers in this book selected?

The doctors in this book represent a cross-section of physician-multiple murderers: the psychopaths, the greedy, the zealots promoting unproven treatments, and those whose nationalistic fervor blinded them to their humanity. These stories are all true and are far more bizarre than any fiction writer would dare to concoct. Without question, these physicians operated outside the law.

Although many societies continue to debate the ethical boundaries of medical practice, such as the physician's role in assisting suicide, most physicians act within the law or, at least, they *and their patients* believe that they are doing the right things for the right reasons. The monsters in this book went far beyond what humanity accepts as just or right.

Predisposing Factors of Multiple Murderers

Past History

- Experience of early violence, such as being a battered child
- No close and trustworthy loved ones
- Poor daily functioning
- Unstable lifestyle, low socioeconomic status, or unemployed
- School dropout, semiliterate, or illiterate
- Live in poor housing or crowded slums
- A long history of being a loner, antisocial, and withdrawn
- Chronic drug or alcohol abuse A history of psychiatric problems with a negative view about seeking help

Psychological State

- Easily aroused to anxiety or panic
- Chronically moody; chronic poor self-image
- Markedly aggressive and angry with poor impulse control (The three childhood traits typical/predictive of later violence— bedwetting, fire setting, and cruelty to other children or animals— are all problems with impulse control.)
- Possesses few coping strategies and, under stress, behaves in socially unacceptable ways
- Lack of contact with reality
- Is unaware of the availability of help or cannot make use of those resources
- History of arrests and imprisonment
- Strong desire never to return to prison
- Has previously assaulted or attempted murder
- Has a plan for murdering
- Has a weapon available

Adapted from Annel NH: "Reflections on Homicides." In: Danto BL, Bruhns J, Kutscher AH (eds.): *The Human Side of Homicide.* New York: Columbia Univ. Press, 1982.

The physicians in this book represent three types of multiple murderers. Most followed the typical serial killer pattern, although they wore the mantle of successful physicians. (See Chapter 10, *Serial Killers: Psychology and Behavior* for in-depth information on serial killers.) Additional notorious physician-serial killers, such as Dr. Michael Swango, who is currently incarcerated and is suspected of killing patients in several countries, have been not been included because their cases are still making headlines. Some of them will be discussed in my next book, *Demonic Doctors: More Physician-Serial Killers*.

The second group is physicians who are political killers. These mass murderers kill, either directly or indirectly, under the auspices of a corrupt and vicious political regime. Chapter 8, *Japan's Inhuman Experiments*, is the sole example in this book of physician-directed killings on a mass scale. Although their story is virtually unknown, unlike that of the Nazi physicians (to be included in *Demonic Doctors*), a similar herd mentality and nationalism gone amok resulted in tens of thousands of murders in the name of medical science. Unbelievably, the world has virtually ignored these deplorable incidents, and many of the perpetrators subsequently prospered.

The physicians in Chapter 7, *The Minor Players*, fall into the third group, episodic killers. This chapter is a compilation of interesting cases about physicians who murdered due to love, hate, psychosis, greed, fear, and anger. They killed for very personal reasons, and most victims were family members, friends, co-workers, or rivals. Their killings made national and international headlines when they occurred, although many have now faded into distant memory.

In two instances, both described in Chapter 5, *The Russian Doctors' Plots*, the physicians involved neither killed nor planned to kill anyone. Even so, Russia's most prominent physicians were accused of fictitious crimes, imprisoned, tortured, and, in some cases, executed. Although the physicians were used as scapegoats by Stalin, many people, especially within Russia, still believe that these physicians were killers. These events are not widely known outside Russia, but they demonstrate the perverse nature of political systems and how physicians can become prime targets for manipulation.

How do physicians kill?

Physician-killers have generally relied on poison to "do in" their victims. Until the mid-nineteenth century, authorities had few methods for detecting poisons or toxins in corpses, but, as the century ended, police developed new methods for investigating such crimes. Sensational murder trials of physician-killers were the result.

Even with their newer methods, police often had a hard time determining if a murder had occurred. Until the 1930s, many over-the-counter medications and other household products contained poisons such as arsenic, antimony, and strychnine, which were the same poisons used by physician-killers. Because of this, it was often difficult to say whether people had been intentionally poisoned or had taken it themselves. Today, there are drugs and poisons far more subtle than those used by poisoners of old. At least one physician in this book—Dr. Debora Green—used an obscure but potent biowarfare toxin: ricin.

Despite improvements in the science of toxicology, physicians can still get away with murder. Cost restraints and changing attitudes have severely decreased the number of autopsies performed over the last decade. And, since doctors determine the causes of death and sign death certificates, they have the opportunity to easily dispose of the evidence. Dr. William G. Eckert, a forensic pathologist who wrote the article that inspired me to write this book, described the various methods that physicians have used to kill in the *American Journal of Forensic Medicine and Pathology*:

> The methods utilized have ranged from poisoning by common substances such as hemlock, arsenic, and strychnine to those using sophisticated and difficult to detect medications such as acontine, morphine, insulin, succinylcholine, curare, pavulon, and innovar. In addition to poisoning, simple blunt trauma, sharp instrument use, and firearms have been commonly used methods, as well as more subtle methods including the injection of toxic materials and virulent microorganisms.
>
> Poison is the obvious weapon of the murdering doctor and murder by poison can be established in many different ways. Death by poison can be established circumstantially, symptomatically, pathologically, chemically, or by experiment, or by all these methods of proof in combination. It is seldom possible to establish murder by poison by direct evidence of administration with intent to kill.

Although less than one murder in 500 is committed in the United States using poison, healthcare providers have more opportunities to use poison than do other killers, thus poisoning is the norm when these individuals kill. Physicians have legitimate access to drugs (which in the right setting or dose are poisons) or can easily steal them from the facilities in which they practice. In addition, physician-killers have routine intimate access to victims that other perpetrators do not: Only in a healthcare setting will normal people allow a stranger to stick them with a needle and administer potentially injurious substances. According to Eric W. Hickey in *Serial Murderers and Their Victims*, today's physician-killers prefer to use easily available drugs such as potassium chloride, pancuronium bromide, succinylcholine, and digoxin. (Although a common plot in fiction, physician-killers rarely rely on *pseudautochiria*, or murder disguised as suicide.)

Of course, physicians are not the only healthcare workers who kill. In the reported cases of medical personnel who murder patients, about 45 percent of the killers are nurses and slightly more than 25 percent are doctors. Other healthcare killers have included dentists, opticians, nurses' aids, nursing home workers, orderlies, and midwives. In the last 50 years, as the sickest and most vulnerable patients have entered hospitals, nursing homes, and other residential facilities, the majority of medically related murders have occurred at those sites. (Dr. Shipman still operated in a culture in which house calls were the norm, and so primarily killed his patients in their homes.) Dr. Robert Forrest, Britain's foremost forensic toxicologist, devised an acronym for medical personnel who kill their patients: CASK, which stands for Carer-Assisted Serial Killings. He describes such incidents as a:

> rare, although possibly underestimated, phenomenon; the systematic infliction of injury, usually with drugs and often with a fatal outcome, to a number of patients by a member of the caring professions ... The numbers of patients involved are not trivial. Typically between five and ten deaths are associated with each case, and the incidence appears to be of the order of one to two reported cases per million health-care workers. This implies that in Britain, cases may be seen every three to six years ... There may be significant under-reporting of cases outside hospitals.

It should be noted that these statistics do not include killings by those who practice euthanasia.

Is there a typical physician-serial killer?

When a doctor does go wrong, he is the first of criminals. He has the nerve and he has the knowledge . . .

— Sherlock Holmes, *The Adventure of the Speckled Band*

On their first day of medical school, medical students are introduced to "their" cadaver, and, for several months, they will intimately explore it with scalpels, scissors, forceps, hemostats, and hands. This gives students an introduction to anatomy, but it also demonstrates, in the most tangible way, that they are now among the select few that society allows to break its most sacred taboos: intimately touching strangers and intentionally mutilating another person's body (often called "surgery"). That physicians feel somewhat apart from lay people should not surprise anyone.

Physicians have another special advantage when it comes to murder: people have been taught to trust them. Doctors are among the last people suspected of murder. Not only are they cloaked in the mystique and prestige of their profession, but they also can intimidate others with their extensive education. As Frank Jones wrote in *Beyond Suspicion: True Stories of Unexpected Killers*:

> When the unthinkable occurs, and such a person turns to murder, it is not surprising that he or she applies all the charm, the skill, and the organizational abilities that ensured success in the legitimate world to secret, nefarious schemes.

An old joke that physicians often tell with some guilty pleasure is about a man who has recently died and is standing in line at the Pearly Gates. He watches as a man in a white coat with a stethoscope runs by and enters heaven. "Who does he think he is?" asks the man. St. Peter answers, "Why, that's God. He likes to play doctor now and then." Although possessing the knowledge, the means, and often the dispassionate demeanor, only a very few doctors actually do begin to "play God" by taking those traits to the ultimate extreme of murder. One physician who did decide to "play God," however, is Dr. Harold Shipman (see Chapter 9, *Harold Frederick Shipman, MBChB*). Mikaela Sitford, who spent a great deal of time observing Dr. Shipman during his arraignments and trial, described the two most significant traits she feels are "typical" of doctor-killers in *Addicted to Murder: The True Story of Dr. Harold Shipman*:

> Above all, and hardest to actually appreciate in its most literal sense, is their utter lack of empathy. They are quite simply incapable of putting themselves in someone else's shoes ... One further feature worthy of comment is the inability to make it to the very top of their profession. Several have been very competent doctors, but none has been outstanding, though they are all inclined to give the impression that they should and would have gone further, were it not for some dastardly injustice not their fault. Then nothing is their fault.

All the doctors profiled in this book have common traits. Aside from their obvious psychopathology, they all seemed to feel that everyone in the world existed only for their own benefit. The philosophical term for this is "solipsism," when individuals perceive themselves as being the only real entity and everything else, including other people, as being illusory.

All these men were also intelligent, which allowed them to enter the medical profession, in some cases despite obvious and documented mental illness. By all accounts, Dr. Petiot was an astute clinician—perhaps on a par with some of the best; Dr. Mudgett/Holmes was a very successful con artist. This suggests, as many others have noted, that intelligence alone should not be sufficient to enter the medical profession.

The paucity of physician-killers who have been apprehended over the past 150 years suggests that either we have not exposed them or they have, indeed, been rare. Once they are caught, however, physician-killers have the same success rate at trials as do other murderers. Robert Furneaux described in *The Medical Murderer* why they might never be caught, and, if they are, what usually trips them up:

> The criminal doctor, a sinister figure with an ingratiating bedside manner and a pocket full of poisons, is a "type" that does not exist outside the pages of fiction. Except in a few isolated cases the murdering doctor is the most prosaic of individuals. He is different from the ordinary murderer only in that he knows, or should know, how to do it successfully . . . Doctors who set out to commit murder should be almost unbeatable, and in all probability the vast majority are never suspected. Their successes far outnumber their failures but, as we know only of the failures, we can get only a lopsided view. It would be a great mistake to conclude that the murdering doctor is always a blunderer . . .
>
> With his knowledge, power, access to poisons, and accepted position, for his is the "trusted hand," the doctor who kills, or who having killed needs to dispose of the body, should be almost unbeatable. He may sign the death certificate, he knows the nature of poisons, the lethal dose, how to time its administration, disguise its effects and stimulate the symptoms of natural disease. He knows how to dismember and what identifiable features to remove. In the sick room his word is law and his opinions are accepted. Who is there to question them? It is remarkable, really, that the murdering doctor should ever fail.
>
> But he does fail because, from the moment death is accomplished, or the body concealed, he becomes just another murderer needing to reap the reward of his crime. He will be treading an unfamiliar path on which he will stumble. His crime is seldom suspected at the moment of death: he creates suspicion by his subsequent behavior or he demonstrates his obvious motive. The trained mind which enables him to commit the perfect crime fails to cope with the situation created by his act for, like ordinary mortals who turn to murder, his horizon is the moment.

All the physician-serial killers profiled in this book were repeatedly caught and sanctioned for misdeeds, mental illness, or sociopathic behavior. Yet they continued to commit murders. This is what makes their stories so scary.

Could the medical profession have prevented these murders?

One disturbing fact is true of most of the physicians in this book: many people in the medical profession recognized their psychopathology along the way and, in some cases, incarcerated them in psychiatric institutions or prisons. This begs the question: Why were they allowed to continue—or even begin—practicing medicine?

Some of the perpetrators got away with multiple murders simply because authorities in various jurisdictions did not communicate with each other. Instead, the authorities failed to pass on information, washed their hands of practitioners when they left the jurisdiction, or simply ignored the pattern. As John Douglas notes ruefully,

> As with most serial killers, it would have been very difficult here to prevent the first murder . . . We have to have an organized, nationwide system for law enforcement to share information on a real-time basis. It won't stop serial murders or spree killers from getting started, but it sure can help stop them in their tracks. And once a violent offender is on the run, that is exactly what we need to do.

Moreover, hospitals, individual physicians, and licensing boards often fail to share vital information with their professional colleagues because they fear legal retribution. This situation allows physician miscreants to move freely from one jurisdiction to another without penalty.

The profession has tried to address this issue, but, thus far, has met with only limited success. An attempt in the United States to compile a unified database, the National Practitioner Data Bank, so that authorities can identify wayward physicians has been fraught with problems. It contains numerous errors, lacks much relevant data, and, regrettably, has become an entity that hospitals shun. In addition, short-sighted "patient advocates" and the legal system have corrupted the process by trying to use the information, meant for professional self-regulation, to malign the profession and individual clinicians.

What about those just entering the profession?

In most countries, medicine is a meritocracy in which those with the intelligence and ability to perform well are allowed to enter and progress in the field. In the United States, the admission pendulum has swung severely toward academic performance and away from valuing the personality traits necessary to become a good clinician. The stories in this book should give pause to that attitude.

Yet, trying to keep potential serial killers out of the medical profession is no easy task. Even after they were identified, some suspected murderers were simply allowed to leave their workplace to protect the institution's reputation. As Forrest warns, "Others in the medical profession simply have to be eternally vigilant, and prepared to think the unthinkable, because there is no way of screening out these people. Working in the medical profession, it is possible to deceive a lot of people for a long time."

Can I find out if my physician has a suspicious past?

Yes, and no. In the United States, state medical boards have only the information provided to them by physician applicants, by the agency that collects information from hospitals (National Practitioner Data Bank), and by local law enforcement agencies. Not all licensing boards make this information available to the public, although an increasing number do so. In other countries, it can be even more difficult to obtain this information.

There are several sources to check for information about whether authorities have caught and/or convicted a doctor of committing a felony. Most have web sites, although the public may not have access to the entire site. You can use a search engine to find the specific web address for the following organizations:

- American Board of Medical Specialties
- American Medical Association
- Federation of State Medical Boards
- State Boards of Medical Examiners
- State Boards of Osteopathic Medical Examiners

There are also private services that check on doctors' credentials, professional history, and criminal records for a fee.

When seeking medical care, the rule is *caveat emptor* (let the buyer beware).

A Sampling of Infamous, Non-Physician Serial Killers

Jack the Ripper is often cited as history's first serial killer for dismembering four, and possibly five, London prostitutes in the late 1800s. But he was a bit player compared to many who preceded him, including Dr. William Palmer, who lived, and killed, decades earlier. The "Ripper" gained fame due to the publicity he garnered, in part, by taunting the police, who never caught him. For example, the August 24, 1892, *London Times* noted:

> The future historian of the latter part of this nineteenth century cannot fail to note the present epidemic of homicide; in the foreground of his picture he will place the dynamiting anarchist, and in the deepest shades of horror the crimes of Deeming, of the Whitechapel "ripper" and of this last, the poisoner of prostitutes; and he will comment on them probably as phases of a curious morbid and dangerous mental phenomenon.

History is replete with serial killers who were caught. Among them are the medieval "wolfmen" Gilles Garnier of France and Peter Stubbe of Germany, both of whom attacked children, ripped them apart, and then cannibalized them. Stubbe's own son, on whose brain he feasted, was one of his victims.

One of history's best-known serial killers was Baron Gilles de Rais, who was reportedly the richest man in France in the early 1400s. The Baron was a proud, young, devoutly Christian military hero and wartime companion of Joan of Arc; he was also known as a scholar, courtier, fashion plate, and patron of the arts. After his service in the Hundred Years' War, he retired to his castle where he delved into alchemy and Satanism. His servants collected children for him to torture and kill in his castle. Hundreds died, as he later said, "entirely for my own pleasure and physical delight, and for no other intention or end." After being tried for these crimes in 1440 by an ecclesiastical court, he was hung and his body was burned.

Evidence exists throughout human history of murderous sprees with patterns similar to those of serial killers. Many of the legends about witches, werewolves, and vampires may stem from early attempts to justify the behavior of serial killers—essentially blaming it on the Devil, since for "God-fearing" humans to have done such cruel things was unthinkable. The Grimm brothers' fairy tales, for example, relate popular myths of ogres and other carnivorous characters that are probably derived from such killers.

Some medieval serial killers drank their victims' blood, and probably initiated the vampire legends; occasionally, modern serial killers, such as Richard Chase, the "Vampire of Sacramento," have done the same. Bram Stoker wrote *Dracula*, in which he described blood-drinking killers. Presaging the modern-day classification, Stoker wrote, "My homicidal maniac is of a peculiar kind. I shall have

continued . . .

A Sampling of Infamous, Non-Physician Serial Killers, *continued*

to invent a new classification for him, and call him a zoophagous (life-eating) maniac: what he desires is to absorb as many lives as he can, and has laid himself out to achieve it in a cumulative way."

The following is a representative sample of history's other infamous non-physician serial killers.

Locusta of Rome

One of the earliest serial killers in recorded history, Locusta of Rome is said to have personally killed hundreds of people in ancient Rome—some for profit and others for enjoyment. She also supplied poison to a well-connected clientele, such as Agrippina, who used the poison to murder Emperor Claudius I, and Nero, who used it to kill his brother Britannicus.

Called "a master creator of potions," she reportedly kept a stable of slaves on whom to try out her potions. She also ran a school for poisoners, and she and her students are believed to have collectively killed as many as 10,000 people. A strange legend says that in 69 A.D., after being publicly raped by a specially trained giraffe, she was torn apart by wild animals.

Albert Fish

He killed and ate at least 15 children between 1917 and 1934. Born in Washington, D.C., in 1870, Fish moved to New York in 1890, after having been involved in masochistic-homosexual relationships. In New York, he began raping children and participated in bizarre sexual acts. He committed his first murder in 1910, mutilating and torturing his victim.

During the 1920s, Fish traveled across 23 states working as a house painter. This provided the opportunity for him to approach, torture, kill, and cannibalize children. He said that godlike voices had commanded him to perform his cruel deeds, which included inserting hundreds of needles around his own genitals. In 1934, after he sent a letter to the family of a 10-year-old girl that he had kidnapped and eaten six years earlier, police located Fish. By then, the newspapers had dubbed him the "Brooklyn Vampire."

In 1935, the 64-year-old Fish was sentenced to death—which he described as "the supreme thrill of my life." He was electrocuted at Sing Sing Prison on January 16, 1936. Several jolts were supposedly needed to kill him, since the needles he had inserted in his body over the years were said to have short-circuited the electric charge.

Peter Kurten

Known as "The Dusseldorf Monster," Kurten killed or attempted to kill more than 50 men, women, and children. For 15 months in 1929 and 1930, 47-year-

continued . . .

A Sampling of Infamous, Non-Physician Serial Killers, *continued*

old Kurten stalked and killed people in Dusseldorf, Germany, beginning with a 9-year-old girl he stabbed, raped, and then partially burned. Kurten killed or tried to kill many more people, using a different method to kill each victim and then mutilating the corpses. He sent police friendly letters and maps detailing the location of some of the undiscovered corpses. In May 1930, police finally caught Kurten when a woman he had attempted to rape identified him.

Kurten said his "chief satisfaction in killing was to catch the blood spurting from a victim's wounds in his mouth and swallow it." Kurten also told police that he enjoyed killing, "the more people the better. Yes, if I had had the means of doing so, I would have killed whole masses of people—brought about catastrophes." He showed no remorse for his actions and said that he might kill again if he were set free. After studying him for a year, Germany's top psychiatrist pronounced Kurten sane, although obsessed with sadism, masochism, fetishism, and pyromania. Even his defense counsel had to admit that Kurten was "a concentrated complex of all sexual abnormalities known, a veritable king of sexual delinquents." He was convicted of nine murders, and was guillotined in Cologne, Germany on July 2, 1931.

Edmund Kemper

As a child, Kemper demonstrated remarkable cruelty to animals. As an adult, he used the same techniques to torture and murder nine women and one man. When Kemper killed his mother, he cut off her head and put it on the mantelpiece, where he threw darts at it. He also cut off her right hand and removed her larynx (voicebox) which he put down the garbage disposal.

He ate parts of his victims and kept their hair, skin, and personal belongings, along with photographs of their bodies as mementos. Kemper generally kept his victims' heads to perform sexual acts with them. One he kept in a box in his mother's apartment, so he could talk to it. After his arrest in 1973, he stated, "If I killed them, they couldn't reject me as a man. It was more or less making a doll out of a human being, carrying out my fantasies with a doll, a living doll."

Ed Gein

Shortly after his mother died in December 1945, 39-year-old Gein began to have strange visions. Voices commanded the bachelor to view women's bodies and to speak to his mother, so he began to disinter recently buried women, taking them home to flay and dismember. For more than a decade, he raided graves in the small farming community of Plainfield, Wisconsin. At some point, he began actually killing women.

continued . . .

A Sampling of Infamous, Non-Physician Serial Killers, continued

When police finally apprehended him, they reportedly found Bernice Worden's naked, headless, and eviscerated body hanging upside down in the barn. Her head and intestines were in a box, and her heart was on a plate in the dining room. Police also found the scattered remains of at least 15 bodies at the farmhouse, although Gein said that he could not remember how many murders he had actually committed. Investigators found preserved skin from 10 human heads and, rolled up on the floor, a vest made from a woman's chest. Other items reportedly found were a chair upholstered in human skin, a skull soup-bowl, newspaper-stuffed faces hanging on the walls, and human organs in the refrigerator.

Gein later confessed that he enjoyed dressing in human-skin garments while pretending he was his mother. (The killer in the movie *Psycho* was based on Gein.) After spending ten years in a mental hospital, Gein was judged competent to stand trial. At trial, Gein was found guilty, but criminally insane. In 1978, he was committed to the Central State Hospital in Waupan, Wisconsin, where he died in the geriatric ward in 1984, at age 77.

Pedro Alonzo Lopez

Known as the "Monster of the Andes," Lopez supposedly killed at least 300 children, mainly Indians from remote jungle villages in Peru, Colombia, and Ecuador. After she caught him fondling his younger sister, his prostitute mother kicked the 8-year-old Lopez out of the house. He lived on the street until his activities landed him in jail, where fellow inmates (whom he later killed) gang-raped him.

Upon his release at age 18, he began killing young girls in Peru. Later, he moved to Columbia and then Ecuador to continue his slaughter. At the peak of his activity, he murdered up to three girls a week. People now refer to him as "the world's most prolific serial killer." He was arrested in 1980 and is currently in prison in Ecuador. If Lopez is ever released, he will then serve prison sentences in Columbia and Peru.

Theodore Robert "Ted" Bundy

A handsome, intelligent, and seemingly charming person, Ted Bundy abducted and killed at least 33 women between 1974 and 1978. He typically stalked young women on college campuses, at shopping malls, in apartment complexes, and at schools. He favored killing dark-haired cheerleader types, first attacking them with blunt objects, then raping and biting them. After 11 years of trials and appeals, he was finally sentenced to death. Bundy was electrocuted at Florida State Prison on January 24, 1989.

continued . . .

A Sampling of Infamous, Non-Physician Serial Killers, continued

Jeffrey Dahmer

As a child, Dahmer decapitated rodents, bleached chicken bones with acid, and nailed a dog's carcass to a tree after mounting its severed head on a stake. As an adult, he murdered and cannibalized 17 men. In June 1978, he began his killing spree by crushing a hitchhiker's skull with a barbell, strangling him, and dismembering his corpse.

When Dahmer was finally arrested on July 22, 1991, police discovered photographs of dismembered corpses in his room, along with human remains. The pictures had been taken at different stages of some of his victim's deaths; some were in various erotic and bondage poses. One showed a man's head lying in a sink. Another showed a victim cut open from the neck to the groin. Some pictures were of his victims before he murdered them. Police found skulls in the refrigerator, and three heads neatly stored in plastic bags in the freezer. A locked room contained a kettle with decomposed hands and a penis, more skulls, and a container with formaldehyde and male genitalia. In 1991, Dahmer was judged legally sane, and he was convicted on multiple homicide charges. On November 28, 1994, while he was in prison, another inmate killed him.

Luis Alfredo Garavito

Garavito claims to have killed 140 children in Columbia; usually he raped them, then slit their throats and beheaded them. He supposedly started his murder spree in 1992, but the search for him only began in 1998, after officials discovered a grave containing 25 of his victims, most of whom were the children of street vendors. Colombian police apprehended him in October 1999.

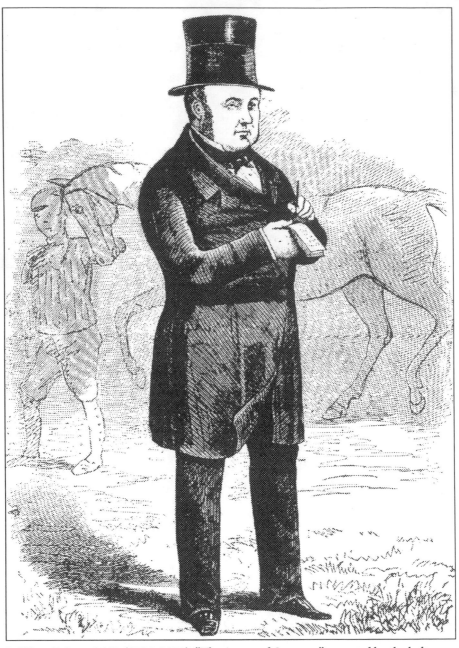

William Palmer, M.D. (1824–1856). "The Accursed Surgeon," executed by the halter on June 14, 1856, in Stafford. (From *The Times Report of the Trial of William Palmer*, 1856)

1

Easy Money, Fast Horses, Dead Women

William Palmer, M.D.

*A*nnie went to bed feeling unwell. Her nausea had increased and the diarrhea would not stop. William, solicitous as ever, gave her a new type of medicine, but her symptoms worsened. Suddenly, her body convulsed as the muscles stiffened like boards and her back arched. The pain was excruciating. She labored to overcome the spasms in her chest, but the short breaths were insufficient to overcome the fear of suffocation. When the seizure ceased momentarily, she was afraid to move or be touched lest it start again.

Was this what her mother had experienced? Had her babies felt this pain and fear as they convulsed and died after William's ministrations? What would happen to her son—was he safe? Tears rolled down her cheeks.

William entered the room and shook his head. "I had to do it, Annie. I love you, but I'm sorely in debt and have no other way out." As her seizure stopped, she stared at him, bitterly recalling the £13,000 life insurance policy William had demanded that she sign a few months back. He put his hand on her shoulder and she seized again, unable to catch her breath. This seizure was short-lived: Annie's face went blue, then her body relaxed.

William Palmer, M.D., closed his wife's eyes and called for Dr. Bamford to pronounce her dead. Then he went to the scullery maid's bedroom for solace.

Early Years

On August 6, 1824, Mrs. Sarah Palmer gave birth to the town's most notorious citizen, William, in a red-brick house named "The Yard" in Rugeley (pronounced Rouge-lee), Staffordshire, England. This was where William, except for the period of his education, would live his entire life.

Rugeley had a population of 4,500 and, according to an inhabitant at the time, was "one of the prettiest places in Europe. Contemporary periodicals described Rugeley as:

> a long straggling town of small houses, kept very clean, and occupied by persons extremely well to do in the world. It is about as large as Twickenham, and seems to have been built up without any apparent design beyond the whim of the bricklayer . . . There is a certain charm in the deserted thoroughfares, when the only persons to be seen are the housewives at the windows, behind the rows of geraniums, plying the needle, whilst the husband is working in the fields . . . It is a very curious little over-grown village, and too pretty to be abused.

The Palmers' home was a large, well-kept two-story structure "standing back, as if in shame, from the road." It was named "The Yard" for the timber yard in back where William's wealthy father reputedly sold stolen timber. After the timber yard closed, the Palmers converted the wharf along the canal into a broad sloping lawn. The gardens and outbuildings on the canal side of the house were not maintained, although those in front were immaculate. (Today the building is called "Church Croft.")

People from the counties surrounding Staffordshire say, in jest, that the region's emblem—the "Stafford knot," which looks like a pretzel with three loops—represents how authorities had to hang Stafford men three at a time because so many scoundrels lived there. William Palmer would do nothing to diminish this reputation.

William was the second of seven Palmer children (five sons and two daughters). Two others were also black sheep: Walter, a corn merchant who went bankrupt and became a drunk, and an alcoholic sister, who married Mr. Heywood of Haywood and "lived badly and died miserably." On the positive side, Thomas became an Anglican minister; Sarah, a "quiet, unassuming, charitable girl," died a spinster; George practiced law in Rugeley; and Joseph, the eldest, became wealthy as a timber merchant and then enhanced his fortune considerably through marriage.

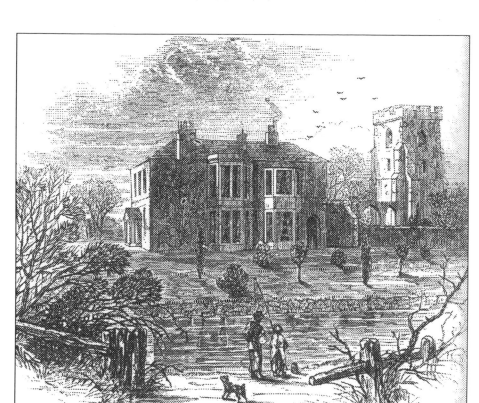

The Palmer house, "The Yard." (From *The Times Report of the Trial of William Palmer*, 1856)

When their father suddenly died in 1837 before signing his will, Joseph inherited the house and grounds. He allowed his mother to use it, but on the condition that she did not remarry. Not one to be outsmarted by her son, Sarah acquired lovers: the first was a strapping linen draper named Duffy (who mysteriously disappeared), and then a young lawyer, Jeremiah Smith. Mrs. Palmer also inherited one-third of her husband's estate, called the "widow's third," which she later used to bail William out of his various legal difficulties.

While Mr. Palmer had been strict with the children and sometimes flogged them, Mrs. Palmer let them run wild. A neighbor described William's childhood behavior:

> [He] was noted for a great display of amiability and kindness, but he was also noted for great cruelty towards animals, and for indulging in general mischief in a sly underhand way; he has been known to torture animals, and even insects, and to play tricks with aged people, when he

thought there was no opportunity of being detected; but in public, he was always officiously helping somebody, as though it were his wish to make himself generally agreeable.

At age 17, the rather obese William graduated from Rugeley Free Grammar School. He was then apprenticed to Messrs. Evans & Sons, Wholesale Chemists of Lord Street in Liverpool.

William Palmer soon became entangled with his landlord's red-haired daughter, Jane Widnall. Claiming that she was pregnant, she demanded that he pay for an abortion. Palmer first tried to get the money by betting on the horses at the Liverpool and Chester racetracks, but, as he would throughout life, lost miserably. He then stole money—about £200 in all—from the mail orders sent to his employers. After several customers complained that their orders had not been filled, his employers began to suspect young William. Following him when he picked up the mail, they saw him rifle through the envelopes in search of cash. He confessed when confronted, and they immediately dismissed him. Palmer would have been prosecuted, but his mother searched for each bilked customer and repaid the stolen money. She also sent William's younger brother, Thomas, to Liverpool to finish William's apprenticeship. It would not be the last time that Mrs. Palmer would make restitution for her wayward son.

William was next sent for a five-year apprenticeship to a local "surgeon" (actually a general practitioner), Dr. Edward Tylecote, in nearby Haywood. Mrs. Palmer agreed to pay him for 18-year-old William's bed and board, plus an additional 50 guineas a year. William enjoyed his work, but had to hurriedly depart after being caught embezzling money again, this time from patients and other townspeople. He was also involved in what Dr. Tylecote characterized as "unruly behavior." In a jealous rage, he poured acid over another apprentice's elegant clothes, and then fled to Walsall with Jane Widnall (who had moved with her mother to Haywood). During this time, William also impregnated at least one other woman and apparently ran his own abortion service, possibly to help dispose of any evidence of his indiscretions.

Mrs. Palmer eventually sent two of William's brothers to Walsall to fetch him. They had to pay his many outstanding debts before his creditors agreed to let him leave. But William still managed to defraud Jane's father of £100, his life savings, before he left. Jane married another man and moved to Australia.

Although Mrs. Palmer tried to force Dr. Tylecote to take William back, he wouldn't accept him. Only after her threats, and a large payoff, did he write a favorable letter so William could resume his medical training in Stafford.

Established in A.D. 219, Stafford was a market town of about 13,000 inhabitants, known for its red bricks, shoes, and salt works. At Stafford Infirmary, Palmer "walked the wards," learning medicine as would a modern medical student on clinical rotations. But he was involved in several incidents and was "advised" to leave after the staff passed a special rule that kept him from dispensing medications.

In 1846, Palmer returned to Rugeley. Shortly after arriving, he challenged Abley, a local shoemaker, to a brandy-drinking contest at The Lamb and Flag. After Abley's second drink—a large bumper of brandy that he finished in one swallow—he stumbled into the courtyard, vomiting profusely. An hour later, patrons found him in the stable, groaning in pain; he died that night. Abley's death was suspicious, and an autopsy was done. However, not enough remained in his stomach to test for poisons, so a coroner's inquest pronounced the death to be from natural causes. The jury's foreman strongly opposed letting Palmer go free—and he reminded his neighbors of this when Palmer was later tried for murder.

Even though Palmer lost his drinking contest with Abley, he won in other ways. He had previously met Abley's wife at the infirmary, where he had treated a burn on her thigh. After her husband's death, he helped the attractive widow relieve her grief in the most intimate of ways. When rumors of their behavior began to circulate, William decided to leave Rugeley and finish his medical training at St. Bartholomew's Hospital in London. He studied there under a well-known instructor, Dr. Stegall, who agreed to act as his "grinder," or mentor and tutor. They agreed that Dr. Stegall would receive 70 guineas if William finished his studies without being expelled and passed his exams to practice medicine.

During this period, Palmer spent much of his time giving extravagant champagne parties, frequenting the racetracks, and consorting with other "sporting men" and "beauties of doubtful reputation." While most medical students of the time had little money, he covered the walls of his lodging with expensive anatomical preparations and models, and he had the finest medical library of any student. Palmer was described by his fellow students as "stupidly good-natured," and he "ate and drank of the best, spent his days and nights in riotous living, and gave but little thought to those severe studies which he was required to surmount to become fitted for his profession."

Even so, he arose early each morning and dressed neatly to attend his lectures and to perform clinical duties. Cohorts recalled that "to the poor patients in the hospital he was very kind; he would frequently get up subscriptions [raise money] for them, when they were on the point of leaving the hospital." His teachers weren't as impressed. Sir James Paget, a famous physician and the first dean of the medical school, wrote:

> [Palmer was] dissolute, extravagant, vulgar and stupid. He scarcely practiced, and was chiefly engaged on the turf ... He was an idle dissipated student, cursed with more money than he had the wisdom or the virtue to use well.

Somehow, on August 10, 1846, Palmer finally obtained his surgical diploma. Although he completed his part of the bargain, Dr. Stegall was never paid.

During the five years he studied medicine, Palmer supposedly sired 14 illegitimate children with various women. Many of these children died from seizures soon after Palmer's ministrations. Yet there was one woman he wanted to marry: Annie Thornton Brookes. His letters suggest that she provided at least some of the motivation for him to complete his medical training and enter a profession. "Good Annie Brookes," as she was known, was born in 1827, and was the illegitimate daughter of Colonel Brookes and his housekeeper-mistress, Ann Thornton. The wealthy debilitated bachelor had retired to Stafford after his service in Britain's Indian Army and there became enamored of his pretty maidservant. As acquaintances wrote, Ann

> soon ceased to be beautiful, and nothing remained of her former self but her ignorance—which was gross, savage, and complete. The beautiful dream of Ann Thornton, the pretty servant maid, had vanished; and Mrs. Thornton, tall, thin and angular—a drunkard and foul-mouthed, loose in her habits, and not even true to her old Colonel—was all that remained ... [she] was in the habit of chasing him round the room with a knife, swearing she would kill him.

The Colonel followed the example of his four brothers and killed himself in 1834. A flaw in his will made his daughter a ward of the court, with Dr. Edward Knight and Charles Dawson, a druggist, as her guardians. It was at the latter's country residence, known as Abbot's Bromley, that Annie met William Palmer.

Unlike her mother, Annie was known for her simplicity, kindness, and engaging manners. Those who knew her said "she was the general favourite of the town, and that, as she grew in years, her virtues kept pace ... at all hours she was present [with ill neighbors] not only to administer medicine and to perform the duty of a nurse, but to give spiritual consolation in the absence of the clergyman." Yet, she was "painfully sensible of her own false position as an illegitimate child, and it is said that she was habituated to look upon herself as an outcast—a being of an inferior order—one who should be deeply grateful to any man who would bestow his name upon a creature unrecognised by the laws, and tainted from her birth."

During his studies at St. Bartholomew's, William wrote her many passionate letters, such as this note:

> My Dearest Annie,—I snatch a moment from my studies to write to your dear, dear, little self. I need scarcely say that the principal inducement I have to work is the desire of getting my studies finished so as to be able to press your dear little form in my arms. With best, best love, believe me, dearest Annie, your own, William.

In August 1846, after passing the tests to enter the Royal College of Surgeons—on his second try—Dr. William Palmer opened a medical practice in Rugeley. His offices were on Market Street, opposite the Talbot Inn (today the Shrewsbury Arms or "The Shrew"). Initially, his practice did well, and he "followed his profession with steadiness and the prospect of success." On October 7, 1847, the bland-faced little doctor married Annie Thornton in the chapel at Abbot's Bromley. At the time, everyone believed that Annie brought a substantial estate with her. The marriage took place under court order, since her guardians objected to the match. Shortly after his marriage, one of Palmer's lady friends, Jenny Mumford, gave birth to a girl that he reluctantly began supporting financially. The baby died shortly after she was seen by Palmer in his office.

Palmer seemed as attracted to the horses—Rugeley's claim to fame—as he was to his new wife. The couple was always in debt, primarily due to Palmer's incessant gambling and continuing losses. Within a few years of his marriage, his medical practice had dwindled to almost nothing. So Palmer became a horse breeder, leasing stables and a paddock and employing several trainers. He spent all his time with others who were involved in the "Sport of Kings." It was claimed, but never proven, that Palmer was a "nobbler," someone who drugged horses to fix races.

Murder in the Family

On October 11, 1848, the couple's first son, William Brookes Palmer, was born. Three months later, Annie's rich, alcoholic, and abusive mother arrived. (Ann Thornton had inherited nine houses and £15,000 when Annie's father had died.) Seeing their troubled financial state, she lent William £20, although he had no way to repay the debt. Unsatisfied with the small sums that his mother-in-law grudgingly doled out to him, William decided to get her entire estate. Less than a week later, Ann Thornton was dead.

Needing a physician to sign the death certificate, Palmer asked an elderly colleague to do so. Dr. Bamford, then 77 years old, obliged, and listed Ann Thornton's cause of death as "apoplexy" (stroke). Dr. Bamford continued to supply Palmer with benign death certificates throughout his killing spree. After her mother's death, Palmer was shocked to discover that Annie would inherit only the rent from her mother's nine houses; the rest of the estate reverted to the Colonel's nephew upon Thornton's death. The rent proceeds were not sufficient to pay Palmer's creditors; he had to get more money.

Shortly thereafter, Leonard Bladon, one of Palmer's gambler friends as well as a creditor to whom he owed £800, visited the Palmer home. He walked in with a large sum in his money belt, died in convulsions several days later, and was carried out without a penny. His relatives thought his death was suspicious—especially since both his money and his betting book (with a list of those owing him money) had disappeared. Dr. Bamford recorded that the death was due to a stable accident that had occurred a few weeks earlier, and Palmer hastily had Bladon buried.

As his debts continued to mount, Palmer became obsessed with money. (Interestingly, witnesses later testified that he became neither elated nor depressed by wins and losses.) By 1853, he was forced to approach moneylenders for funds, and agreed to pay up to 60 percent interest annually. Even so, Palmer took out a second £2,000 loan with Padwick, a notorious moneylender and racing man. As he usually did, he forged his mother's signature on the loan, so it was readily accepted.

Between 1849 and 1854, William and Annie had four more children: Elizabeth, Henry, Frank, and John. To keep down expenses, Palmer murdered these four, as well as several of his illegitimate children. William, his first son, was the only one to survive him. After the last of his children with Annie died in convulsions, their nurse, Ann Bradshaw, ran into a nearby inn, crying:

> I'll never go back to that wretch Palmer's house again ... The poor dear child was as well and as hearty as possible, when Palmer comes upstairs and says to me, "You can go down, Bradshaw; I'll nurse the child for a few minutes." But in a few minutes the poor child's screams made me run up again, when I found the poor baby had just died in violent convulsions.

To keep up a respectable front during this period, Palmer regularly attended church services—a behavior that marked him as a gentleman, rather

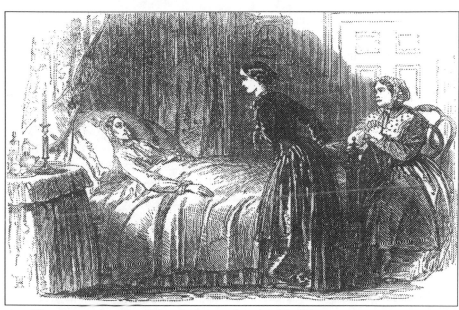

Ann Thornton, Palmer's mother-in-law, on her deathbed. (From *The Illustrated Life & Career of William Palmer*, 1856)

than as a believer. What he *believed* was that he needed more money—and he had a plan to get it. On September 29, 1854, six months after reluctantly signing life insurance policies worth £13,000 (equivalent to more than $1.5 million in 2002) that Palmer had taken out on her, Annie mysteriously died. Both Palmer and Dr. Bamford attributed her death to "English cholera," now called dysentery or food poisoning. Although Annie had no history of seizures, she died in convulsions, similar to other deaths involving Dr. Palmer.

The insurance company at first hesitated to pay on the claim because of suspicions concerning Annie's death. They finally paid after Thomas Pratt, Palmer's solicitor (and principal creditor who was to become deeply involved in Palmer's sordid life), approached them. With the insurance money, Palmer paid £8,000 to Pratt and £5,000 to lawyer-moneylender Herbert Wright. This temporarily eased—but did not eliminate—his debt. He still owed at least £2,000 that he had fraudulently obtained from Padwick. Palmer sent William, his only living child, to live with a local physician, Dr. Salt, and his wife, saying "I wish to carry out my dear wife's last injunction, which was to place him under your care." Apparently, he could not be bothered with a child.

Three months later, deep in debt again, Palmer decided to cash in on the impending death of his brother Walter, who was bankrupt and in the last stages of alcoholism. Walter had barely survived an attack of *delirium tremens* and his recent suicide attempt. William offered to insure his life and to give him £400, knowing that the money would buy more liquor and provide an even faster demise. With Pratt's assistance, he attempted to secure a total of £82,000 of life insurance on his brother from six insurance companies. Dr. Waddell, a Stafford surgeon, completed the insurance physical, writing that Walter was "healthy, robust, and temperate." He then added a note for only the insurance companies to read: "*Most confidential.* His life [insurance request] has been rejected in two offices. I am told he drinks. His brother insured his late wife's life for many thousands, and after first payment she died. *Be cautious.*" [original italics]

All but one insurance company refused to write a policy on Walter. The Prince of Wales Company agreed to issue a policy for £13,000. Pratt received a £106 12s commission on the sale, and William gave him the policy as collateral for the £12,500 in loans he had received. Typically, Palmer had forged his mother's name for these loans as well. Interestingly, all the loans were due between September 28, 1854, the day before Annie's death, and January 5, 1855.

With some of his debts paid, Palmer bought two top-ranked horses, *Chicken* and *Nettle*, for several thousand borrowed pounds. Although *Chicken* won a handful of races, Palmer's horses generally didn't perform well. In an 1855 race at the Oaks, *Nettle* stumbled and fell, breaking the jockey's leg and completely bankrupting Palmer. (He had backed her so heavily that she started as a 2-to-1 favorite.) He sold her for 430 guineas, but this financial disaster and the claims of creditors precipitated his next desperate acts.

In May 1855, his 29-year-old friend, John Parsons Cook, vouched for a £200 loan from Pratt so that Palmer could pay off another debt. Cook was a solicitor but, after inheriting "some £12,000 or £15,000, he abandoned the laborious profession of the law, and betook himself to the turf." Being about the same age, Palmer and Cook gravitated toward each other, although Cook was a more successful gambler. When the debt came due, Palmer refused to pay and Cook had to repay the money. Palmer then intercepted a £440 loan check from Pratt to Cook and forged the endorsement so he could cash it. Cook would have learned of the deception when the debt came due—if he had lived that long.

On August 14, William spent the day in Stafford with Walter, who was clearly dying. Just as his brother died, William got a hot tip on a horse and placed a bet, which he lost. He was once again desperate for money and waited for the insurance proceeds from Walter's policy. Palmer wrote a consolation letter to his sister-in-law:

> Ah poor fellow. I often think of him, and only wish I could have done more for him while he was alive; and I assure you I did a very, very great deal for him—perhaps a great deal more than you are aware of.

By September 1855, Palmer was still waiting for the money. Moreover, at any time, either Pratt or Padwick could reveal that he had forged his mother's name on the loans. So he hatched a new plan and persuaded young George Bates, who had fallen on hard times and was then a regular fixture at Palmer's stables, to sign papers so that Palmer and Cook could apply for £25,000 life insurance on him. Reluctant at first, Bates was finally persuaded when Cook, who also planned to benefit from this transaction, said, "You had better do it; it will be for your benefit, and you'll be quite safe with Palmer." However, the Solicitors and General Insurance Office declined to write the policy. They may have been hesitant because Palmer was listed as the physician and Cook as the witness on the application. The pair then tried to get a £10,000 policy with another company, but were again refused.

About this time, the Prince of Wales Company became suspicious about Walter's death and sent investigators Messrs. Field and Simpson, both retired policemen, to look into the case. They became convinced that Dr. Palmer was a scheming, and probably homicidal, character, and refused to pay on the insurance policy. They even threatened to begin criminal action against Palmer. Negotiations with the insurance company dragged on until Cook's death, at which time, the company closed the case without paying.

After Annie's death, the citizens of Rugeley became wary of Dr. Palmer, whose medical practice had dwindled as his racing debts mounted. When he entered the pub, they would shout, "Here comes the poisoner," which Palmer would shrug off with the retort, "What's your poison, boys?" It didn't help that on June 26, 1855, exactly nine months after Annie's death, Eliza Tharm, Palmer's pretty housemaid, gave birth. In addition, after his wife's death, Palmer had arranged an abortion for another lady friend, Jane Bergen, with a practitioner "who would be silent as death" about the procedure. Unfortunately for Palmer, Ms. Bergen would only be silent for a price—and she began blackmailing him.

On November 13, Palmer sent Jane Bergen a note saying that he could not pay what she was demanding for the return of his letters. "I should not mind giving £30 for the whole of them," he wrote, "but I am hard up at present." On the 19th, he offered £40 "to split the difference," and, the next day, he sent half of eight £5 notes, sending the other half of each note on November 24. She never returned the letters (which disappeared in 1933).

Meanwhile, Pratt was becoming more suspicious of the wily doctor. Throughout October 1855, he wrote to Palmer numerous times demanding payment on loans that were either coming due or overdue. It must have scared Palmer when, in one of his letters, Pratt wrote, "I have your note acknowledging receipt by your mother of the £2,000 acceptance due the 2nd October. Why not let her acknowledge it herself!" Finally, on November 6, Pratt had two writs for £4,000 issued, one against Palmer and the other against his mother—who was still unaware that her name had been forged on promissory notes. Pratt delayed service on the writs to give Palmer time to pay. But the Palmers owed him another £1,500 on November 9—and Pratt wanted his money. Palmer did manage to pay Pratt £600, but the moneylender was still hounding him for the balance.

John Parsons Cook

On Tuesday, November 13, after writing the letter to Ms. Bergen, Palmer went to the Shrewsbury races with John Parsons Cook. That same day, Pratt wrote to Palmer saying that he needed to be paid on Walter's life insurance policy. William's life was getting complicated, but things seemed to be looking up for Cook when his horse, *Polestar,* won £2,050 in the Shrewsbury Handicap. After *Polestar* won, Cook "was so excited" according to his friend and personal physician, Dr. William Henry Jones, "that for two or three minutes he could not speak to me." Cook, already carrying about £750 that he had won the prior week, would now get the £381 stake, the money he had won betting at the racetrack, and an additional £1,020 in bets that he could collect at Tattersall's in London on Monday.

The following night at the Raven Hotel in Shrewsbury, Cook and Palmer sat drinking brandy and water when two betting agents, Ishmael Fisher and George Herring, joined them. Before Cook sipped his drink, a witness saw Palmer hold the tumbler up to a light "with the caution of a man who was watching to see what was the condition of the liquid." He then went to his room with the glass, came back, and gave Cook the drink. Cook said to Palmer, "You'll have some more, won't you?" Palmer replied, "I shall not have any more till you have drunk yours." To which Cook rejoined, " 'I will drink mine,' and he took up his glass and drank it at a drop," leaving only a few sips. He imme-

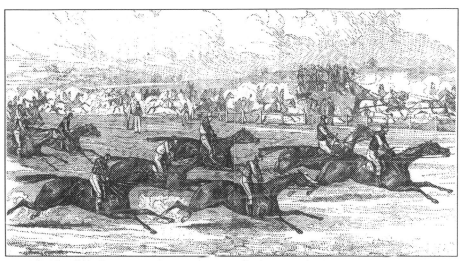

The Shrewsbury horse races. (From *The Illustrated Life & Career of William Palmer*, 1856)

diately cried out, "Good God! There's something in it; it burns my throat dreadfully."

That was not surprising, given that Palmer had probably added antimony, in the form of tartar emetic, to the drink. The poison, used as a medication at the time, is soluble in fluids. It would have affected the brandy's taste, if given in large quantities, but would not have affected the color. Palmer, gulping the little remaining in the glass, declared, "Nonsense, there's nothing in it." He then pushed the glass toward the other two men and said, "Cook fancies there is something in the brandy-and-water—there's nothing in it—taste it." They replied, "What is the use of handing [us] the glass when it is empty?"

Cook immediately fled the room, yelling that he was ill. He vomited repeatedly and was forced to retire to his bed. He said to Fisher, who looked in on him later, that "he thought that Palmer had dosed him," and he gave Fisher about £800 for safekeeping, which was returned to him the next day. He continued to have violent stomach pain, accompanied by severe retching and vomiting. About midnight, Mr. Gibson, a physician's assistant, was called to attend Cook. He said, "I treated Cook as if he had taken poison. I took him at his word, that he had taken poison." Several hours after he received treatment, Cook's symptoms began to subside, and he fell asleep about 2 A.M. Palmer later said that he thought that Cook was drunk, although everyone else in attendance disagreed.

The next day Cook's vomiting had stopped, although he still looked and felt very ill. He returned to the track, where Palmer lost an enormous amount of borrowed money when *Chicken* failed to place. Palmer now had no funds; he had even borrowed the money to get to Shrewsbury racetrack. Cook and Palmer returned to Rugeley about 10:30 P.M. Cook took a room at the Talbot Arms Hotel. Palmer went to his house across the street.

On Friday, November 16, Cook dined with Palmer and their friend, Jeremiah Smith. Smith was the Palmer family lawyer and was also involved in some of the insurance schemes. Cook had regained his usual state of good health. Why would Cook continue to associate with Palmer even though he suspected that Palmer had tried to poison him? The answer might be that Palmer's unsavory reputation, his confident air, and his experience drew the young gambler to the dangerous killer.

Saturday morning, Palmer visited Cook in his hotel room, where he ordered coffee to be sent up. Palmer handed it to Cook, who drank it immediately and "the same symptoms set in which had occurred at Shrewsbury." Palmer then sent Cook a bowl of "reviving broth" that Palmer's servant, Anne Rowley, got from the Albion Inn and brought to Palmer's kitchen, where the doctor himself was sitting, to warm it. Palmer then told her to take it to Cook, but instructed her to tell him that it was from Smith. Later, he learned that Cook hadn't eaten the broth, so he asked the servant to take it back to Cook. After he ate only one spoonful of it, Cook immediately began retching. Cook was too ill to leave his room, and Palmer attended to him, administering everything that he ate or drank. Even the "toast and water was brought over from [Palmer's] house, instead of being made at the hotel, as it might have been, and again the sickness ensued."

Dr. Bamford then was called and arrived about 3 P.M. Palmer told him that Cook had taken too much champagne the night before and was suffering a gallbladder attack. When Bamford examined him, "he found Mr. Cook suffering from violent vomiting, and the stomach in so irritable a state that it would not retain a tablespoonful of anything." Cook's symptoms persisted, and Dr. Bamford prescribed two pills, each containing one-half grain (32 mg) of morphia acetate (morphine), one-half grain of calomel, and four grains of rhubarb.

Cook's illness continued on Sunday, but Dr. Bamford found no trace of bile or fever. Palmer was in constant attendance, administering food, drink, and medicines. On Sunday, and again Monday, Palmer wrote to Cook's friend, Dr. Jones, who practiced in Lutterworth:

November 18, 1855.

My dear Sir,—Mr. Cook was taken ill at Shrewsbury, and obliged to call in a medical man; since then he has been confined to his bed here with a very severe bilious attack, combined with diarrhœa, [sic] and I think it advisable for you to come and see him as soon as possible.

Palmer had his gardener bring another cup of broth to Cook, but he refused it. Another servant at the hotel, "thinking that it looked nice, took a couple of tablespoonfuls of it; within half an hour she also was taken severely ill . . . She was obliged to go to bed, and she had exactly the same symptoms which manifested themselves in Cook's person after he drank the brandy and water at Shrewsbury." It was noted later that every time Cook ingested anything that Palmer could have altered, he immediately became ill. However, when he took anything that Palmer could not affect, he had no difficulty.

About this time, Palmer sent for his illegitimate child by Eliza Tharm, who was being kept a few miles from Rugeley. He said he wanted to be sure that the child was well. Palmer's examination did not take long but, on the way back home, the child died in convulsions.

On Monday, November 19, Palmer traveled to London. Before leaving, he asked the hotel's housekeeper to make coffee, which he gave to Cook himself. Cook immediately began to vomit after drinking the coffee. Palmer left and Dr. Bamford arrived and gave Cook some medication. By 1 P.M., Cook had improved enough to wash, shave, dress, and sit up in a chair. Although weak, he met with two of his jockeys and his horse trainer.

Meanwhile, in London, Palmer pretended to be Cook's partner and met Mr. Herring, a bettor's agent to whom he also owed money. Herring and similar agents were authorized to receive bettors' winnings

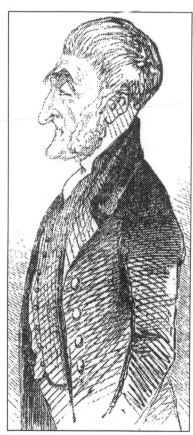

Dr. Bamford, of Rugeley. (From *The Times Report of the Trial of William Palmer*, 1856)

when they could not appear in person. Palmer told Herring that Cook "is all right; his medical man has given him a dose of calomel and recommended him not to come out, and what I want to see you about is the settling of his accounts." He dictated the list of who Herring was to collect from and how much each owed—since such a list in his own handwriting could later provide evidence of fraud.

Herring was to collect about £1,020 of Cook's winnings and, at Palmer's instructions, immediately pay Palmer's moneylenders, Pratt and Padwick, to keep them quiet about the forgeries. But Herring did not pay Padwick, instead pocketing the sum as payment on the debt Palmer owed him.

Palmer returned to Rugeley about 9 P.M. and went to Dr. Salt's office, where the assistant, Charles Newton, sold him three grains of strychnine. (For a description of strychnine and its actions, see Chapter 2, *Thomas Neill Cream, M.D., C.M.*) He then returned to Cook's room and gave him some pills that supposedly were from Dr. Bamford. Observers later said they looked just like the strychnine pills Palmer had purchased from Newton.

After leaving Cook around 11 P.M., Palmer returned to his house. About midnight, Cook awakened the hotel's occupants with violent screaming. Elizabeth Mills, a maidservant who rushed to his room, later said:

> I found him sitting up in bed . . . and beating the bedclothes, with both hands and arms stretched out. He said, "I cannot lie down. I shall suffocate if I do! Oh, fetch Dr. Palmer!" His body, his hands, and neck were moving then—a sort of jumping or jerking. His head was back. Sometimes he would throw back his head upon the pillow, and then he would raise himself up again. This jumping and jerking was all over his body.
>
> He appeared to have great difficulty in breathing. The balls of both the eyes were much protruded. It was difficult for him to speak, he was so short of breath. He screamed three or four times while I was in the room. He called aloud "Murder" twice.
>
> He asked me to rub one hand. I found the left hand stiff. It appeared to be stretched out as though the fingers were something like paralysed. It did not move. It appeared to me to be stiff all the way up his arm. I did not rub him very long. The stiffness did not appear to be gone after I had rubbed him.

Dr. Palmer arrived and instructed Mills to give Cook a dark fluid and some pills. She described what happened next:

> When I gave him from the spoon, his body was then jerking and jumping. He snapped at the spoon with his head and neck, and the spoon was

fast between his teeth. It was difficult to get it away. He seemed to bite it very hard. While this was going on the water went down his throat and washed the pills down. Mr. Palmer then handed him the draught from the wineglass. It was something liquid, and the wineglass was three parts full with a liquid of a dark, heavy-looking nature. Cook drank it. He snapped at the glass just the same as he did at the spoon. He swallowed the liquid, which was vomited up immediately.

The attack lasted about 30 minutes before subsiding. Palmer stayed at Cook's bedside until about 4:45 the next morning.

On Tuesday, Mills arrived in Cook's room about 6 A.M. and found him to be "comparatively comfortable, though still retaining a vivid impression of the horrors he had suffered the night before. He was quite collected, and conversed rationally with [her]." Mills later said that Cook asked her "if I had ever seen any one suffer such agony as he was in the last night, and I said no, I never had. I asked, 'What do you think was the cause of all that, Mr. Cook?' and he said the pills that Palmer gave him at half-past ten."

Just before noon, Palmer went to Mr. Hawkins's chemist shop and purchased two drachms of prussic acid, two drachms of Batley's solution of opium (a common sedative), and six grains of strychnine from the assistant, Charles Joseph Roberts. As he was paying, Newton walked in. It was unusual for Palmer to be buying medications from Mr. Hawkins's shop—he usually purchased them from Mr. Thirlby—so Newton was suspicious and asked Roberts what Palmer had bought. Palmer next visited William Cheshire, the Rugeley postmaster and an old school friend and racing buddy. According to Cheshire, Palmer

asked me to meet him at his house and bring a receipt stamp with me. I did so. He said he wanted me to write out a cheque, which, he said, was for money Mr. Cook owed him. He produced a copy from which I was to write, and I copied it. He gave me as a reason why he wanted me to write it that Mr. Cook was too ill, and he said Charles Weatherby would know his writing. After I had written it I left it with him, and he said he was going to take it over for Mr. Cook to sign.

The £350 check was sent to Charles Weatherby, secretary to the Jockey Club, who received bets for "gentlemen who own racers (horses)." He returned it, noting that the organization would not honor the document.

That afternoon, Palmer returned to the hotel and gave Cook more coffee. Cook started vomiting, and his illness continued throughout the afternoon. Dr. Jones came around 3 P.M., and he and Palmer examined Cook. Dr. Jones

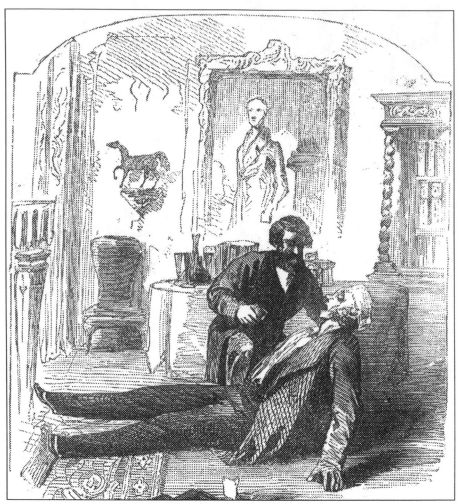

Dr. Palmer "treating" John Cook. (From *The Illustrated Life & Career of William Palmer*, 1856)

commented, as would a practitioner of the time, "this is not the tongue of bilious fever," contradicting Dr. Palmer's prior diagnosis.

Around 7 P.M., Drs. Jones, Bamford, and Palmer discussed Cook's case and agreed that he should take morphine pills before retiring. Palmer had not told them about the prior night's attack. Cook suddenly turned and said, "Palmer, I will have no more pills or medicine tonight." The three physicians, however, decided that Cook should still take the medication. Although on previous nights, a messenger retrieved the pills, that evening Palmer called on Dr. Bamford himself. Since Palmer was to administer the medication, Dr. Bamford found it unusual when Palmer asked him to write the directions on the box, but he wrote "Night pills, John Parsons Cook, Esq." Palmer had the pills in his possession for about 45 minutes—easily enough time to substitute them with something more deadly.

At about 10:30 P.M., Palmer opened the box with the pills and, pointing to Bamford's directions, exclaimed, "What an excellent hand for an old man upwards of 80 to write." Up to that point, Cook was described as being "easy and cheerful, and presented no symptoms of the approach of disease, much less of death." Cook at first refused to take the two pills, but Palmer insisted, and Cook ultimately swallowed them. Palmer then left for his own house. Dr. Jones, who was to spend the night in Cook's room, retired just before midnight. About 20 minutes later, he was aroused by Cook screaming:

> "Doctor get up; I am going to be ill; ring the bell for Mr. Palmer"... He asked me to rub his neck. I rubbed the back part of his neck and supported him with my arm while doing so. There was a stiffening of the muscles; a sort of hardness about the neck.

Elizabeth Mills was in the hotel's kitchen when

> the bell of Mr. Cook's room rang violently... I went upstairs to Mr. Cook's room on hearing the bell. He was sitting up in bed, and Mr. Jones appeared to be supporting him. Mr. Cook said, "Oh, Mary, fetch Mr. Palmer directly." He was conscious at the time. I went over for Mr. Palmer. I rang the surgery bell at the surgery door... I asked him to come over to Mr. Cook directly, as he was much the same as he was the night before. I then went back to the hotel. Palmer came two or three minutes afterwards.

Cook was "gasping for breath, screaming violently, his body convulsed with cramps and spasms, and his neck rigid." Cook asked Palmer to give him the pills that had relieved his symptoms the night before. According to Dr. Jones:

> [Palmer] gave Cook two pills, which he said were ammonia pills. Directly he swallowed them, he uttered loud screams, threw himself back in the bed and was dreadfully convulsed... [Cook] said to me, "Raise me up or I shall be suffocated"...
>
> When he called out to me to raise him, I endeavored to do so with the assistance of Mr. Palmer, but found it was quite impossible owing to the rigidity of the limbs. When he found I could not raise him up he asked me to turn him over, which I did... The head was quite bent back by spasmodic action. The body was twisted back like a bow; the backbone was twisted back. If I had placed the body at that time upon the back on a level surface, it would have rested upon the head and heels.

> After I turned him over I listened to the action of his heart. I found it gradually to weaken . . . He died so very quietly that I could hardly tell when he did die . . . From the time when he raised himself in bed and called upon me to go for Palmer to the time when he died, would be from ten minutes to a quarter of an hour. In my judgment, as a medical man, he died from tetanus, or in ordinary English parlance, lockjaw.

According to Palmer's diary, Cook died at 1 A.M. on Wednesday, November 21. Although Dr. Jones first suspected tetanus as the cause of death, he later thought the convulsions were due to "overexcitement" because his horse had won so much money.

Just after Cook died, Palmer turned to Dr. Jones and said, "It is a bad thing for me, as I was responsible [Cook owed him] £3,000 or £4,000, and I hope Mr. Cook's friends will not let me lose it. If they do not assist me, all my horses will be seized." When Elizabeth Mills entered the room to lay out Cook's body, she saw Palmer searching the pockets of Cook's clothes. (According to testimony presented at the trial, several people saw him search Cook's clothes and other belongings several times after his death.) Some of Cook's missing belongings, including £600 and his betting book in which he recorded all his transactions (including the money Palmer owed him) were never found. Although destitute a few days earlier, Palmer now deposited money in the bank and, on Thursday, paid Pratt £100.

The next day, William Vernon Stevens, Cook's stepfather, arrived in Rugeley and met with Palmer to discuss Cook's affairs and funeral. Palmer told Stevens that he had a legal paper showing that Cook had owed him £4,000 and, to speed interment, Palmer had already ordered the coffin. Stevens was appalled and responded that "there would not be 4,000 shillings" for those Cook owed. When he asked to see Cook's betting book, Palmer told him, "The betting-book would be of no use to you if you found it, for the bets are void by his death." Stevens now had grave misgivings about his stepson's death and returned to London to consult a lawyer.

On Saturday, November 24, Palmer also went to London to pay Pratt another installment on his debt. Palmer would later write to Pratt:

> (Strictly private and confidential.) My dear sir,—Should any of Cook's friends call upon you to know what money Cook ever had from you, pray don't answer that question or any other about money matters until I have seen you.

Stevens ran into into Palmer on the train to London and said that he intended to request a post-mortem examination and would hire a solicitor to investigate.

On Sunday, at Palmer's request, Dr. Bamford completed a death certificate for Cook listing "apoplexy" as the cause of death. Bamford expressed surprise at being asked to do this, but Palmer persisted and Bamford completed the form. Palmer then discussed with Newton the strychnine dosage needed to kill a dog and how much residual would be found in the stomach after death. Palmer also visited with Cheshire, the postmaster, and asked him to witness a document Cook purportedly had signed, acknowledging a debt of £4,000 to Palmer. Cheshire refused, exclaiming, "Good God! The man is dead!" Palmer replied, "It is of no consequence; I dare say the signature will not be disputed, but it occurred to me that it would look more regular if it were attested."

Autopsy and Aftermath

On Monday, November 26, Palmer wrote in his diary, "an autopsy was performed on poor Cook." He insisted, both as a physician and as Cook's friend, that he be present. Dr. Bamford also attended, and Dr. Harland, a local physician, supervised the procedure. On his way to the autopsy, Harland met Palmer and "asked him what the case was; that I heard there was a suspicion of poisoning. He replied, 'Oh, no! I think not; he had an epileptic fit on Monday and Tuesday night, and you will find an old disease in the heart and in the head'"

At the autopsy, Mr. Devonshire, a London University medical student, did the manual work, assisted by Charles Newton. Newton had never before seen an autopsy—and so fortified himself in advance with two wineglasses of brandy. He was, however, intimately involved in the case, since it was he who had supplied Palmer with three grains of strychnine the night before Cook's death. He was also aware that Palmer had purchased six grains more of strychnine on November 20, and he had discussed strychnine poisoning with Palmer the previous evening.

Dr. Harland stated that "about the whole body generally there was no appearance of disease that would account for death." This would not be surprising: strychnine leaves no typical post-mortem traces other than engorgement of the lungs and the vessels of the brain and spinal cord. These are also found in deaths from many other diseases (and could be due to delaying the autopsy for six days). He also noted that "the body seemed to me to be stiffer than bodies generally are six days after death. The muscles were strongly contracted and thrown out, which showed there was a strong spasmodic action in the body before death. The hands were clenched; firmly closed." The autopsy report read:

Post-mortem examination of John Parsons Cook, Esq., Rugeley, Nov. 26th, 1855.—

The body is moderately muscular; the back and most depending parts of the body are discoloured from blood having gravitated there. Pupils of the eyes neither contracted nor dilated. No serum in the peritoneal cavity; the peritoneum slightly injected; no adhesions—stomach as now exposed is rather distended, and the course of some of its vessels is seen beneath the peritoneal coat. The stomach, on being removed, contained some ounces of a brown fluid—the large curvature resting on the spleen was of dark colour. The internal mucous membrane of the stomach was without ulceration or excoriation.

On the inferior surface of the cardiac extremity were minute yellowish-white specks, of the size of mustard seeds. The small intestines contained some bilious fluid in the duodenum; they were altogether small and con-tracted, but presented no other remarkable appearance. The large intestines contained some fluid feculent matter. The spleen and pancreas seemed to be healthy. The right kidney was rather large, soft, and its whole texture full of blood; there were no granulations, nor coagulable lymph. The left kidney was of less size, but its appearance was the same as the right, in less degree.

Between the base of the tongue and epiglottis were numerous enlarged follicles like warts. The œsophagus [sic] and epiglottis were nat-ural. The larynx was stained with dark blood, which had penetrated through all its tissues. The lungs contained much fluid blood in their poste-rior parts, which would be accounted for by gravitation. The lungs every-where contained air. The pleura were healthy, the heart was of natural size, and in every part healthy. In the aorta, immediately behind the valves, were some yellow-greyish-white patches like soft cartilage. The heart pre-sented no remarkable appearance.

The skull was of natural thickness. The dura mater had its arteries injected with blood. There was no excess of serum, nor adhesions. The pia mater and arachnoid, as well as the brain, appeared altogether healthy; all the blood was fluid and uncoagulated.

Signed, J. T. Harland, M.D.

Dr. Harland later testified that "when the intestines and stomach were being placed in the jar, and while Mr. Devonshire was opening the stomach, I noticed Palmer pushed Mr. Newton onto Mr. Devonshire, and he shook a por-tion of the contents of the stomach into the body." To avoid losing any more evidence, they tied the stomach and sealed it in the jar. Palmer later admitted he had handled the jar, and put it by the door. He commented privately to Dr. Bamford, "We ought not to have let that jar go." Palmer tried to bribe the carriage driver to give him the jar, but he refused. Law clerk John Boycott delivered the jars to toxicologist Dr. Alfred Swaine Taylor at Guy's Hospital in London.

Dr. Taylor said that "on opening the jar we found the stomach cut open from end to end, turned inside out, with its mucous membrane lining in contact with the intestines." There were no contents remaining and no ligature was apparent, although Dr. Harland stated that they had tied the stomach. Taylor also received a second jar with some viscera and, in their midst, a corked bottle with some blood. After studying this case, modern forensic pathologist John Glaister said:

> Viewed by present-day standards, the whole investigative procedure was grossly mismanaged. It therefore becomes impossible to express any worthwhile opinion as to whether or not strychnine was originally present in the material submitted for analysis. This aspect of the case provides a model for the teaching of what not to do in the medico-legal investigation of poisoning cases.

On November 29, physicians reopened the body to remove the liver, kidneys, and spleen for analysis. (On January 25, they decided to exhume Cook's body to examine his spinal cord, and found it normal and healthy.) On December 5, the results of the autopsy requested by Cook's stepfather were returned to Rugeley by mail. Postmaster Cheshire steamed open the letter and notified Palmer that neither strychnine nor prussic acid (the two suspected poisons) had been found. Dr. Taylor had found only traces of antimony. When later asked if strychnine can be detected in tissues post-mortem, Taylor said,

> There is no process I am acquainted with when it [strychnine] is in a small quantity; so far as I know it cannot be detected . . . After the post-mortem examination on the body of Mr. Cook, some portion was sent up to me . . . The part which we had to operate upon was in the most unfavourable condition for finding strychnia if it had been there.

Nevertheless, he testified that he knew of no other cause to which Cook's symptoms and death could be attributed except for strychnine poisoning.

On December 8, Palmer foolishly wrote to the Stafford coroner, a lawyer named William Webb Ward, detailing the contents of Professor Taylor's letter (which had not yet been released) and professing his innocence. Hoping to sway the inquest verdict, Palmer sent Ward a gift package (which he never paid for) with a 20-pound turkey, a brace of pheasants, a codfish, and a barrel of oysters. Although Palmer was not named as the donor, the coroner had no doubt about the package's origin. In retrospect, Palmer could not have done more to point an accusatory finger at himself. Ward immediately gave police the note.

On December 14, Professor Taylor gave evidence at the coroner's inquest, where the verdict came back "willful murder." Palmer was already in custody because Padwick had had him arrested for overdue debts. After the indictment, he was taken to Stafford's jail. Police then found evidence of Palmer's forgeries and possible other poisonings. Both Annie's and Walter's bodies were exhumed. While Walter's body was too decomposed to perform toxicological tests, Annie's was found to be saturated with antimony. The investigation also led to Postmaster Cheshire, who was jailed for tampering with the mail.

Normally, Palmer would have been tried by an Assize court in Staffordshire. But he engendered so much hatred among the citizenry that every time he left the jail for a court appearance, he was greeted by a booing, spitting crowd. The situation deteriorated to the point that Parliament hastily passed a special law (*19 Vict. Cap. 16*) permitting Palmer's trial to be held in London's Central Criminal Court at the Old Bailey, rather than in the obviously "poisoned" atmosphere of Staffordshire. That action set the precedent for allowing a change of venue for a trial if there has been publicity that would undermine the possibility of a fair hearing.

Palmer was indicted not only for Cook's death, but also for those of his wife Annie and his brother Walter. The trials were to proceed in sequence. In jail, a disheartened Palmer went on a hunger strike, intending to cheat the hangman. He began eating again only after the jailer said that he would force-feed him through a tube into his stomach.

Palmer's creditors auctioned his 17 remaining thoroughbreds and his personal effects. (Prince Albert, the Queen's husband, bought *Trickstress* for 230 guineas.) Some creditors dunned Mrs. Palmer for payment; since her signature had been forged, she maintained that she had no responsibility to pay. On January 21, 1856, William Palmer was brought in to testify at a creditor's trial against his mother. Anticipating his appearance, "the court was crowded to suffocation, and most of those present were nervous with excitement, in their eagerness to obtain a view of this individual . . . In a perfectly cool and collected manner, [he] surveyed leisurely the crowded audience, to some of whom he nodded in a familiar way." William readily admitted getting his wife, Annie, to sign the note for £2,000 using Mrs. Palmer's name—and, if it was to believed, on other notes as well.

Sir James Stephen, a judge who knew Palmer, came to a conclusion that also is true of many contemporary serial killer physicians:

His career supplied one of the proofs of a fact which many kind-hearted people seem to doubt, namely the fact that such a thing as atrocious wickedness is consistent with good education, perfect sanity, and everything in a word, which deprives men of all excuse for crime. Palmer was respectably brought up; apart from his extravagance and vice, he might have lived comfortably enough.

He was a model of physical health and strength, and was courageous, determined, and energetic. No one ever suggested that there was even a disposition towards madness in him; yet he was as cruel, as treacherous, as greedy of money and pleasure, as brutally hard-hearted and sensual a wretch as it is possible even to imagine. If he had been the lowest and most ignorant ruffian that ever sprang from a long line of criminal ancestors, he could not have been worse than he was.

The Trial

William Palmer, M.D., was charged with murdering John Parsons Cook using strychnine, and the trial began on May 14, 1856. The trial itself was complex; three judges presided, which was very unusual in criminal proceedings. The judges were there to control the powerful and talented lawyers on both sides and to provide balance to the high-profile case. The panel was led by 77-year-old Lord Chief Justice John Campbell, who was thought to be talented but overly ambitious and self-serving. The defense attorneys were not pleased with his conduct during the trial. One later wrote in his memoirs:

> Lord Campbell had prejudged him [Palmer] and was determined to convict. On the first day of the proceedings he showed an unfairness which gradually increased, until his conduct can be justly described by no other word than infamous . . . During Shee's speech for the defense, everything in Palmer's favour was met by frowns and by dagger looks from Campbell, while he made a point of writing down fully everything against, noting scarcely anything to the prisoner's advantage.

Palmer, likewise, did not appreciate Chief Justice Campbell's behavior on the bench. While they were in court, he wrote to his lawyers, "I wish there was 2½ grains of Strychnine in ole Campbell's draught solely because I think he acts unfairly."

Baron Alderson and Justice Cresswell assisted Chief Justice Campbell. Sir Edward Hall Alderson, 69 years old, was a brilliant but undistinguished judge. He was, however, known as a humane jurist who desired to restrict the use of capital punishment. Sir Cresswell, 62 years old, was seen as a strong, learned jurist. He would become the first judge appointed to the new Probate and Divorce Court in 1858.

Sir Alexander James Edmund Cockburn, Britain's attorney general and an excellent orator, was the prosecutor. Lord Cockburn was best known for his high-profile, successful defense of Daniel M'Naughten in 1843, which established his client's innocence by reason of insanity. The plea was known as the McNaughten Rule: a perpetrator was innocent if, at the time of the act, he or she could not distinguish between right and wrong due to mental disability. Cockburn ultimately was elected to Parliament and became Lord Chief Justice of England.

Four distinguished barristers assisted Lord Cockburn. The first was John Edwin James, who subsequently was elected to Parliament, mishandled his finances, fled to America, and returned later to die in poverty. The second was Sir William Henry Bodkin, a distinguished criminal attorney who was also later elected to Parliament and became a specialist in the "poor laws." The team also had William Newland Welsby, a specialist in criminal law, and Sir John Walter Huddleston, who later became a member of Parliament, a judge, and a prominent socialite.

Sir William Shee, a brilliant Irish barrister, led the defense team. Palmer, however, was his first murder defendant. "Serjeant (at law)," the term usually associated with his name, was a title granted to those who excelled in the legal profession. Fifty-two years old at the time of the trial, he later became a member of Parliament and the first Roman Catholic judge in Britain since the Reformation. Serjeant Shee was not Palmer's first choice as lead counsel; he had first employed Serjeant Wilkins, a noted attorney. However, Wilkins had fled the country just before the trial to avoid his own creditors, and Shee was called to fill in.

Shee had three assistants: Sir William Robert Grove, best known as a scientist, was a legal specialist in patent and scientific cases; Edward Vaughan Hyde Kenealy was a poet, legal scholar, activist, and (later) politician; and John Gray, who later became the attorney for the Treasury.

Palmer, sitting quietly in the dock, looked at least ten years older than his 31 years. Confident that he would be acquitted, he showed no emotion throughout the 12-day trial. The *Illustrated London Times* noted that "his features are of a common and somewhat mean cast. There is certainly nothing to indicate . . . the presence of either ferocity or cunning." Another reporter said, "Shrewd observers, however, will notice a remarkable discrepancy between the ruddy coarseness of his face and the extreme prettiness of his hands." Mr. Kenealy of his defense team described Palmer:

> His face bore the impress of honesty, calm, passionless, and truthful . . .
> He displayed the greatest composure on every occasion. His manners
> were courteous, bland, and sympathetic. Yet there was something in their
> very smoothness which reminded me of some creeping reptile; not repul-
> sive, on the contrary, attractive, but suggestive of the gliding, stealthy
> movements of a snake . . . His voice was low and unctuous, almost tender.

In his opening remarks, Lord Cockburn summed up Palmer's motivation:

> Being in desperate circumstances, with ruin, disgrace, and punishment
> staring him in the face, which could only be averted by means of money,
> he took advantage of his intimacy with Cook, when Cook had become the
> winner of a considerable sum, to destroy him, in order to obtain posses-
> sion of his money.

This characterization didn't sit well with William's younger brother, the Reverend Thomas Palmer, and his sister, Sarah Palmer, who attended the trial.
After an early outburst from the reverend, Chief Justice Campbell warned, "Sir,
if you respect my wig, I'll undertake to respect your cloth." No further disrup-
tions occurred.

Prosecution and Defense

As the first of the Victorian doctor-poisoner trials, the Palmer affair attracted
much public attention. It was a "hot ticket," and many of London's rich and
famous attended as spectators. As the prosecutor said, "The peculiar circumstances of this case have given it a profound and painful interest throughout
the whole country." This was the first time that an individual had been accused
of murder using "strychnia" (strychnine) although, almost simultaneously, a
Dr. Dove of Leeds was accused of using the same poison to kill his wife. The
Illustrated London Times published a special edition about the trial that sold an
unprecedented 400,000 copies. As a betting man, Palmer would have been
impressed that the public wagered £200,000 ($11.4 million in 2002) on his
possible conviction.

There were 39 technical witnesses: 24 physicians and scientists for the
prosecution and 15 for the defense. The prosecution alone paraded a total of
66 witnesses before the jury. These witnesses frequently contradicted each
other and their testimony can best be characterized as inconsistent, incom-
plete, and, at times, bizarre. In some cases, however, this simply reflected the
rudimentary medical knowledge and scientific capabilities of the time. Among
the alternatives to strychnine poisoning that the experts suggested were

"general convulsions, arachnitis, epilepsy proper, and epilepsy with tetanic complications." They even mentioned angina pectoris as the cause of death!

Tetanus was the most common alternative suggested, and witnesses described varieties of tetanus that had never existed. Not knowing that microorganisms cause tetanus, practitioners waxed eloquent about "traumatic" and "idiopathic" tetanus, the latter actually nonexistent. As London Hospital's surgeon, Thomas Blizzard Curling (famous for describing "Curling's ulcers"), said, the term implies that tetanus "originates, as it were, as a primary disease, without any wound." Curling, along with most other prosecution experts, said that Cook's symptoms did not fit the picture of tetanus, adding that "a medical practitioner who saw a case of convulsions would be able at once to know the difference between symptoms of general convulsions and of tetanus."

The physicians who attended Cook, however, either could not or did not want to identify his symptoms as anything else. In fact, there was little scientific knowledge about tetanus in 1856. It was not until 1884 that Carle and Rattone successfully induced tetanus in an animal from a tetanus wound, 1885 when Nicolaier produced tetanus in an animal from garden soil, and 1889 when Kitasata successfully isolated the tetanus bacillus. The clinical course of most tetanus cases is gradual, with early fixation of the lower jaw. Strychnine's effect is rapid, and jaw clenching is only part of the general contraction of the body's muscles.

Decades later, when testifying in the case of Dr. Thomas Neill Cream, Dr. Thomas Stevenson, a noted lecturer on medical jurisprudence at Guy's Hospital and an "analyst" (toxicologist/chemist) employed by the British government, observed that they tried the William Palmer case

> in the infancy of our knowledge of strychnine ... It was the first homicidal case in which it was used, and some time after I had the first suicidal case ... If the patient died in one of the paroxysms, I should expect rigidity of the body after death, and that that rigidity would last for some time. It would generally disappear in a week or two after death, but in Palmer's case some portions of the body [of Cook] remained rigid from 21st November, when he died, to early January, when the body was exhumed.

Dr. Bamford initially did not testify in person, since he was ill, and sent a deposition instead. Dr. Robert Bentley Todd of King's College Hospital in London, known for his description of Todd's (post-seizure) paralysis and of *tabes dorsalis* (advanced syphilis), disputed Dr. Bamford's pronouncement of "apoplexy" or "epilepsy." He believed the cause of death to be from strychnine poisoning.

The differences between tetanus, which the defense proposed, and strychnine poisoning were aptly summarized by Lord Cockburn in his opening remarks:

> Tetanus the disease commences with the milder symptoms, which gradually progress towards the development and final completion of the attack. When once the disease has commenced, it continues without intermission, although, as in every other form of malady, the paroxysms will be from time to time more or less intense. In the case of tetanus from strychnine [he meant tetanic spasms] it is not so. It commences with paroxysms which may subside for a time, but are renewed again; and whereas other forms of tetanus almost always last during a certain number of hours or days, when we deal with strychnine we deal with cases not of hours but of minutes—in which we have no beginning of the disease, and then a gradual development to the climax; but in which the paroxysms commence with all their power at the very first, and terminate, after a few short minutes of fearful agony and struggles, in the dissolution of the victim.

Palmer himself wrote a more succinct description in his copy of *Manual for Students Preparing for Examination at Apothecaries' Hall*: "Strychnia kills by causing tetanic fixing of the respiratory muscles." Palmer seems to have been very well-versed in this poison's mode of action, in contrast to one of his defense witnesses, who demonstrated an appalling lack of medical knowledge—even for the mid-1800s:

> I think all forms of convulsions arise from a decomposition of the blood, if a person has probably an incipient tendency to disease of the brain, that it always may be affected, and that the decomposition of the blood might set up the diseased action.

So frustrated was the prosecutor with some of the bizarre medical testimony that he delivered these scathing closing remarks:

> I cannot help saying, to me it seems that it is a scandal upon a learned, a distinguished, and a liberal profession, that men should come forward and put forward such speculations as these, perverting the facts, and drawing from them sophisticated and unwarranted conclusions with the view of deceiving a jury. I have the greatest respect for science—no man can have more; but I cannot repress my indignation and abhorrence when I see it thus perverted and prostituted to the purpose of a particular cause in a Court of Justice.

While the prosecution's toxicologists admitted that they could not find any trace of strychnine in the body parts that had been analyzed, they suggested that Cook might have received a dose of strychnine too small to be detected, even though enough to be fatal. The prosecution did show that no natural disease, including tetanus (which was then common), could provoke Cook's symptoms; only strychnine poisoning would explain them.

Palmer's defense relied primarily on the fact that strychnine was not found in Cook's body and that some scientists, including Dr. Herepath, Professor of Chemistry at Bristol Medical School, believed it could be found, with proper chemical analysis, in any victim. On cross-examination, some defense witnesses, however, had to admit that the symptoms did sound a lot like those of strychnine poisoning.

Serjeant Shee's closing speech for the defense grated on those who heard it. The leading legal journal wrote:

> The defence of Mr. Serjeant Shee was clever, ingenious, and eloquent, but wanting in judgment and taste. The peroration was a striking instance of this defect, for the allusion to the family of the prisoner, and to his supposed affection for his wife, grated sorely, and almost ludicrously, on the sense of propriety in the face of the undisguised fact, known to all his audience, that he was accused of murdering his wife, that he slept with his maidservant on the very night she died, and that he had confessed himself guilty of forgery upon his mother. Equally injudicious was the philippic against the insurance offices. In worse taste still was his solemn assertion to the jury that he was convinced by the evidence of the prisoner's innocence.

In his closing arguments, Lord Cockburn gave a long and impassioned speech without notes. Palmer wrote a note in racing language to his lawyers, complimenting Cockburn on his speech's deadly effect: "It was the riding that did it."

Chief Justice Campbell spent two days delivering his summary of the trial and instructions to the jury. In part, he said:

> If you are satisfied of his guilt—it will be your duty to return a verdict of guilty; for if the poisoner were to escape with impunity, there would be no safety for mankind, and society would fall to pieces ... In a case of this kind you cannot expect that witnesses should be called to state that they saw the deadly poison administered by the prisoner or mixed up by the prisoner openly before them. Circumstantial evidence as to that is all that can be reasonably expected; and if there are a series of circumstances leading to the conclusion of guilt, then, gentlemen, a verdict of guilty may satisfactorily be pronounced ...

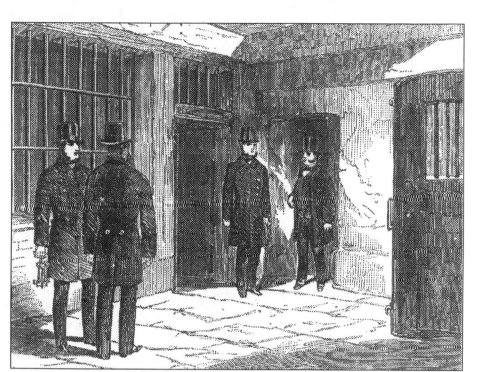

Cells below the Central Criminal Court. (From *The Times Report of the Trial of William Palmer*, 1856)

You will look at the medical evidence to see whether the deceased, in your opinion, did die by strychnia or by natural disease; and you will look at what is called the moral evidence, and consider whether that shows that the prisoner not only had the opportunity, but that he actually availed himself of that opportunity, to administer to the deceased the deadly poison of which he died.

Punishment

Throughout his trial, Palmer remained confident of an acquittal, even after the judge's prejudicial instructions to the jury ended on May 27. After two days of listening to instructions, when the jury took only an hour and 18 minutes to reach their verdict, Palmer realized he had been wrong. He later wrote, "I saw the cocked-up nose of the perky little foreman, I knew it was a gooser with me!" The jury pronounced him guilty. Palmer was asked why the Court should not sentence him to death; he remained mute. Chief Justice Campbell then pronounced sentence:

> William Palmer, after a long and impartial trial you have been convicted by a jury of your country of the crime of wilful murder. In that verdict my two learned brothers, who have so anxiously watched this trial, and myself entirely concur, and consider that verdict altogether satisfactory. The case is attended with such circumstances of aggravation that I do not dare to touch upon them. Whether it is the first and only offence of this sort which you have committed is certainly known only to God and your own conscience. It is seldom that such a familiarity with the means of death should be shown without long experience; but for this offence of which you have been found guilty your life is forfeited. You must prepare to die; and I trust that, as you can expect no mercy in this world, you will, by repentance of your crimes, seek to obtain mercy from Almighty God . . .
>
> I will content myself now with passing upon you the sentence of the law, which is, that you be taken hence to the gaol of Newgate, and thence removed to the gaol of the county of Stafford, the county in which the offence of which you are justly convicted was committed; and that you be taken thence to a place of execution, and be there hanged by the neck until you be dead; and that your body be after-wards buried within the precincts of the prison in which you shall be last confined after your conviction; and may the Lord have mercy upon your soul. Amen!

Lord Campbell later wrote in his diary:

> My anxiety was over on the last day, when the verdict of *guilty* was pronounced and I had sentenced the prisoner to die, for I had no doubt of his guilt, and I was conscious that by God's assistance I had done my duty. Such was the expressed opinion of the public and of all the respectable part of the Press.

Over the years, it has been suggested that Cook's stepfather, Mr. Stevens, paid some witnesses to provide false and damaging testimony. But, as toxicologist John Glaister wrote [quoting from an unnamed source], "William Palmer was not convicted upon loose coincidences but, irrespectively of all medical theories, he led to his own conviction by a series of acts which, in the mind of every unbiased person, were perfectly inconsistent with his innocence." Glaister came "to the definite conclusion that they [these episodes] were fully consistent with strychnine poisoning."

Prosecution of an individual for homicidal poisoning has always been difficult. There are three basic problems that must be overcome:

1. There are generally no witnesses.
2. It may be difficult to positively identify the poison or the substance used to deliver the poison, such as food, in what remains of the body.
3. Circumstantial evidence matching the poison's actions to those of the victim's symptoms is often the only testimony available.

While in prison, Palmer was quoted as saying, "I am innocent of poisoning Cook with strychnia." Whether Palmer murdered his friend with strychnine or another poison did not matter, however, for he had been found guilty and, at the time, no procedure existed for appealing criminal convictions.

On June 14, 1856, after only a few hours of sleep, Palmer was awakened by the prison chaplain. He was allowed to shave and wash up before eating breakfast. Then he emerged from the Stafford jail to face a vast throng of spectators who had been arriving for days to watch his execution. Witnesses described the scene:

In the more immediate vicinity of the gaol raised platforms were erected on every available spot from which a sight of the gallows could be obtained . . . the charge for admission to some of the front seats was as high as a guinea for each person; half a guinea was the ordinary rate, but back standing places were attainable for less money . . .

Long before five o'clock [A.M.], every avenue leading to the gaol was choked up . . . Upwards of 20,000 strangers had assembled in the town . . . The scaffold was a huge affair, somewhat resembling an agricultural machine, and hung with black cloth. Contrary to the usual custom in small country towns, it was not built upon the top of the prison, but was brought out in front, so as to encroach upon the road, and thus circumscribe the points occupied by the spectators. It was brought out from the jail about four o'clock in the morning.

Another report indicated:

Between his conviction and his execution Palmer entertained no thought of confession, and exhibited no feeling, not even the slightest, of compunction or remorse . . . Lord Brampton obtained the following account from the Governor of the gaol of his [Palmer's] procession to the "fatal tree" . . .

On the morning of the execution the path from the condemned cell to the gallows was wet and muddy, it having rained during the night, and Palmer minced along like a delicate schoolgirl, picking his way and avoiding the puddles. He was particularly anxious not to get his feet wet. He was received on the scaffold with a deafening round of curses, shouts, oaths, and execrations from a crowd of twenty to thirty thousand people.

At the time, it was expected that the condemned prisoner would speak to the crowd before his execution, often confessing to the crime. Palmer looked briefly at the vast multitude as if ready to address them. But he turned away, the long cap was drawn over his face, and he was heard to murmur "God bless you" to the executioner. The drop fell, and William Palmer, M.D., age 31 and the first of the Victorian doctor-poisoners, died dangling at the end of a rope.

Epilogue

After Palmer's death, the Rugeley town council petitioned the Prime Minister to change the town's name so it could disassociate itself from Palmer's legacy. Prime Minister Palmerston agreed, but on the condition that they name the town after him! (The name-change idea was dropped.) Palmer's impressive Tudor house eventually became a video store. Palmer was buried in an unmarked grave in the prison where he was hanged.

The epitaph on Cook's grave reads:

Sacred to the memory of John Parsons Cook whose life was taken away from him on the night of 20 November, 1855 in the 29th year of his age. Amiable and affectionate in his disposition and generous in his conduct, he was sincerely beloved and will long be lamented by his kindred and friends.

This was the legacy of William Palmer, M.D.

How Much Was A Pound (£) Worth?

William Palmer killed at least two people for £13,000 and murdered his final victim for about £2,500. It doesn't sound like enough to spark such heinous crimes. Or was it? The answer lies in the confusing British monetary system of the nineteenth century and the changing value of money over the past two centuries.

Victorian Britain used a monetary system with units that still have a familiar ring because of their use in the popular literary works of Charles Dickens, Arthur Conan Doyle, and their contemporaries. Yet, even modern Brits have difficulty explaining the likes of a *farthing* or a *groat*, common coins of that period.

The monetary units were, to say the least, a bit complicated. The basic unit was the *pound Sterling* (£). A gold coin worth £1 was a *sovereign*. They also had *half-sovereign* coins. Each pound was divided into 20 *silver shillings* (s), also called a *bob*. The silver *crown* was worth 5s; a *half-crown* was worth half that much. Each shilling, in turn, was divided into 12 *pennies* (d) or *pence*, so 240 pence made one pound. (The "d" for pence comes from "denarius," the Roman silver coin. It was initially used for the English silver penny, which was no longer in general circulation in Victorian times.)

Pennies were made of copper until 1860, when the government switched to bronze. Copper coins, referred to as "coppers," included the *halfpenny* and the *farthing* (worth a quarter of a penny). One-third and one-quarter farthing coins were also minted, but were used mainly in the British colonies. Silver *sixpence* and *threepence* coins, sometimes called "thrupp'ny bits," were also in circulation, as were silver *groats*, also called "Joeys," worth four pence.

A more gentlemanly method of payment was the *guinea*. Each guinea was worth £1-1s (£1.05) and was abbreviated 1*g* or 1*gn*. The government also issued *half, third,* and *quarter guineas*. While the lower classes such as tradesmen expected to be paid in pounds, professionals such as lawyers, doctors, writers, and artists expected their pay in guineas. For example, when barristers (lawyers) were paid in guineas, they kept the pounds for themselves and gave the shillings to their law clerks. Although the coins were not minted after 1813, this tradition remained intact far longer.

In a first step toward decimalizing their coinage, the British government issued the *florin* in 1849. Worth two shillings, exactly one-tenth of a pound, it was also called the "two-shilling piece" or "two-bob-bit." The *double florin* was issued in 1887. Money changes value, usually buying less with each passing year. So what was this money worth in today's currency? According to data compiled by the Economic Policy and Statistics Section of the British House of Commons, the equivalent of the pound in various years would be:

£100 (1850) = £7,200 or $11,448 (2002)
£100 (1855) = £5,700 or $ 9,063 (2002)
£100 (1877) = £6,200 or $ 9,858 (2002)

continued . . .

How Much Was A Pound (£) Worth?, continued

In 1855, £1,000 would buy the equivalent of $90,630 (U.S.) in 2002, while £13,000 would now be worth about $1.2 million!

In the United States, while the dollar has always been the standard currency, its value has also changed over time. According to the U.S. Department of Labor Statistics and the Bureau of Living Conditions' statistics, $100 in 1890 would be equivalent to $1,871 in 2002.

What is $1 worth in constant 2002 dollars? If you had $1 in any given year since 1820, it would be worth the following in 2002:

1820–1850	$16.73	1965	$5.43
1850–1875	$16.56	1975	$2.96
1875–1900	$18.71	1985	$1.59
1900–1925	$14.34	1991	$1.26
1935	$12.49	2002	$1.00
1945	$ 9.53		

Obviously, neither the dollar nor the pound go quite as far as they once did.

Nineteenth-Century English Monetary Units

Name	Symbol	Value
Guinea	g or gn	1 1/20 pound
Pound Sterling	£	1 pound
Sovereign	£	1 pound (gold coin)
Half Sovereign		1/2 pound (gold coin)
Silver Crown		1/4 pound or 5 shillings
Double Florin		1/5 pound or 4 shillings
Half Crown		1/8 pound
Florin or Two-Bob-Bit		1/10 pound or 2 shillings
Shilling or Bob	s	1/20 pound or 12 pence (silver coin)
Sixpence		1/2 shilling
Silver Groat or Joey		1/3 shilling or 4 pence
Threepence		1/4 shilling
Penny or Pence	d	1/240 pound or 1/12 shilling
Halfpenny		1/24 shilling
Farthing		1/48 shilling or 1/4 pence

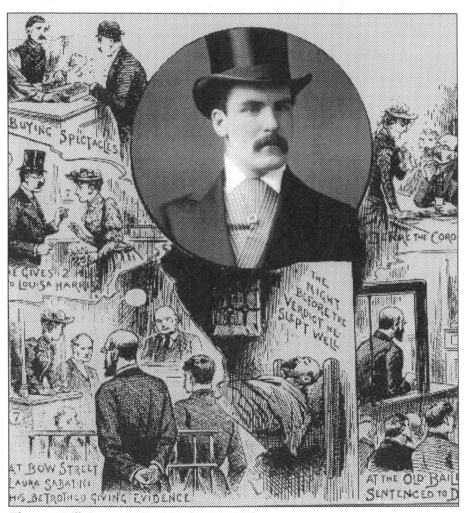

Thomas Neill Cream, M.D., C.M. (1850–1892).

2
Seed of a Poisonous Tree

Thomas Neill Cream, M.D., C.M.

"*He warn't a bad trick, for a medical man,*" she thought. "*We 'ad a good time at the Music Hall before, and the dinner and food warn't bad aftarward. And to boot, he gave me them there pills to ward off the clap.*" The 19-year-old prostitute had swallowed the capsules with the last of her beer and started for home. She suddenly felt anxious, her nerves on edge. Muscles started twitching in her face. Feeling weak, she leaned against a wall, then fell flat on her face. Another trick was approaching with "that look" in his eyes.

"*Not now, I carn't go with 'im now,*" she thought. As the man approached, she moaned, "*Someone 'as given me a drink. Take me home.*" He helped her to her feet, but she had trouble keeping her balance. "*I must look pretty bad,*" she thought. "*He's taking me home.*"

"*What happened, dearie?*" asked her landlady.

"*A tall gentleman with cross eyes, a silk hat, and bushy whiskers gave me two drinks out of a bottle with white stuff in it.*"

Ellen Donworth made a piercing cry as her back suddenly arched and her arms went rigid—only her feet and head were touching the floor. Her eyes were wide with fear, her face turning bluer with every second.

"*I'll get the police and a doctor,*" said her landlady.

Between spasms, she gasped for breath, dreading the sound or movement or touch that would set it off again. "*Let me die at home, don't leave me,*" she pleaded. But they bundled her into a waiting cab, the horse jittery with the commotion.

She seized again in the cab, her arms and legs crashing against its thin walls. As she gasped, straining for air that wouldn't come, the world faded into a gray mist, and she found peace.

~

Early Years

Born in Glasgow, Scotland, on May 27, 1850, Thomas Neill Cream was the oldest of William and Mary Elder Cream's eight children. Nothing is known of his mother, but his father was an industrious and well-liked man. The family moved to Canada when Thomas was four years old, and his father managed Gilmour & Company, a Quebec shipbuilding and lumber firm.

Only sparse information exists about Thomas Cream's childhood years. He was apprenticed as a youth to the shipbuilding firm of Baldwin & Company, and later worked with his father when William became a wholesale lumber merchant in Quebec City. Meanwhile, he attended the company school and also taught Sunday school. This life did not appeal to Thomas, and he left to study at the university, although he did return every summer to work with his father.

Cream entered McGill College in Montreal on October 1, 1872, and he formally enrolled as a medical student on November 12. He seemed to be a competent, but not brilliant, student. As a harbinger of things to come, Cream was said to have gained distinction in school for writing an essay on chloroform. While his landlady in Quebec remembered him as a gentleman, he earned a reputation among fellow students and the faculty for living the high life, with his expensive clothes, jewelry, and horses and carriages. His father kept him supplied with sufficient funds for this lifestyle. Also known for his ingratiating manner, Cream dabbled in music, participated in sports, and continued to teach Sunday school.

In September 1874, Cream took out $1,000 of fire insurance on the personal goods he kept in his lodgings. Two weeks after he graduated, a small fire broke out in his room. Firemen responding to the blaze discovered a charred medical school skeleton in his bed. Cream filed a claim for $978.40, but the Commercial Union Insurance Company smelled a rat and refused to pay. After arbitration, they settled on a payment of $350—arson and insurance fraud were probably Cream's first unpunished crimes.

He graduated in less than four years, receiving the degrees of Doctor of Medicine (M.D.) and Master of Surgery (C.M.) on March 31, 1876. His class photograph shows Cream with short bristling hair and long sideburns. By the end of his life, he would be bald and have a full beard. Upon graduation, Cream became, in the words of a McGill professor, "a man who may fairly be regarded as McGill's most infamous medical graduate." At his commencement, Professor Thomas Roddick addressed the class, saying, "I stand here, Gentlemen, on this account more than on any other, to implore you in the name and for the sake of this great University, in the name and for the sake of our common humanity, on behalf of all that is near and dear to yourselves, to pursue a course of prudence, sobriety and honour." Cream obviously paid little heed to these words, quickly embarking on what has been described as a "terrible career of debauchery and crime."

It was claimed that after Cream's first murder conviction, McGill University removed his name from its alumni rolls. McGill history professor Edward Bensley set the record straight:

> No doubt McGill would have been glad to wash its hands of Thomas Neill Cream but in fact it never managed to do so. His name was not struck from the alumni roll. It appears in the *1924 McGill Directory of Graduates*, the last to include deceased as well as living graduates . . . On the contrary, his name remains with those of his classmates in the various registers of graduates.

Bensley did point out that despite McGill's possible miscalculation in granting Cream a medical degree, Quebec never granted him a license to practice medicine in that province. Other jurisdictions made that error.

Not long before he graduated from medical school, Cream met Flora Eliza Brooks, from Waterloo, about 70 miles from Quebec. The daughter of the major hotel owner in that city, they met when she visited Montreal, and soon were a couple. On the night of September 6, 1876, Flora became very ill. The family doctor told her father that her illness was due to a recent abortion—a procedure that Cream had, in fact, performed. At that time, abortions were relatively common, since condoms, diaphragms, and douches were very expensive. *Coitus interruptus*, little better than Russian roulette, was the only practical method available to most couples.

Her father was livid and raced to Montreal, where he confronted Cream and threatened to shoot him if he did not immediately marry Flora. Flora became Mrs. Thomas Cream on September 11. The day following his shotgun wedding (he actually was taken to Waterloo at gunpoint), Cream announced that he was going to England to complete his medical training. Such postgraduate work was not unusual at the time, but, for Cream, escaping Waterloo and his new spouse seemed a prudent thing to do.

Lambeth and St. Thomas's Hospital

Cream arrived in London in October 1876, and lodged on Lambeth Palace Road while he attended lectures across the street at St. Thomas's Hospital and served as a resident ("temporary clerk") in obstetrics. The narrow streets of Lambeth smelled of fish shops, jam factories, and hop yards. The sidewalks were clogged with swarms of dirty, sore-eyed children, who, along with the adults, died at a much higher rate than elsewhere in London: one out of every five Lambeth infants died in the first year of life.

It was a rough area, and the pervasive cart peddlers (coster mongers) united to stave off the police. (A policeman was called a "bobby" or "peeler," after Sir Robert Peel, who established London's Metropolitan Police Force in 1829.) Lambeth's only beauty was Lambeth Palace, the London home of the Archbishop of Canterbury, and its claim to fame was Charles Morton's Canterbury Music Hall.

St. Thomas's Hospital, founded in 1552 and newly rebuilt in 1871 with eight pavilions on nine acres, stretched along the Thames River directly across from the House of Commons. Florence Nightingale established her nursing school at the hospital and, subsequently (at the same time Cream returned to the area, supposedly to attend lectures at the hospital, but actually to continue his killing spree), the physician-novelist Somerset Maugham also trained there in obstetrics. He would later write about his experiences in his first novel, *Liza of Lambeth* (1897):

> The messenger led you through the dark and silent streets of Lambeth, up stinking alleys and into sinister courts where the police hesitated to penetrate, but where your black bag protected you from harm. You were taken to grim houses, on each floor of which a couple of families lived, and shown into a stuffy room, ill-lit with a paraffin lamp, in which two or three women, the midwife, the mother, the "lady as lives on the floor below" were standing round the bed on which the patient lay.

Located as it was in an area of indigents and manual laborers, St. Thomas's received a steady stream of patients burned at the gasworks, cut by chisels, maimed by pottery machinery, crushed on the docks, and hurt in carriage accidents.

Lambeth women had few opportunities to work. They could serve as domestics, fur pullers, or in one of the jam, pickle, or sweets factories. But, given the numerous pubs, railway lines, and music halls in the area, many women opted to become an "unfortunate," trading sexual favors for money.

Cream already seemed to be familiar with, if not expert in, abortions, as evidenced by his work on Flora. Yet he won no prizes at St. Thomas's, perhaps because he spent inordinate amounts of time "paying his addresses" to women. On April 16, 1877, he failed the Royal College of Surgeons' anatomy and physiology examinations. Cream may have moved across the ocean, but he had not entirely forgotten Flora. As a Scotland Yard detective later wrote after interviewing Flora's physician, Dr. Phelan:

> Subsequent to the marriage when Mrs. Cream became ill, [Dr. Phelan] was scarcely able to understand her symptoms and he asked the deceased if she had been taking anything and she said she had taken some medicine her husband sent her. He told her not to take anything except what he himself prescribed and she promised not to do so and the symptoms he had not understood gradually passed away. Dr. Phelan says he never saw any of the medicine Cream had sent his wife but he strongly suspected him of foul play.

On August 12, 1877, Mrs. Flora Brooks Cream died of what was diagnosed as tuberculosis. Neither an autopsy nor toxicological analysis was done. Although Cream had abandoned his new wife immediately after their wedding, he filed a claim with his father-in-law for $1,000 still due under his marriage contract. He later settled for $200.

On April 13 of the following year, he passed the examinations to qualify for membership in both Edinburgh, Scotland's, Royal College of Physicians and Royal College of Surgeons. Cream's time at St. Thomas's had ended and, armed with some of the best medical education of the time, he was ready to begin his deadly career.

Murder in the Americas

Cream returned to Canada and set up practice above Bennett's Fancy Store in London, Ontario. He specialized in obstetrics just as the specialty was becoming marginally recognized within the field of medicine. Perhaps the stirrups, straps, and invasive equipment of the gynecological examining room attracted him, especially when legally used on unwilling prostitutes for disease monitoring.

Not long after his arrival, on May 3, 1879, a young hotel chambermaid, Kate Hutchinson Gardener, was found dead in an outhouse behind Cream's offices. Her face had been mutilated with chemicals and a bottle of chloroform lay by her side. She had seen Cream repeatedly about getting an abortion and, for the week prior to her death, she had been living in a boarding house rather than in her room at the hotel.

Cream claimed that Kate Gardener had told him that a prominent businessman had impregnated her and declared that she must have committed suicide. Gardener's roommate testified at the coroner's inquest that Cream not only had given her an abortifacient (medication, often a poison, to induce an abortion), but also had suggested that she blackmail a wealthy hotel guest by saying that he was the child's father. Expert medical testimony concluded that no one could commit suicide by holding a chloroform-soaked rag over their own face. The coroner's jury ruled that "the deceased died from chloroform administered by some person unknown."

Years later, when Cream was awaiting execution in England, he confessed to his lawyer that "he made a practice of poisoning dissolute girls in Canada." Kate Gardener may have been the first. In fact, either by intention or through malpractice, Cream may have murdered countless women who sought his medical assistance as a physician-abortionist. Although it could not be proven, everyone in London, Ontario, suspected that Dr. Cream was an abortionist, blackmailer, and murderer. His practice ruined, he fled to the United States.

In August 1879, Thomas Neill Cream, M.D., obtained an Illinois medical license and opened an office in the 400 block of Chicago's West Madison Street. Chicago had been designated the "wickedest city in the world," and Cream did his part to uphold the title. His office abutted the West Side, where many of the city's 3,500 prostitutes worked for 50¢ a trick. Word on the street was that Dr. Cream was primarily an abortionist. A young black midwife, Hattie Mack, who lived six blocks from his office, often assisted him.

On August 20, Miss Mack's tenant became suspicious when, after seeing her quickly leave, he smelled a "horrible stench." He called the police, who broke down Mack's door and found the rotting remains of a young woman who was later identified as Mary Anne Faulkner from Ottawa, Canada. They also found a letter Mack had written to Cream saying that since the woman was dead, she was leaving. An autopsy confirmed that Faulkner had died after an abortion.

Chicago police arrested both of them on August 23, 1880, for murder. Mack was willing to testify that she had boarded Mrs. Faulkner only because she owed Dr. Cream money. She said that Faulkner, whose husband had recently deserted her, felt that she had to abort the fetus so she could support herself. She had given another doctor her gold watch just to get Cream's name as a doctor who was "in the business" of doing abortions. Cream was, indeed, in the business, and had told Mack that "he had treated 500 like cases either at the St. Johns or some other hospital in Canada." Mack also said that Faulkner had told her that Cream was well-known by prostitutes as an abortionist and that he had operated on "as many as 15 cases in one sporting house [brothel] with success."

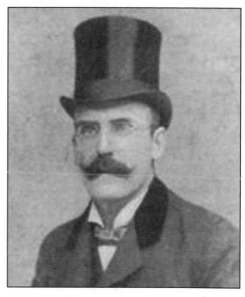

Yet, Mrs. Faulkner became septic after her abortion and was desperately ill. Cream visited her frequently, but he could not help her. As Faulkner lay in critical condition, Cream suggested that Mack burn down the house to destroy any evidence; she declined to do so.

Thomas Neill Cream, M.D., C.M.

The public was furious. The *Chicago Tribune* editorialized, "Let the law be invoked to its utmost limit. If Earl [Cream's abortionist cellmate] and Cream be the guilty persons, as seems to be the case from all the evidence at hand, let them hang. This is the surest remedy against the prevalence of abortion as a practice."

Cream was tried for Mary Anne Faulkner's murder on November 16, 1880. He was acquitted primarily because the all-white male jury would not accept a "coloured" woman's word against that of a white male physician. The contrast between the two also played a role. Cream, according to the *Chicago Tribune*, was the best-dressed and best-looking defendant to appear in a Chicago courtroom for years. In contrast, the *Tribune* reported that Hattie Mack, "tripped downstairs in an exceedingly dirty gown, to say that 'she didn't know nuffin' 'bout nuffin'." Cream's lawyer asserted that Mack probably caused the death, "since it was a bungling piece of work and could not have been done by an experienced physician." His defense counsel, A. S. Trude, later revealed that he knew that Cream's "mania was to get rid of women who were in a condition in which they were a menace to society."

In December 1880, a Miss Stack died after taking a medication Dr. Cream prescribed. Starting a practice that he would repeat, in early 1881, Cream sent blackmail letters to the pharmacist who had prepared the prescription. The pharmacist went to the police, but they dropped the matter, leaving the pharmacist with a tarnished reputation. During Cream's trial for Daniel Stott's murder, the truth became known and the pharmacist's reputation was restored.

Sex, Lies, and Strychnine: The Stott Case

Cream tried to augment his income by promoting his own nostrum to cure epilepsy. The doctor not only made extra money from his bogus medicine, but also met Julia Stott, the pretty, 33-year-old wife of Daniel Stott. The 61-year-old Daniel was a railway station agent in Boone County, Illinois. Mr. Stott suffered from epilepsy, and his wife made frequent visits to Dr. Cream's office on the pretext of obtaining fresh medicine for her husband. Actually, she was having an affair with Dr. Cream.

On June 11, 1881, she picked up her husband's medicine at the pharmacy, then returned to Cream's office. While there, as she later testified in court, she saw Cream put a white powder into the medicine and also into some rhubarb pills she had bought. On June 14, Daniel Stott took the medication; 20 minutes later he was dead. No one thought much about his death, since it could easily be ascribed to epilepsy. But Cream could not let well enough alone; he had unsuccessfully tried to insure Stott's life just before he died. In addition, after the death, he contacted the Boone County coroner, saying that Stott's death was probably due to the pharmacist putting too much strychnine in the man's medication. (Strychnine, a white powder, was used in small quantities in some medications of the time.) Meanwhile, Cream persuaded Mrs. Stott to give him the legal power to sue the pharmacist.

While this complicated scheme involving murder, sex, fraud, and blackmail was in progress, Cream had already been arrested for sending "the vilest sort of postal cards through the mails" to Joseph Martin, whose family Cream had been treating. Cream alleged that Martin owed him $20, a charge Martin denied. The *Chicago Tribune* reported:

> [Cream] informed Martin that his (Martin's) wife and children were suffering from diseases which, he said, they had contracted through Martin himself. He then proceeded to threaten him with an exposure of the matter unless his bill were paid, and, to be more circumstantial, added that the proofs of his allegation consisted of certain prescriptions on file at one Knox's drug store.

The second letter was similar in its tone, but wound up with the threat, "I will learn [teach] that damned vixon of a low wife of yours to speak ill of me."—from which it might be inferred that Mrs. Martin had perhaps been somewhat free in the use of her tongue ... Cream has added the crowning infamy of attempting to blast that which every man holds dearest—the fair name of his wife and children.

Mary McClellan, an elderly English woman, posted the $1,200 bail necessary to free Cream. He immediately jumped bail and fled to Canada.

While Cream was embroiled in his libelous activities, the county coroner took a sample of Daniel Stott's medication and injected it into a dog. The dog seized and died 15 minutes later. That provided a reason for him to exhume Stott's body. Cutting out the corpse's stomach, he sent it to Professor Walter S. Haines at Rush Medical College for analysis. Dr. Haines found nearly 4 grains of strychnine (1 grain equals 64.8 milligrams) in Stott's stomach and more than 2½ grains in each of the pills Stott had received after Cream's tampering. Police arrested Dr. Cream on July 27 near Windsor, Ontario. They brought him back to Chicago, where both he and Mrs. Stott were jailed for murdering her husband.

Cream's trial began on September 20, 1881, the day after U.S. President James Garfield, who was wounded by an assassin in July, finally succumbed to his wounds. This time, Cream did not have the money to hire the best defense attorney and his father refused to pay. Mrs. Stott turned state's evidence and, according to the *Chicago Tribune*, "tried to convict Dr. Cream to save her own neck." Her 10-year-old daughter, who was described as "very brilliant for her age," testified that "Dr. Cream told me he loved my mother, and would like her as his own."

Mrs. McClellan testified that "on the night of the death of Daniel Stott, Cream was at her house in Chicago, and that he told her he expected to hear of Daniel Stott's death at any time, as he knew he had been poisoned." She also admitted that she had lost the money that she had put up for Cream's bail when he fled the country. What she did not say (although the police knew it) was that Cream had seduced, impregnated, performed an abortion on, and then abandoned her daughter.

On September 23, the jury announced its guilty verdict and imposed a sentence of life imprisonment, which was to include one day each year in solitary confinement. "Cream," said the *Chicago Tribune*, "took the verdict very coolly." His lawyer immediately moved for a new trial, but, as the *Tribune* reported:

general opinion is that the case is at an end, and that, even if new trial could be obtained, it would do Cream no good, but that if another jury were to pass on the case, the death penalty might be inflicted.

On November 1, 1881, Cream was sent to Illinois State Penitentiary in Joliet. Mrs. Stott remained in the county jail awaiting her own trial, but no trial ever took place. She then disappeared so completely that even the Pinkertons could not locate her.

Joliet Prison housed 1,500 inmates and was known for its corruption. Said one man who worked there, "Everything connected with the prison administration was rotten to the core." As a result, although Cream had been sentenced to life in prison, on June 12, 1891, the governor of Illinois commuted his sentence to 17 years. Allowed time off for good conduct, he was released on July 31, 1891—after serving fewer than ten years. Cream's brother, who believed that he was innocent, later admitted that "leading politicians" helped him secure his brother's release shortly after the Cream children came into an enormous inheritance from their father. Cream's defense lawyer would later say that his release was primarily due to political influence that the family purchased.

After his release, Cream returned briefly to Canada to collect his inheritance of $16,000. Upon his arrival, his family was shocked to find that prison had turned Cream into a frightening drug addict; some family members even voiced suspicions that he was insane. With his newfound wealth, and after the cool reception from his family, he decided to return to England "for his health." Once there, he quickly resumed his evil ways.

Jolly Old England

On October 1, 1891, Cream landed in Liverpool aboard the *Teutonic*. By October 5, he had made his way to London, eventually again taking lodgings on the sordid Lambeth Palace Road, which he would make infamous.

Cream preferred to spend his days reading and writing in his residence. At night, he frequented the music halls that offered not only vaudeville acts but also a plethora of women willing to show him a good time. On October 6, Cream met two such women, Eliza Masters and Elizabeth May (who eventually would be damning witnesses against him). They described Cream as having a squint. This was confirmed by a local optician who fitted him for glasses. Cream actually suffered from hypermyopia in his left eye, making him cross-eyed and giving him a pronounced squint.

Three days after their meeting, Masters received a letter saying that Cream would call on her that afternoon between 3 P.M. and 5 P.M. In the letter, he asked her "not to be as cross" with him as she was during their first meeting. At the appointed time, she and May sat at the window waiting for him. When they spied their intended client with another prostitute, Matilda Clover, the women followed the pair until they entered Clover's residence together. Although they waited a half-hour, neither Cream nor Matilda reappeared.

A few days later, Cream went to a local pharmacy and purchased *nux vomica*, a "scheduled drug" that required physician-purchasers to register their name and address. (Although the pharmacy assistant could not find Cream's name in the register of licensed physicians, he apparently assumed that he was simply a not-yet-licensed medical student. The test was "whether the man could write a Latin prescription or not.") The drug contained two chemicals: the alkaloids of brucine and strychnine. When the pharmacy assistant asked why he needed that dangerous drug, Cream said that it was for a medical course at St. Thomas's that he was attending. (He took no such course, as the registrar from St. Thomas's Hospital would later testify.)

Cream continued to buy quantities of the drug, along with a supply of small Number 5, or Planter's, capsules—presumably in which to put the drug. As the pharmacy assistant said, "they are used for putting powders and solids into, in order as far as possible to render the medicine tasteless . . . they are not commonly used by medical men in London. We have different kinds of capsules prescribed . . . English people prefer English capsules and foreigners prefer foreign ones." Soon, Cream began to use his deadly purchases.

On October 13, Ellen Donworth, a 19-year-old prostitute, received a letter asking her to meet someone that evening. Ellen lived a few blocks from Masters and May, and had recently lost her only child. She became a prostitute after finding work in a bottle-labeling plant too boring. After having dinner with Ernest Linnell, the soldier with whom she lived (and whose last name she sometimes used), she met a man at the York Hotel. Later, as she leaned against a wall, James Styles, who was thinking of using her services, saw her suddenly fall on her face. He helped her stand up, but she staggered, trembling severely. "Take me home," she moaned. Styles and another man took her home, where her landlady said that she initially thought Donworth was drunk, as she could smell alcohol on her breath. Even though her facial muscles kept twitching, Donworth was able to tell her, "A tall gentleman with cross eyes, a silk hat, and bushy whiskers gave me a drink twice out of a bottle with white stuff in it." Donworth then had such severe convulsions that it took several people to restrain her.

A physician was summoned, and described Donworth's symptoms as "tetanic convulsions as would be caused by an overdose of strychnine." During one of her few lucid moments, she told Police Inspector George Harvey of L (Lambeth) Division that she had received two letters from the gentleman she had seen that evening, but she had returned them to him at his request. Knowing, as do most people poisoned with strychnine, that she was dying, she begged, "Let me die at home, don't leave me, doctor." They rushed her to the hospital, but she was dead before they arrived. An autopsy was negative until the contents of her stomach revealed the presence of strychnine.

Less than a week later, in what seemed a compulsion to publicize his crimes, Cream wrote to the deputy coroner asserting that he could produce evidence that would lead to the arrest and conviction of Ellen Donworth's (according to the letter, "*alias* Ellen Linnell") murderer—"provided your Government is willing to pay me £300,000 for my services." He signed the letter "A. O'Brien." (In this letter, he gave a clue to his identity that the police eventually noticed. An Englishman would have written "the government" or "our government" rather than "your government.") The coroner declined this offer and ruled that the cause of death was "poisoning by strychnine and morphia by a person unknown." Until that time, police did not think there was the "slightest evidence of foul play," and had "little doubt that she took the poison herself knowing as she expected to die, and wished to expire at home." The populace was justifiably agitated by what the press called "The Lambeth Mystery."

Two weeks later, on November 6, 23-year-old Frederick Smith, a prominent lawyer who had recently inherited his father's book-selling empire and seat as a Member of Parliament, received a letter from "H. Bayne" (later shown to be in Cream's handwriting). The letter purported to be from a barrister with information about the Donworth murder. Enclosed was a letter to "Miss Ellen Linnell" warning her that Frederick Smith was trying to poison her with strychnine. "Bayne's" letter gave instructions for Smith to follow if he wanted to meet and discuss the issue and, in cooperation with police, he followed them; nobody showed up. Ten days later, Cream sent a letter to the local magistrate stating that he had enough evidence to hang Mr. Frederick Smith and that he "would make it hot for the police" if they did not take action in the matter.

Matilda Clover

During this period, Cream was not merely writing letters. During the night of October 20, he revisited 27-year-old Matilda Clover. Clover, described as a woman with somewhat prominent teeth, a pockmarked face, and long dark-brown hair, lived in two rented rooms on Lambeth Road and worked as a prostitute. She had a two-year-old child, but the child's father, who had been a regular visitor, had left a month earlier after he and Matilda quarreled. Matilda was "cut up" about the breakup and wanted a reconciliation.

She was also being treated for alcoholism, a condition not uncommon in the trade. As a contemporary observer, Reverend G. P. Merrick, concluded, the prostitute's lifestyle led her to drink, rather than the other way around. As he was told, "We could not go out if we didn't drink. We must drink, and that is how we get a taste for it."

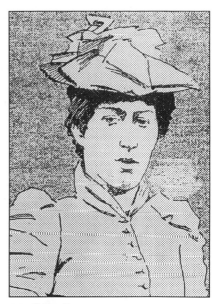

Matilda Clover. (From *Illustrated Police News*, The British Library)

Apparently, Cream had sent Clover a letter asking her to meet him—if she could "come clean and sober." As in other cases, he asked her to return the letter to him when they met. When he left her room, neighbors heard her call out "Good-night, Fred," a name Cream used with many of Lambeth's prostitutes.

About 3 A.M., the household was awakened by screams of agony from Clover's room. Rushing in, they found her naked and lying on her back across the foot of the bed. Her head was between the mattress and the wall, "obviously suffering the greatest agony." Those in attendance tried to give her some tea (the British remedy for everything that ails), but she vomited it up. According to the servant, Miss Clover "complained of her throat; said she seemed as if she had something sticking in her throat. If she could get it up she thought she would be better." Mrs. Phillips, her landlady, ran to fetch the doctor.

Dr. Robert Graham had seen Clover for alcoholism eight or nine times in the twelve days before her death. (She belonged to a treatment "club," a kind of early HMO.) He prescribed bromide of potassium and sedatives, the standard treatment for that condition. When Mrs. Phillips arrived to retrieve him, he was first out on a house call and then on his way to attend a complicated childbirth. He sent her to Dr. McCarthy, who, in turn, sent his assistant,

Mr. Francis Coppin, to see Clover. Coppin later described Matilda Clover's condition:

> She was lying on the bed. She was not in a fit at the time I saw her first. She had a quick pulse, was bathed in perspiration, and trembling. I was with her about 10 or 12 minutes. She had a convulsion while I was there. There was a twitching of the body. She had vomited previous to my being there . . . I gave her some medicine to stop the vomiting. I concluded that she was suffering from epileptic fits, convulsions due to alcoholic poisoning. [Assuming that this was delirium tremens, the result of alcoholism, he prescribed carbonate of soda to help stop the vomiting.]
>
> When I saw her at seven in the morning I thought she would die, but not so quickly. I thought she was in a dying condition. About an hour after I saw her, soon after eight, Mrs. Phillips [the landlady] came round to ask me to go again immediately. I sent a messenger to Dr. Graham to tell him to go, as he had been attending her for 12 days previously. I did not go myself.

After suffering for over five hours, Matilda Clover died at 8:45 A.M. on October 21.

Dr. Graham signed a death certificate "under the grossest culpability" according to the attorney general, since "he certified that he had attended Matilda Clover during her last illness, but he really had not attended her at all on that occasion." Nevertheless, Graham wrote, "to the best of my knowledge and belief the cause of her death was, primarily, delirium tremens; secondly, syncope (passing out)." Although England's rules for completing a death certificate, including viewing the body, had existed since 1874, Graham was not prosecuted for this lapse in professional duties, because of his "good character."

Matilda Clover was interred in pauper's grave #22154 at Tooting Cemeery on October 27. Her child was put up for adoption at the local workhouse and subsequently found a home. As was said at Cream's trial, Clover

> was lying in a pauper's grave, thought of and remembered by few. Only one person living could know that a fearful tragedy had been enacted in her case, and that person was the one who had administered to her the fatal dose of strychnine which resulted in her death.

Since everyone believed that Clover had died as the result of alcohol, her death was not reported to the police. Some of the neglect in this case can also be attributed to the general feeling, as the *St. James's Gazette* reported, that "the woman Clover was only a miserable street outcast, whose life was of no particular value to anybody." The case was closed—except that Dr. Cream could not keep quiet.

Cream first spoke of the case to his landlady's daughter, mentioning the "young girl in Lambeth Road, a young girl with a child, who, he suspected, had been poisoned." (No one else had as yet suggested any foul play, let alone poisoning, in the case.) He then sent a letter to Countess Russell, who was staying at London's Savoy Hotel. In it, he accused her husband, Lord Russell, of murdering a woman on Lambeth Road. The Russells were involved in a messy and very public divorce at the time, and had caught Cream's attention when his landlady read him an article about them from the *Daily Telegraph*. The countess ignored the letter.

On November 30, Cream wrote to Dr. William Henry Broadbent, an eminent cardiologist and the royal family's physician, declaring that he had proof that Broadbent "not only gave her the medicine which caused her [Clover's] death, but that you had been hired for the purpose of poisoning her." If Broadbent wanted a way to save himself "from ruin," Cream would sell the evidence to him for £2,500. Broadbent was to put a "personal" in the *Daily Chronicle* saying that he would pay "Malone," Cream's alias in this letter. Cream would then "send a party to settle this matter." He ended by writing, "I am not humbugging you. I have evidence enough to ruin you for ever." Broadbent turned the letter over to Scotland Yard, who inserted the ad in the paper's "Agony" section and then waited in the doctor's house for someone to arrive; no one did. They told Broadbent that the letter was probably the "handiwork of a lunatic" and dropped the matter.

When he was later arrested, police found a handwritten note in Cream's lodgings with the initials "M.C." adjacent to three dates; the last was October 20, the date he poisoned Clover. On the same page was "E.S." (Emma Shrivell, a subsequent victim) next to the date April 11, which was the day she died.

More Murders and Blackmail

In his more lucid moments, Cream apparently sought a normal, middle-class life. To achieve that goal, Cream made the acquaintance of Laura Sabbatini, a proper young woman from Berkhamstead who had moved to London to learn dressmaking. By the end of 1891, they were engaged to be married. But Cream told her that he had to go to America to check on his father's estate. He sailed for Canada on January 7, 1892, after writing out a will in which he left Miss Sabbatini all his possessions. Cream, according to fellow passengers, was inebriated during most of the trip, supposedly using alcohol to wean himself off morphine.

This trip was notable for a few odd occurrences. While in Quebec, Cream befriended grocery representative John Wilson McCulloch, and showed him a bottle with white crystals that he described as "poison I give to the women to get them out of the family way." As McCulloch later said, Cream "always had a loose tongue about women" and bragged that he had slept with as many as three prostitutes in a five-hour period. He also noted that Cream repeatedly displayed pornographic pictures and often seemed stupefied from the "morphia" (probably opium) he continually took for severe headaches. When Cream returned to England, acquaintances there also described him as "constantly taking drugs" such as morphia, strychnine, and opium.

On the trip, Cream also encountered Mr. M. A. Kingman, a pharmaceutical representative from whom he first ordered 500 strychnine pills and then even more. In Canada, he also ordered 500 "Metropole" circulars that read:

Ellen Donworth's Death
To the Guests of the Metropole Hotel

Ladies and Gentlemen,

I hereby notify you that the person who poisoned Ellen Donworth on the 13th last October is today in the employ of the Metropole Hotel and that your lives are in danger as long as you remain in this Hotel.

Yours respectfully,
W. H. MURRAY
London, April 1892

Cream then returned to England, arriving in London on April 2. He had the flyers sent to him there; he planned to distribute them to the hotel's guests. Why he would do this and who, if anyone, was the intended target, remains unclear. During the first week of April, he again visited the Sabbatinis in Berkhamstead, where he asked that a Bible be put in his room and attended "song services" with Laura.

On April 11, back in London, Cream spent the evening with two prostitutes, 21-year-old Alice Marsh and 18-year-old Emma Shrivell. Both women came from working class families and had worked at a Brighton biscuit factory before moving to London. The women took their new profession seriously and even purchased business cards printed with their address and "Please ring middle bell."

The women had separate rooms on the second floor of Charlotte Vogt's boarding house on Stamford Street. The area was described as "full of dirty so-called hotels and disreputable apartment houses, and is the headquarters of theatrical and music hall agents." Aside from their more intimate activities, Cream and the two women ate a dinner of Acme Flag brand tinned salmon. After dinner, he gave each of them three long thin capsules, presumably to avoid "catching the disease." At the time, mercury was used to treat venereal disease. Unfortunately, there was no guarantee of a cure—and mercury poisoning was as bad or worse than the disease.

At 1:45 A.M., Constable Comley saw a man he later identified as Cream leave the residence as he passed by on his beat. Mrs. Vogt stated that at 2:30 A.M.:

> [I] was awakened by a screaming and shrieking outside my door. In the passage I saw Marsh, who was screaming and appeared to be in great agony. I sent my husband for a cab and a policeman. I then heard Shrivell screaming upstairs for "Alice!" Going up to her room I saw her on the floor at the foot of the sofa, leaning against the sofa. She appeared to be in great agony. I spoke to her, and she answered me.
>
> I then heard Marsh screaming below again, and I went down to her and found her lying on her stomach in the passage and her body twitching as if in great pain ... [The twitching] continued to come on and pass off and then come on again. I spoke to her, and when the twitching was not in operation she spoke to me; she was quite conscious. I asked her a question and she answered it.
>
> My husband came back with a cab and the police, and the girls were carried after a little while and put into the cab and taken to the hospital. I first tried to give them an emetic, some mustard and water. They were carried out of the house and I never saw them alive again.

The constables put both women in a cab and rushed them to St. Thomas's Hospital, with constable Comley riding on the outside. House surgeon Cuthbert Wyman continued the tale:

> On 12th April, about 3 A.M., I was at the hospital when Marsh and Shrivell were brought in. Marsh was dead. Shrivell was suffering from tetanic convulsions; she showed all the symptoms of strychnine poisoning. I gave her an emetic [medication to induce vomiting], and afterwards chloroform. She died about eight the following morning. I made a post-mortem examination afterwards; I found no organic disease to account for death. The stomach and viscera of each girl were sealed up in jars and handed by me to George Hackett [post-mortem assistant at St. Thomas's Hospital], to be conveyed to Dr. Stevenson.

At an inquest on April 14, the treating physician said that the symptoms were consistent with strychnine poisoning. The police, however, believed that the women's deaths were probably "another case of poisoning by eating tinned salmon." Even though the police chemists (pharmacists) confirmed that the food the women ate at dinner had not been contaminated, police launched a nationwide hunt for contaminated cases of Acme Flag salmon. Finally, police accumulated enough evidence so that everyone had to agree that the women died from strychnine poisoning. But they never confirmed how it had been administered. Meanwhile, the bodies of Alice Marsh and Emma Shrivell were returned to Brighton for a humble burial.

On April 17, two prostitutes visited Lambeth Mortuary, where a wake was being held for Marsh and Shrivell. They mentioned that they knew the decedents and that they had seen them with a man named "Fred" at a local pub. Police did not hear about this conversation until April 28, and then tried to find these witnesses.

Continuing to stir up trouble, Cream told his landlady on April 18 that another of her tenants, Walter Joseph Harper, was responsible for the two murders and that the police knew it. Harper knew Cream by sight, but had never spoken with him. Perceptively, his landlady said that Harper, a quiet 26-year-old medical student, "was the last man in the world to do such a thing; that he (Cream) must be mad." A week later, Cream sent a letter to Dr. Joseph Harper, Walter's father, saying that he had incontestable proof that Walter had poisoned the two women. For some reason, he enclosed a newspaper clipping describing Ellen Donworth's death, rather than one describing Marsh and Shrivell's murders. He said he would suppress the evidence for £1,500 and signed the letter with his common alias, "W. H. Murray." Dr. Harper immediately took the letter to his lawyer. They waited for his son to return home before deciding whether to contact "Murray." When the police received a similar letter a few days later, they tried to contact the sender, without success.

Now that three Lambeth-area prostitutes—Donworth, Marsh, and Shrivell—had died suddenly, apparently murdered using strychnine, the police became interested. They questioned chemists and prostitutes throughout London. The chemists supplied them with names of those who had recently purchased strychnine. From this list, their prime suspect appeared to be William Slater, a traveling salesman who was known to have attacked a woman. He was ultimately exonerated. Another suspect was Joseph Simpson, a wealthy stockbroker who had tried to "rescue" Emma Shrivell from her life of prostitution by periodically sending her money (he knew her family). The most unlikely suspect was an American doctor, Thomas Neill (Cream often went by his middle name, as the prosecutor later mentioned in his opening remarks).

When police began interviewing London's prostitutes, they heard about Matilda Clover's death, which had occurred within days of Donworth's. After questioning the servant girl who had been present at her death, they felt they had a fourth death fitting the same pattern. The only difficulty was that the two pairs of deaths—Donworth and Clover;

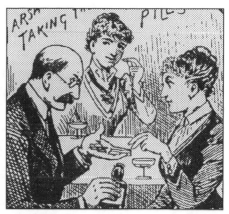

Dr. Cream handing out his deadly pills to Alice Marsh and Emma Shrivell. (From *Illustrated Police News*, The British Library)

Shrivell and Marsh—were separated by a six-month interval, two in October and two in April. This suggested that a sailor was involved, so they began watching the docks for men called Fred who met the suspect's description. (Cream had been in Canada in the intervening period.)

The Lambeth Division surgeon agreed that Clover's death also sounded like strychnine poisoning and the Home Secretary ordered her body examined. On April 30, her body was exhumed. Given the haphazard method of burials in potter's fields, 14 coffins were removed before Clover's was eventually identified by the nameplate: "M. Clover, 27 years." Remarkably, since embalming was not used, they found "the body, except as regards the face, neck, and fingers, was in an unusual state of preservation."

Dr. Thomas Stevenson, the Crown's toxicologist, performed an autopsy and found "no indication of any disease in the vital organs that went to account for her death." After he had removed various organs and fluid samples for chemical analysis, it took him three weeks to analyze, distill, and test the material for poisons. Ultimately, he found a bitter-tasting, white crystalline substance that mimicked the effects of strychnine when injected into a frog. His diagnosis was death by strychnine poisoning. Scotland Yard was now searching for the killer of at least four women.

The same day as Clover's exhumation, Cream again visited Laura Sabbatini and asked her to write some letters for him. He did not explain why he was not writing them himself. The first was to the coroner and asked him to forward an enclosed note to the foreman of the Marsh-Shrivell inquest. The note accused Walter Harper of the women's murders, as well as the murder of a Lou

Harvey. Miss Sabbatini also wrote a third letter at Cream's request. This letter was inexplicably sent to a detective who, up until that time, had no knowledge of Cream or of these cases. All three letters were signed "W. H. Murray."

Laura Sabbatini subsequently testified that Cream had dictated these letters. She also confirmed that a handwritten will had indeed been written by Cream and given to her. This allowed investigators to compare the handwriting with the blackmail notes and other letters he had sent. At trial, Cream's lawyer did not contest either that the letters were in Cream's handwriting or that the paper had a unique American watermark unavailable in England. (This was unfortunate for Cream, since the Crown's two handwriting experts initially said that the letters Laura Sabbatini had written were in Cream's handwriting. The police "suggested" to these experts that they were someone else's work and they revised their reports.)

Constable Comley had spent almost a month on plainclothes duty while looking for suspects in the Marsh-Shrivell murders. On the evening of May 12, he saw a man enter Canterbury Music Hall who closely resembled the one he had seen leaving the women's residence the night they died. Based on Comley's identification, Scotland Yard began shadowing Cream the next day, and his neighbors began noticing them. When a neighbor, Mr. Armstead, questioned Cream, he replied that he was mistakenly being watched because of the murders committed by "the same unconscionable villain, Harper, who had killed Donworth, Clover, and Lou Harvey." With the police now watching him, Cream began to dress differently and alter the course of his walks in the area.

On May 18, Cream met Detective Sergeant McIntyre, who was investigating the murders. Cream was on edge and said, "I am going away today at three o'clock. Will I be arrested if I do so?" McIntyre replied, "I cannot tell you. If you walk across with me to Scotland Yard, I will make inquiries." As they walked across Westminster Bridge, Cream suddenly stopped and said, "I will not go any further with you. I am suspicious of you, and I believe you are playing me double [double-crossing me]." He left McIntyre on the bridge. But events were rapidly overtaking him.

By June 1, young Dr. Harper had finished medical school and started his practice in Devonshire. Police Inspector Tunbridge met with both Dr. Harper and his father to review the letters that had presumably come from Cream. Recognizing that he had the opportunity to arrest Cream for blackmail, since the handwriting matched, Tunbridge obtained an arrest warrant from Bow Street Police Court on June 3 and arrested him that evening. They nabbed Cream just in time—he had booked passage back to America.

"The Prisoner Neill"

On October 24, 1892, while Cream was in jail charged with murder, the *St. James Gazette* published an article titled "The Prisoner Neill," written by "One Who Knew Him." It presents a chilling picture of a fiendish physician-poisoner. Cream met the anonymous author at a local restaurant and talked about women, his favorite topic, as well as music, money, and poisons. He spoke, said the writer, with "a soft voice, though strong American accent; dressed with taste and care, and was well-informed and travelled as men go." The writer noted that Cream was addicted to gin, "tobacco and cigars," and chewing gum, and that he seldom laughed or smiled.

> He was of an exceedingly restless temper, always pacing about, even when drinking at a bar; and, when sitting, was always moving his legs like a dog dreaming, or fiddling with something on the table, and moving his head and rolling his eyes to watch everyone who moved . . . He appeared to hate being alone, for though he never seemed to enter with anybody, when my table was full he never went and sat by himself, but always managed to go and sit at an occupied table.

> Women were his preoccupation, and his talk of them far from agreeable. He carried pornographic photographs, which he was too ready to display. He was in the habit of taking pills, which, he said, were compounded of strychnine, morphia, and cocaine, and of which the effect, he declared, was aphrodisiac. In short, he was a degenerate of filthy desires and practices . . .

> Almost from the time the question of the Lambeth poisoning case began to attract attention and, at any rate, from the time he knew he was watched and guessed he was suspected, Neill became a changed man. Every trait in his character became exaggerated. He became more nervous and excitable. He turned round and stood to see if men were following him . . . He had the air of a hunted man, and it would seem as if he was haunted in the night by the faces of the seven women and one man whom he had murdered, for he kept a candle alight in his room all through the night.

Dr. Cream's Last Trial

On June 4, 1892, Dr. Thomas Neill Cream was arraigned at Bow Street Police Court for attempting to extort money from Dr. Joseph Harper. He was placed in a lineup with 20 other men, and Eliza Masters tried to identify him, but could not. Elizabeth May then came in and quickly spotted Cream. Masters came in again (May was not present) and identified Cream after he removed his top hat. Yet the Home Office Secretary of State wrote the same day, "The moral proof of his guilt is ample, but my utmost efforts have so far failed to procure any direct evidence connecting him with these crimes."

Scotland Yard then searched Cream's room on Lambeth Palace Road, and found incriminating scrawls on an envelope that listed the dead women's initials and dates of death. The envelope contained 500 opium pills and 500 pills of *Cannabis indica* (marijuana) extract. On June 22, Cream appeared before a coroner's inquest concerning Matilda Clover's death. He was represented by counsel, and had been instructed not to answer any questions, and he obeyed, even refusing to confirm his identity. Nevertheless, after 20 minutes of deliberation, the jury declared:

> We are unanimously agreed that Matilda Clover died of strychnine poisoning, and that the poison was administered by Thomas Neill (Cream) with intent to destroy life. We therefore find him guilty of wilful murder.

On July 18, Cream learned that he was now charged with murder. "What, in the Clover case?" he asked. "Is anything going to be done in the other cases?" Cream still had not learned when to keep quiet. But the inquest continued. Although Cream had admitted poisoning "Lou Harvey" at a music hall, the police had been unable to locate her body or find anyone who knew her. During the course of the hearing, the magistrate received a letter from a Mrs. Harris, stating that she had read her name in the papers and was prepared to come forward. (Louisa "Lou" Harris was Charles Harvey's common-law wife and often used his last name.) Harris's tale revealed her narrow escape from death, due to her caution and quick thinking. The letter detailed her meeting with Cream on October 20, 1891:

> [I] went with him from St. James to an hotel in Berwick St. Oxford St. Stayed there with him all night left about 8 oc. in the morning. Made an appointment with him to meet the same night ... he gave me two capsules. [Cream gave them to her to supposedly clear up some marks on her face.] But not liking the look of the thing, I pretended to put them in my mouth. But kept them in my hand. And when he happened to look away, I threw them over the Embankment. He then said that he had to be at St. Thomas's Hospital, left me, and gave me 5s. to go to the Oxford Music Hall ...
>
> I never saw him again till about 3 weeks after ... So I said to him don't you remember me. He said no ... He then said what's your name. I said Louisa Harvey. He seemed surprised, said no more, and walked quickly away ... I had not troubled to read the case particular till Friday night ... I got the *Telegraph* next morning, saw my name mentioned. So I was

almost sure. He being under the impression that I took the capsules, and either dropped dead in the street, or music hall.

On July 21, a hearing was held to arraign Cream for the murders of Matilda Clover, Ellen Donworth, Alice Marsh, and Emma Shrivell and for attempting to murder Lou Harvey. He would be tried simultaneously for blackmailing Drs. Broadbent and Harper.

On September 13, the grand jury issued a "true bill" against Cream (an indictment that a grand jury believes is supported by sufficient evidence). The "Lambeth Poisoning Mystery" trial began on October 17, 1892, at Central Criminal Court. Although he had been indicted for multiple murders and two counts of blackmail, the trials were to proceed separately. Cream was first tried for Matilda Clover's murder. While the blackmail cases were solid, all the murder cases were individually weak. The only chance the Crown had of convicting Cream of murder was if evidence from all the murders could be introduced at one trial. Justice Henry Hawkins (later Sir Henry Hawkins), the presiding magistrate, held that since Cream had grouped all the cases together in his letter to Dr. Harper (accusing his son), he would allow evidence from all the murders to be admitted. With that decision, Cream's fate was sealed.

Cream's luck had clearly run out when Judge "Hanging Hawkins" was assigned to his case. Justice Hawkins, who seemed to like only dogs and racehorses, was justifiably feared for his liberal application of the death penalty. Lawyers of the time felt that he was biased and unfair; a peer could say only that he was "a wicked judge and a wicked man." The prosecutor in the Cream case was the attorney general for the Gladstone government, Sir Charles Russell. Cream's barrister, Gerald Geoghegan, was known as brilliant but erratic, due to his fondness for alcohol. The high-profile case drew an enormous, predominantly female, crowd inside and outside the courtroom. According to witnesses:

> At first Cream sat composedly on a chair in the corner of the dock, but during the Attorney-General's opening speech his attitude became one of keen and close attention, his mouth twitched and his hands shifted uneasily. At the time of the trial he wore a full moustache and beard of reddish-brown; his face was pale.

A long parade of witnesses testified for the prosecution. But Geoghegan called no witnesses for the defense. Cream did not testify because, at that time, the defendant in a capital case was not permitted to take the stand. If Cream had testified, he would have had to explain his criminal record for murder in America, as well as the other cases in which he had been involved.

After his lawyer's closing argument, Cream was ecstatic, singing and dancing in his cell, confident that he would be acquitted. Indeed, his lawyer had tried to cast doubt on each element of the Crown's case. Geoghegan questioned the credibility of the witnesses, emphasized that no one could place Cream at the scene of any crime, and suggested that the lineup in which Masters and May had identified him had been rigged (it probably was). He also said that the pornography and alleged blackmail were merely evidence of Cream's macabre sense of humor, adding that these were influenced by his unfortunate addiction to drugs. Hoping to sway the jurors, Geoghegan concluded with an image that Cream should have taken to heart:

> I remember . . . trying to picture to myself what those people must have felt as they lay under that sentence [of death]. I cannot help thinking that when you come to consider what a sentence of death means, you will agree with me that it is the most awful position in which a fellow creature can be placed. That sentence means separation from one's fellow-men; it means being immured in a prison cell; it means that the condemned is about to stand on the threshold of the most awful of all mysteries, and that, when that mystery is solved, his name shall be a hissing, a byword, and an abomination even to his nearest and dearest.

On October 21, the trial ended and Justice Hawkins gave his charge to the jury. Clearly biased, he again laid out the prosecution's case, ordering the sequence of events and highlighting the most damning evidence. He described Matilda Clover as "an unfortunate, [who] seemed to have been a quiet, well-conducted girl, following her calling, but had given way to habits of drink." He also, probably unfairly, lambasted Miss Clover's caregivers, saying, "For the sake of their own feelings, I hope that each of these gentlemen had something like a legitimate excuse for not attending that unfortunate girl in her last moments." (Dr. Graham was attending a woman in childbirth with a prolonged and difficult labor, and Mr. Coppin, the assistant, was convinced that he had already done everything possible.)

Most damning of all was that while Geoghegan had told the jury that they had to be convinced of Cream's guilt "beyond a shadow of a doubt," the usual standard in criminal proceedings, Judge Hawkins told them that in such cases eyewitness testimony was often not available and that it "was not to be expected in every case that there should be mathematical proof of the commission of the crime."

A Lasting Punishment

The jury took only ten minutes to convene, find Cream guilty of murder, and return to the courtroom. After hearing the jury's verdict, Cream was asked if he had "anything to say why the Court should not give you judgment to die according to law?" Cream remained silent. Justice Hawkins declared:

> Thomas Neill [Cream], the jury, after having listened with the most patient attention to the evidence which has been offered against you in respect of this most terrible crime, and having paid all attention to the most able arguments and the very eloquent speech which your learned counsel addressed to them on your behalf, have felt it their bounden duty to find you guilty of the crime of wilful murder, of a murder so diabolical in its character, fraught with so much cold-blooded cruelty, that one dare hardly trust oneself to speak of the details of your wickedness. What motive could have actuated you to take the life of that girl away, and with so much torture to that poor creature, who could not have offended you, I know not. But I do know that your cruelty towards her, and the crime that you have committed, are to my mind of unparalleled atrocity.
>
> For the crime of which you have been convicted our law knows but one penalty—the penalty of death ... The crime which you have committed, I have already said, can be expiated only by your death. I proceed, therefore, to pass upon you the dread sentence of the law, which is, that you be taken from hence to the place whence you came, and thence to a lawful place of execution, and that there you be hanged by your neck until you be dead, and that when you are dead your body be buried within the precincts of that prison within the walls of which you shall have been confined last before the execution of this judgment upon you. And may the Lord have mercy upon your soul.

As was typical, the hanging was to take place after three Sundays had passed. (After 1859, to avoid working on Sunday, gallows were erected on Monday and the executions held on Tuesday.) Geoghegan asked for a delay so that evidence showing that Cream was insane could be sent from America. However, it is unlikely that that defense tactic would have been successful, because the modified 1843 McNaughton Rules required the accused to be totally incapable of distinguishing between good and evil, or at least to have a "defect of reason." (Between 1884 and 1893, only 8 of the 256 people sentenced to death for murder in England were declared insane and committed to the asylum, even though some of those who were hung had a long documented history of incarceration for mental illness.) Cream's evidence arrived and was reviewed. Geoghegan received official notice on November 12 that the Secretary of State was "unable to discover any sufficient grounds to justify him, consistently [sic] with his public duty, in advising Her Majesty to interfere with the due course of the law."

That same day, this macabre advertisement appeared in the *Illustrated Police News*:

Execution of Dr. Neill Cream
Next Week (November 19th)
Illustrated Police News
(Unless the respite is extended)
Will Contain a Full Page Illustration of the
EXECUTION OF
DR. NEILL CREAM
Give early orders. An enormous sale is expected.
All unsold copies exchanged.

Any doubt about Cream's guilt was erased when he boasted to a close acquaintance that he had killed prostitutes. When asked, "Do you really say you have killed women?" he replied, "Yes, all of that class are to be killed." The lead article in *The Times* on October 22, 1892, summarized why they thought that Cream's sentence was more than proper:

> Nobody who has read the evidence can doubt the justice of his doom; all right-minded persons, as we believe, must experience a feeling of satisfaction that a villain so inhuman is soon to meet his deserts. That feeling is, in our opinion, legitimate and praiseworthy. It springs from an instinct implanted in our nature, and which constitutes one of the strongest and most valuable of the great permanent bulwarks of society—the instinct that justice ought to be retributive and that abominable crimes rightly deserve the hatred of the community.
>
> Neill has been convicted of one murder only, but it is morally certain that he is guilty of all the four murders for which he was indicted, and of an attempt to murder the woman Harvey.
>
> The history of his career, or rather of the brief portion of his career which was discussed in the witness-box, is of a kind which is not easy to discuss in decent language, but it is not without its own terrible lessons. It reveals ... the depths of depravity and cruelty which exist in the human heart. It demonstrates what too many amiable persons, who have no practical acquaintance with misery and with crime, are in these days inclined through a false and misguided benevolence to doubt and to deny, that there does exist amongst us a certain number of moral monsters whom it is the first duty of society to hunt down and to destroy.

With keen perception, a contributor to the socialist *Clarion* suggested that society would do well to look at the reasons that people like Dr. Cream (the term "serial killer" had not yet been invented) performed their heinous acts:

> We are entitled in self-protection, I suppose, to hang him. Hang him at any rate we shall. But if we would prevent the future propagation of such distorted fiends, let us cease to plague our minds with futile efforts to divine the workings of such misshapen minds, and reserve our attention for careful and more profitable research into the social causes which favour their loathsome production.

Cream was kept under close watch for fear that he would commit suicide. In part, this was due to his statement after his sentence had been read, "They shall never hang me." But the lead officer overseeing Cream did not think he would kill himself, saying, "he is utterly reckless of other people's lives, but he is particularly careful of his own neck. He does not mind how many he kills, but he won't kill himself."

The *Morning Advertiser* described Dr. Cream's last hours:

> On the Monday night, his last night, he was very restless, uneasy, silent; pacing up and down the cell for nearly an hour, as though endeavouring to tire himself out. When at last he lay down he was unable to sleep, tossing restlessly from side to side; occasionally falling into a doze broken by moanings. He rose soon after six o'clock, haggard and worn; his cheeks bloodless, his eyes incessantly moving, his face and hands twitching nervously. He ate no breakfast. He wore the clothes in which he had appeared at the trial, black coat and dark trousers. He neither confessed his crime nor admitted the justice of his sentence.

Others present at the execution disagreed, stating that he admitted killing many more women and that his sentence was just. Aside from the guards, seven others watched or participated in the November 15 execution. Observers noted:

> The culprit's demeanour was calm and composed, and it is understood that he made a short statement thanking the officials for their kindness to him since he had been under their charge. The length of the drop was five feet. A crowd assembled outside the prison to witness the hoisting of the black flag, the appearance of which was greeted with cheering.

The drunken throng watched as, in the fine drizzle, Dr. Cream was hanged. As a Canadian newspaper wrote, "Probably no criminal was ever executed in London who had a less pitying mob awaiting his execution."

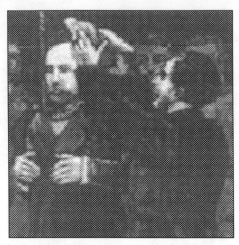

Dr. Cream's hanging. (From *Illustrated Police News*, The British Library)

Cream's was only 1 of 22 death sentences (20 men and 2 women) handed out in England that year. Of those, 18 men, including Cream, were executed. The others had their sentences commuted to life in prison.

Even before his death, Dr. Cream became a part of Madame Tussaud's exhibition in London and faced down visitors for 70 years. After he was hung, the museum paid £200 for his clothes—his lawyers got the money. A preposterous tale arose that in the seconds before he dropped to his death, Cream murmured, "I am Jack . . ." (He had been in jail during some of the Ripper killings and, more important, he was a poisoner-blackmailer, not a lurker-slasher.) Still, over time, the memory of his crimes faded as the relative magnitude of his iniquity diminished, and his bust was replaced by others who had performed more recent and even greater horrors.

After studying the case, W. Teignmouth Shore wrote:

> [Cream's] actions were probably governed by a mixture of sexual mania and sadism. He may have had a half-crazy delight in feeling that the lives of the wretched women whom he slew lay in his power, that he was the arbiter of their fates. It is, of course, possible, but I think not probably, that he wreaked vengeance on these "unfortunate" women because he had acquired in early life disease from contact with a prostitute. Sensuality, cruelty, and lust of power urged him on. We may picture him walking at night the dreary, mean streets and byways of Lambeth, seeking for prey, on some of whom to satisfy his lust, on others to exercise his passion for cruelty; his drug-sodden, remorseless mind exalted in a frenzy of horrible joy. Whatever exactly he was, the halter was his just award.

Thomas Neill Cream, M.D., C.M., had his killing spree halted at the end of the hangman's rope.

Strychnine

Aside from his occasional use of chloroform, Dr. Cream's modus operandi was to kill his victims with strychnine, a truly vicious weapon. Strychnine ($C_{21}H_{22}N_2O_2$) is the principal alkaloid in *nux vomica*, the dried seeds of *Strychnos nux-vomica*, a small tree native to Sri Lanka, Australia, and India. The term *nux vomica* has been mistakenly translated as "emetic nut." It actually means a nut with a cavity in it, describing its physical features. (Small quantities of strychnine do not induce vomiting.)

Europeans first used strychnine in sixteenth-century Germany, where it was used to poison rats and other animals. Physicians used it as a medication as early as 1540, although it only became popular in the 1700s. The drug has a long history of medicinal use, even though it has no demonstrated therapeutic value. It has been used as an antiseptic, an aphrodisiac, a stomach tonic, a general medication for alcoholism, a circulatory and nerve stimulant, and a treatment for constipation. It can still be found in products used to kill insects and pests such as birds and rodents, especially in cracked-corn bait.

Strychnine comes either as an odorless, colorless crystal or as a bitter white powder. It is readily absorbed from the stomach, nose, and injection sites and rapidly spreads to the tissues. Effects can be seen within 15 to 20 minutes of administration. Absorption can be slowed if it is administered in a thick capsule or a hard pill. Approximately 75 percent of a strychnine dose is eliminated from the bloodstream and passed into the urine within 100 minutes after being absorbed.

Strychnine works by inhibiting glycine, which is a chemical at nerve junctions that blocks unneeded nerve signals. When strychnine removes this blockade, all impulses travel to all nerves and cause a stimulatory overload.

Strychnine is used as much to torture as to kill. Victims first experience anxiety and stiffness or twitching in their face and neck muscles. This is quickly followed by muscle spasms and pain, muscle swelling, heightened reflexes, increased sensitivity to pain, and, rarely, eye jerking (nystagmus). Victims remain awake until just before death, when they are wracked with horrendous seizures as their muscles repeatedly contract. Any stimulus, such as light, noise, or touch, produces violent spasms. These "tonic" seizures extend the body—the person remains conscious—to produce an arched torso, with only the head and heels touching the ground (opisthotonus). These "tonic" seizures are due to the action of the body's most powerful muscles, the extensors, which cause the limbs to straighten, the jaw to clench, and the back to arch. If untreated, death usually results after no more than five seizures. Death is due to a lack of oxygen, because the generalized seizures, especially contraction of the chest wall, make it impossible to breathe.

continued . . .

Strychnine, continued

The horror of dying from strychnine results from the victim's awareness of impending death, the severe pain, and the inability to control one's body. Dr. Thomas Stevenson, lecturer on medical jurisprudence (now called forensic pathology) at Guy's Hospital and the Crown's toxicologist for Dr. Cream's trial, explained:

> In strychnine poisoning after twitching the whole body, as a rule, becomes rigid and often arched backwards; the patient has a sense of being suffocated, due to a fixing of the muscles of the chest, and generally in half a minute, or more often in two or three minutes, all the spasm passes off, the patient is perfectly sensible, bathed in perspiration and free from spasms . . . there are those violent agonies and spasms followed by minutes of freedom from pain, calmness and collectedness, that would be a symptom of and would point to strychnine poisoning.

In Victorian times, strychnine was sold to physicians and pharmacists as a powder or as pills containing either 1/16 or 1/22 of a grain (3 to 4 mg). At the time, the maximum medicinal dose was 5½ mg. Dr. Cream put up to 20 of the pills, or even more powder, into gelatin capsules. This way, he could administer 60 to 80 mg of strychnine with one capsule. Expert testimony at the trial indicated that only about 33 mg was required to kill an adult.

Over time, scientists developed sophisticated methods to test for strychnine's presence in the body. As early as Dr. William Palmer's trial in 1856 (see Chapter 1, *William Palmer, M.D.*), scientists could detect minute quantities of strychnine through colorimetric tests. That is, when they added certain chemicals to a solution made from tissue containing strychnine, it turned a specific color. However, their knowledge of strychnine poisoning and the chemical analyses for poisoning cases were rudimentary, for several reasons.

First, scientists needed an adequate sample. Urine would be best, since strychnine is quickly excreted; however, urine was not routinely used for testing in the nineteenth century. Second, they often did not perform the tests correctly. Finally, they were often fooled by the presence of similar substances. For example, brucine, which is also found in *nux vomica*, gives a different color reaction and masks the presence of strychnine.

Dr. Alfred Swain Taylor, lecturer on medical jurisprudence at Guy's Hospital and the author of the standard textbook on poisoning and forensic medicine, described just how inadequate toxicological testing was at that time. For four animals he had intentionally poisoned with strychnine, the color test was positive in only one; tasting the liquid demonstrated a bitter taste in another.

The analytic techniques had improved when Dr. Cream went to trial, but researchers still needed a large sample to perform the colorimetric test. In contrast,

continued . . .

Strychnine, continued

modern toxicologists test for strychnine with minute samples of urine and tissues from a decedent's kidneys and liver, using High Performance Liquid Chromatography (HPLC).

For Dr. Cream's trial, the limited tissues (stomach, liver, and kidney) examined from Alice Marsh yielded 440 mg of strychnine, and those from Emma Shrivell (vomitus, stomach, liver, and kidney) yielded 211 mg. Dr. Stevenson testified that these quantities represented much more than a fatal dose. Samples from Matilda Clover (stomach, 1/3 of the liver, 1/4 of the brain, and 1/2 of the chest fluid), recovered after her body had been buried for six months, contained only 4 mg of strychnine, probably because of decomposition. (One adult has survived after ingesting 15,000 mg, but was immediately treated using modern life-support.) Two more Cream victims were autopsied and strychnine was found in their stomachs: Daniel Stott had more than one gram and Ellen Donworth had more than 16 mg remaining.

There was no treatment available for victims of strychnine poisoning in Victorian times. The best that physicians could do was to administer chloroform to allay the pain of the contractions, but, as one witness at the Cream trial said, this would only prolong the death. Modern treatment for strychnine poisoning includes giving medications to stop the seizures and artificial airway support and ventilation to keep patients breathing.

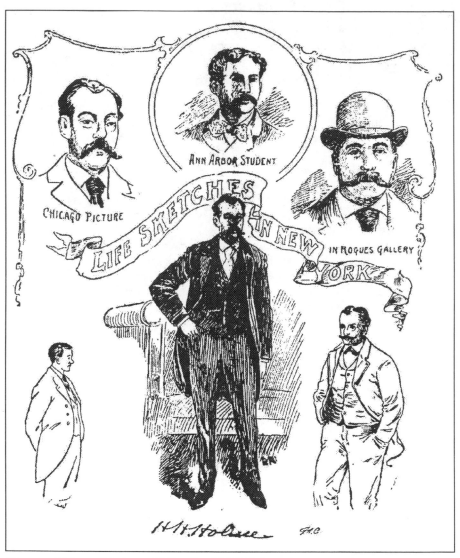

Herman Webster Mudgett, M.D., alias H. H. Holmes (1860–1896). (Sketches circa 1895)

3
Nightmare on 63rd Street

Herman Webster Mudgett, M.D., alias Dr. H. H. Holmes

The young woman was becoming tiresome. No longer an exciting lover, she had also begun to interfere with his other dalliances—she even suggested that she knew what he was doing in the basement. It was time to end this relationship—permanently. She wouldn't willingly accompany Holmes to his dungeon, but that was no problem. Waiting until she was asleep, he draped a chloroform-soaked rag over her face. When she was unconscious, he dragged her body to the greased chute and pushed her. She slid to the bottom, the next subject of his torturous experiments to produce a race of giants.

Awakening groggily, she found her arms immobilized and stretched over her head. Her feet were secured to the table. And there was Holmes standing above her, his eyes brighter than she had ever seen them. He moved to adjust some machinery, and she felt her arms slowly being pulled tight as her body was stretched by Holmes's self-made rack.

"Not too fast," he mumbled, "not too fast." He stripped off her night-clothes, and ran his hands over her live, intact body for the last time. Then, picking up a scalpel, he carefully began to cut the ligaments that held her joints tight, just as he had learned to do during his medical training. His mustache twitched as he smiled when she begged him to stop, screaming as the blade sliced neatly through her alabaster skin.

Holmes enjoyed watching them suffer. He asked her if she would like him to prolong her agony. She stared at the man she loved, and screamed again. He paused only long enough to feel his excitement build before continuing the dissection. Ever so slowly, her body lengthened as Holmes cranked the rack's gears; she lapsed into unconsciousness, a specimen pinned to the table. It was time to gratify his urges on his mistress.

At last he was satisfied, and now had a little pity. "Chew this," he said as he stuffed a cyanide tablet in her mouth. Her eyes widened with horror as the death spasms commenced. Wracked with pain, she died. Now she was just a piece of meat to cook in the crematory. There were more where she came from.

It is not possible to find in the annals of criminal jurisprudence, a more deliberate and cold-blooded villain than the central figure in this story.

– Detective Frank Geyer, the man who
finally caught Mudgett/Holmes

*H*erman Webster Mudgett, M.D., alias Dr. H. H. Holmes, was the greatest serial killer in U.S. history. He killed more than 150 men, women, and children—many of them in his infamous "Murder Castle" on Chicago's South Side during the grand World's Columbian Exposition of 1893. A large number of young women answered the employment ads placed by this smooth con artist, only to end up in his chamber of horrors. After killing his victims in a variety of ways, Holmes dissected and sold or discarded their bodies. He was ultimately convicted and hanged for only one murder, that of his longtime accomplice, Benjamin F. Pitezel. Holmes took the full truth of his fiendish crime spree to his grave.

In a "confession" commissioned by William Randolph Hearst, Holmes wrote:

My head and face are gradually assuming an elongated shape. I believe fully that I am growing to resemble the devil—that the similitude is almost completed. In fact, so impressed am I with this belief, that I am convinced I no longer have anything human in me . . . I couldn't help the fact that I was a murderer, no more than a poet can help the inspiration to sing. And I was born with the Evil One standing as my sponsor beside the bed where I was ushered into the world. He has been with me ever since.

Having been given a name that could have come from a Dickens novel, Herman Webster Mudgett sensed that he needed something more dashing to present to the world. He assumed the alias of "Harry Howard Holmes," the name he most commonly used during his adult years. Never one to simplify matters, he also used many other names to disguise his nefarious deeds and to promote his various scams. These included: Dr. Henry Howard Holmes, Henry Mansfield Howard, D. T. Pratt, Harry (Henry) Gordon, Edward Hatch,

J. A. Judson, Alexander E. Cook, A. C. Hayes, George H. Howell, G. D. Hale, and Mr. Hall.

This physician and pharmacist appeared to be an intelligent, handsome, and charming ladies' man. Those who dug deeper, however, discovered a swindler, bigamist, inventor, horse thief, and arsonist, as well as a sadistic killer.

Without a doubt, Dr. Mudgett/Holmes was evil incarnate.

Early Years

Herman Webster Mudgett was born on May 16, 1860, in tiny Gilmantown Academy in the Lake District of southern New Hampshire. It was "so remote from the outside world," he later wrote, "that daily newspapers were rare and almost unknown." Neighbors described him as being slightly built with blue eyes, brown hair, and a grown-up manner. The little that is known about his home life corresponds to that of other serial killers. He was regularly beaten by his drunken father, who was a farmer and the town's postmaster, inadequately protected by his pious, submissive mother, and abused by neighborhood bullies. Quiet, aloof, and studious, he regularly attended the Methodist Sunday School.

As an adult, Holmes said that one experience punctuated his childhood: During his first year of school, when he was only five years old, bullies dragged him into the local doctor's office while the doctor was on a house call. They pulled the struggling, petrified Mudgett into the office and toward the object he feared most: an articulated skeleton hanging on its stand. At the last moment, the doctor returned and "rescued" him. Holmes later wrote,

> . . . nor did they desist until I had been brought face to face with one of its grinning skeletons, which, with arms outstretched, seemed ready in its turn to seize me. It was a wicked and dangerous thing to do to a child of tender years and health, but it proved an heroic method of treatment, destined ultimately to cure me of my fears, and to inculcate in me first, a strong feeling of curiosity, and, later, a desire to learn, which resulted years afterwards in my adopting medicine as a profession.

One must wonder whether this incident helped propel Holmes along his twisted path, since, by the time he was 11, he was capturing animals—first salamanders and frogs, then rabbits, cats, and dogs—for use in gruesome experiments. He delighted in operating on them while they were alive, and developed a method to disable the animals without killing them, a talent he later used on his human victims. Hidden in a metal box in his cellar were his "trophies": rabbit skulls, cat paws, and other animal parts.

A loner, Holmes had only one close friend, Tom, during his school years. One incident illustrates his pervasive anger toward others: When a farmer refused to pay the boys for clearing a field of weeds, Holmes sowed the field with seeds from the weeds they had pulled. He later said:

> It is, perhaps, a small matter to speak of here, but it so well illustrates the principle that many times in my after life influenced me to make my conscience become blind.

His friend Tom died a short time later, under mysterious circumstances, after he fell from an upstairs landing while exploring an abandoned house with Holmes.

Exceptionally bright, Holmes finished high school at 16 and immediately began teaching school. Detective Geyer would later write that he had "a sagacity, which would have served him well, had he chosen to earn an honest living." At 18, he eloped with Clara A. Lovering. Since he never divorced her, she remained his legal wife and bore his only legitimate child. Using her money, he attended the University of Vermont, in Burlington, and completed his studies at the University of Michigan Medical School in Ann Arbor in 1884, at age 24. Although he completed medical school in only two years, students at that time could graduate in as little as one year with prior experience.

Holmes skipped many medical school lectures, but spent inordinate amounts of time in the anatomy lab. Morbidly intrigued by dissection, he once took an infant's corpse home so he could continue his work while the lab was closed for a holiday. Throughout his school years, he stole cadavers from the University's hospital, disfigured them with acid, planted them around the town, and then collected on life insurance policies he had fraudulently taken out in their names. While he later admitted that he was involved in "many quaint and some ghastly experiences" during that period, he maintained that

> they stopped far short of desecration of country graveyards, as has been repeatedly charged, as it is a well-known fact that in the State of Michigan all the material necessary for dissection work is legitimately supplied by the State.

(This was not true in a number of other states, where body snatching to supply anatomical cadavers continued into the 1920s.)

While in medical school, Holmes perpetrated other schemes and, as noted in a University of Michigan press release, "some professors here recollected him as being a scamp." They had good reason. In what he later called "the first really dishonest act of my life," he cheated a Chicago textbook publisher out of the funds he had gathered one summer while acting as their agent in northwestern Illinois. On another occasion, he contracted to build a barn but absconded with the money. He spent the money from a student boarding house that he managed, mollifying the owner by sleeping with her and then promising to marry her. Months later, she finally discovered that he was already married.

After graduating as a physician, Holmes nearly went bankrupt when he combined medical practice with schoolteaching in Mooers Forks, New York. Giving up on medicine, Holmes then took a rapid succession of odd jobs: bankruptcy receiver, tree salesman, schoolteacher, and, in Norristown, Pennsylvania, an insane asylum administrator. At this last position, a wealthy inmate offered the destitute Holmes $5,000 to help him escape. Shortly thereafter, the inmate was found drowned in a pond on the asylum's grounds, with his wallet empty. A scandal erupted and Holmes was forced to flee to Philadelphia, where he briefly worked as a druggist until a client died from one of his potions. He next fled to the Chicago area with newfound wealth, presumably acquired by nefarious means. It was then that he changed his name from Mudgett to Holmes.

Merriment, Mayhem, and Murder in Chicago

When Holmes moved to Chicago in 1886, the city was the epicenter of what Mark Twain described as America's "Gilded Age," a period that celebrated enterprise and gaudy excess with, in Twain's words, a "mania for money-getting." Less than 15 years earlier, on October 8, 1871, most of Chicago, including its business district, had been destroyed in the day-long Great Fire that started in Mrs. O'Leary's barn. The city quickly recovered from "The Greatest Calamity of the Age," rebuilding itself in a grand style. By 1885, Chicago boasted the nation's first skyscraper and, by 1889, had a population of one million. The dynamic growth attracted a swarm of young innocents from small towns and rural areas—perfect prey for those with dark motives.

Holmes settled in the well-to-do suburb of Englewood. According to the 1882 *Englewood Directory:* "located 12 feet above the level of the lake, with a perfect water, sewerage and gas system, and an excellent police and fire

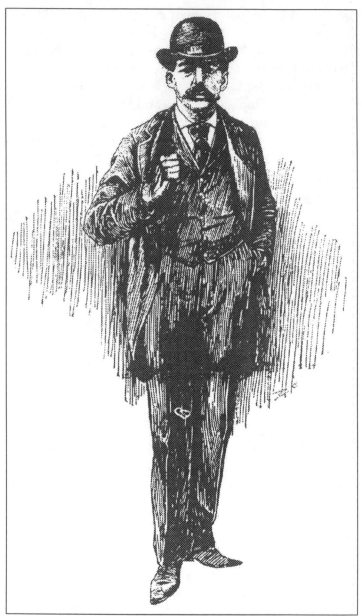

Dr. Mudgett/Holmes. (Sketch circa 1895)

department, Englewood combines all of the conveniences of the city with the fresh, healthful air of the country." From fewer than 20 families in 1868, Englewood grew to nearly 2,000 residents by 1882, and had increased to more than 45,000 by the time Holmes arrived.

In July 1886, Dr. E. S. Holton's Drugstore was thriving in the heart of Englewood's business district. Dr. Holton, though, was dying of prostate cancer as his 60-year-old wife struggled to keep the business afloat. Not a pharmacist herself, she was out of her depth in an age when patients expected the neighborhood apothecary to compound many of their medicinal powders and potions. She was delighted, therefore, when a dapper young doctor offered to work for her as a pharmacist, and she hired Holmes on the spot. Initially, Holmes seemed to be an excellent assistant, and was clearly at home with medicinal chemicals. Apparently, she never learned of his hasty flight from Philadelphia or of the reason behind it. She would later suffer dearly for this ignorance.

Dr. Holton died in August, and Holmes arranged to purchase the pharmacy from his widow, with the stipulation that she could continue to live in her apartment above the store. True to his nature, Holmes repeatedly promised to pay Mrs. Holton the money due her, but failed to do so. She threatened legal action. When this produced no results, Mrs. Holton filed suit; she was never heard from again. Holmes claimed that she had become despondent and moved to California to be near her relatives. Yet years later, when everyone who had ever known Holmes came forward to talk with the police and the press about the nation's most notorious criminal, Mrs. Holton was not among them.

The Holton pharmacy was only a small stepping stone on a path toward a more flamboyant lifestyle. In 1890, after completing work on his "Castle," Holmes sold the pharmacy to young newlyweds in what was, for Holmes, a typical scam. After hiring "clients" to make it appear that the shop was much busier than it really was, he sold the business for the entire amount of the couple's inheritance. The shop was actually a thriving establishment—until Holmes opened a pharmacy across the street in the Castle. His new shop made the old one look like a poor cousin: Holmes attracted nearly all the local business and the couple went bankrupt. Holmes had triumphed again.

Holmes maintained his lavish lifestyle through an unending stream of "cons." Most commonly, he bought merchandise on credit, immediately resold it for cash, and hid the money in a variety of ways. He also sold a bogus cure for alcoholism (actually tablets of sugar and bismuth), dabbled in real estate scams, and attempted more outlandish cons.

On one occasion, he tried to dupe Canadian investors into purchasing the patent on his "Chemical-Water Gas Generator," which was supposed to turn tap water into natural gas. The device he showed them was described as "a washing machine on stilts." Nevertheless, they became believers after they poured in a cup of water, adjusted some knobs, and flammable gas flowed out of the machine. The gas actually came from the Chicago Gas Company's public gas main that Holmes had tapped into. The gas company discovered the ruse, confiscated his machine, and dug up part of his cellar to remove the pipes. For some reason, they declined to prosecute Holmes, a tale that was to be repeated interminably.

Taking adversity in stride, Holmes capitalized on the new hole in his basement by claiming it contained an artesian well from which he extracted an elixir of youth, "Linden Grove Mineral Water." Actually, it was city tap water flavored with vanilla and an extract of herbs and roots. He sold his elixir for 5 cents a glass or 25 cents a bottle. It took the city water department three tries to discover where he was tapping into their system and to halt this profitable venture. Somehow, he avoided prosecution again.

Among government authorities and businessmen, Holmes gained a reputation as a consummate liar and get-rich-quick schemer. The *Chicago Herald* described him as

> one of the boldest and shrewdest swindlers in the country. He left scores of victims in Chicago, where firms and individuals right and left were swindled out of various sums through all sorts of fantastic methods . . . He swindled with a dash and vim that must have won the admiration of most of those who lost.

The day after he was finally arrested in Philadelphia, more than 50 victims of his swindles called Chicago's Central Police Station to find out how they could retrieve their money (they couldn't). But money was not his only objective—his actions resulted in much more sinister endings.

Soon after he arrived in Chicago, Holmes arranged to have his parents notified that he had died. Despising them, especially his brutal father, he would not return to his hometown or see his parents again until just before his arrest in November 1894.

During a business trip to Minneapolis in late December 1886, Holmes met Myrta Z. Belknap, a tall, buxom, fun-loving woman with long blond curls, brown eyes, and a baby face. After a rapid courtship, they were married in January 1887, even though Holmes had never divorced his first wife. After the couple returned to Englewood, the shrewd and able Myrta worked as a salesclerk in the pharmacy for several months. But Myrta's presence cramped the style of the ever-flirtatious Holmes, and he forced her out of the store with angry outbursts.

By the summer of 1888, Myrta, pregnant and still in love with Holmes, went to live with her parents in Wilmette, Illinois, just north of Chicago. Her father reportedly was less than fond of Holmes, believing (probably correctly) that his "son-in-law" was poisoning him to get his estate. With Myrta out of town, Holmes was alone again and ready to pursue his nightmarish dreams.

Holmes must have felt some affection for Myrta, because he agreed to both financially provide for her and visit regularly. She was undoubtedly involved in his furniture scams and, most likely, in several insurance scams, under the alias "Lucy Belknap" (Lucy was their daughter's name). Even after Holmes had been arrested and some of his macabre secrets had been revealed, she remained loyal, saying,

> I have no doubt he will clear himself of all accusations if given a fair opportunity . . . As for having another wife, I do not believe it. I have the utmost confidence in him . . . I hear from my husband two and three times a week and he continually sends me money for my needs and wants. That does not look like there being trouble between us, does it?

Holmes's affection for Myrta was most clearly demonstrated, however, by the fact that she was allowed to outlive him—a fate not granted to most of the young women who had contact with him. It seems that she also acquired most of Holmes's money after his arrest, including Hearst's payment for his story.

"Murder Castle"

In the fall of 1888, Holmes began building his Castle, filling every inch of the 50' x 162' double lot at the corner of Sixty-third and Wallace Streets. The brick and clapboard structure contained more than 100 rooms in three stories aboveground and two below. It was topped by a turreted roof with sham battlements, which made it look like a medieval castle. An impressive edifice, this enormous Gothic structure eventually became known as "Bluebeard's Castle," "Murder Castle," "Nightmare Castle," and "The Castle of Horror."

A structure that should have taken 6 months to build took 18 months. Although labor was cheap at that time, construction was hampered by

Holmes's lack of funds and his need for secrecy about the special features included. Although more than 500 craftsmen and laborers were employed, few knew much about the structure's floor plan. Holmes was able to conceal the layout by acting as architect, general contractor, and construction foreman; he supervised his eerie project from his pharmacy across the street.

The laborers he chose were either extremely close-mouthed or were people who would not be missed if they disappeared. Perpetually short of funds, Holmes often fired craftsmen for "poor workmanship" just before they were to be paid. If they threatened legal action, the wily Holmes would force them to go to court. If they physically threatened the small Holmes, Benjamin F. Pitezel, his large and constant companion, dissuaded them.

By the time the building was completed, the mechanics' liens and mortgages on the Castle exceeded its value. As one tenant said, "If all the writs of mechanic's lien that have been levied on this structure were pasted on these three walls, the block would look like a mammoth circus billboard. But I never heard of a lien being collected." Holmes, even while he continued to collect rent, "sold" the completed building to a succession of non-existent individuals and directed creditors to them. At least once, Holmes even tried to combine his construction project with a life insurance scam. As one workman later described it:

> Why, I hadn't been working for him but two days before he came around and asked me if I didn't think it pretty hard work, this bricklaying. He asked me if I wouldn't like to make money easier than that, and of course I told him yes. A few days after he came over to me and, pointing down to the basement said, "You see that man down there? Well, that's my brother-in-law, and he has got no love for me, neither have I for him. Now, it would be the easiest matter for you to drop a stone on that fellow's head while you're at work and I will give you $50 if you do." I was so badly scared I didn't know what to say or do, but I didn't drop the stone and got out of the place soon after.

Undeterred, Holmes simply proceeded with his other murderous schemes.

As construction progressed, Holmes purchased a huge walk-in safe on credit. He placed it on the third floor and built a room around it with a tiny doorway, through which the safe would not fit. When Holmes did not pay for the safe and creditors came to repossess it, he encouraged them to take their safe but threatened them with legal action if they damaged the room. Holmes kept the safe.

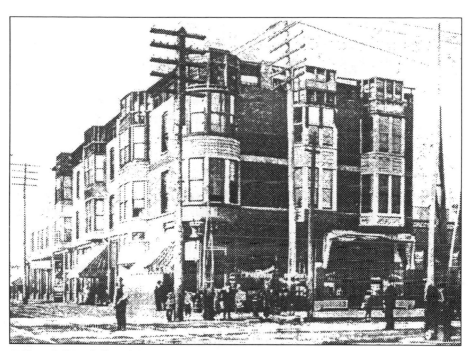

Holmes's "Castle." (From the Illinois State Historical Society)

He acquired most of his other supplies and equipment in a similar fashion. For example, to furnish the Castle, he bought one set of furniture on credit, sold it for cash, and then used the money for a down payment to purchase more furniture. He repeated that scheme until the entire structure contained the requisite beds, tables, chairs, couches, lamps, and bath items—and his basement had its equipment as well. He got away with his scams because, as one employee said:

> He was the smoothest man I ever saw. Why, I have known creditors to come here raging and calling him all the names imaginable, and he would smile and talk to them and set up the cigars and drinks and send them away seemingly his friends for life. I never saw him angry. You couldn't have trouble with him if you tried.

One firm was able to beat Holmes at his own game. The Tobey Furniture Company, which sold Holmes furniture on credit, purchased secret information about the Castle's layout from a workman. That information allowed them to find a secret storage space hidden behind a wallpapered partition in one of the Castle's vacant rooms. They also discovered that the freight elevator in the rear of the building provided access to the room—but only if it was stopped between floors and some boards were removed. They retrieved their furniture. Few other creditors were as resourceful.

The Castle was a labyrinth of secret passages, concealed staircases, false walls and ceilings, airtight and soundproof rooms, and trapdoors. An 8-foot-square concealed room was accessed through a trapdoor hidden under a heavy rug in Holmes's bathroom, with a human-sized, greased chute leading to the basement. The room also had a stairway to the street—in case a rapid escape became necessary. Doors opened to brick walls, stairs led nowhere, hallways took unexpected turns or came to dead ends, and one elevator had no shaft while another shaft contained no elevator. All the second- and third-floor bedrooms had peepholes. Holmes could fill them with either sleep-inducing gas or lethal gas through pipes that he controlled from a cabinet in his bedroom closet. He had some rooms lined with asbestos-covered sheet-iron plates, making them fire-resistant, in case the occupant should somehow catch fire.

The street-level floor contained offices and shops, including a pharmacy. Holmes ran some of the shops, including a jewelry store, restaurant, and barbershop; local merchants leased the remainder. He also ran the new pharmacy; its magnificent wooden sign depicted a mortar and pestle proclaiming in gold letters that it was the "H. H. Holmes Pharmacy." The elegant shop had a semi-hexagonal entrance topped by massive curved glass windows, marble countertops, brass soda fountain spigots, and a black-and-white tile floor. The multitude of glass cases and walnut shelves were stocked with elixirs and other nostrums.

According to his public statements, the second floor would serve as his living quarters and the third floor was to be a boarding house for visitors to Chicago's 1893 World's Columbian Exposition. The third floor actually contained Holmes's private office, as well as three dozen rooms scattered along a network of dimly lit hallways. The office contained a stove that was eight feet high and three feet in diameter, and a door, as one witness noted, that was "sufficiently large to admit a human body." When police searched the stove and its chimney, they found human bones and hair and the remnants of women's clothes. While most of the rooms were unexceptional and comfortably furnished like most other Chicago boarding houses, other rooms were always locked.

The second floor's layout was even more convoluted than that of the third. Six shadowy hallways, running in a haphazard pattern, contained

51 doors and 35 rooms. While a few rooms held normal furnishings, most were fitted with more ominous accouterments. As historian Herbert Ashbury wrote:

> The second floor contained thirty-five rooms. Half a dozen were fitted up as ordinary sleeping-chambers and there were indications that they had been occupied by the various women who had worked for the monster, or to whom he had made love while awaiting an opportunity to kill them. Several of the other rooms were without windows, and could be made air-tight by closing the doors . . .
>
> Some had been sound-proofed, while others had extremely low ceilings, and trapdoors in the floors from which ladders led to smaller rooms beneath. In all of the rooms on the second floor, as well as in the great safe, were gas-pipes with cut-off valves in plain sight. But these valves were fakes; the flow of gas was actually controlled by a series of cut-offs concealed in the closet of Holmes's bedroom.
>
> Apparently one of his favorite methods of murder was to lock a victim in one of the rooms and then turn on the gas; and the police believed that in the asbestos-lined chamber he had devised a means of introducing fire, so that the gas-pipe became a terrible blow-torch from which there was no escape. Also in Holmes's closet was an electric bell which rang whenever a door was opened anywhere on the second floor.

The second floor also contained at least one dissecting room, sliding panels that concealed secret closets, and a greased shaft leading to the cellar. Police later found human bloodstains and bloodstained clothing in some bedrooms and bathrooms and in the secret stairways. In one secret room, they found a child's clothing wedged into the plaster.

As a physician, Holmes had access to chloroform, which he bought in massive quantities to use on his human guinea pigs. A local druggist would later state:

> He always wanted so much chloroform. During the time I was there, it was only a few months, I sometimes sold him the drug nine or ten times a week and each time it was in large quantities. I asked him what he used it for on several occasions, but he gave me very unsatisfactory answers. At last I refused to let him have any more unless he told me, as I pretended that I was afraid that he was not using it for any proper purpose.

Detective Geyer wrote, "As every step of Mephistopheles is marked by a track of fire, so do the devious paths of Herman Webster Mudgett, alias Holmes, bear the scent of the deadly chloroform."

When Chicago Fire Department chemists later analyzed the unusual oil found spilled in Holmes's huge office safe, they discovered that an instantaneously suffocating gas would form if they added petroleum, benzine, gasoline, or kerosene to it. They theorized that Holmes put some of his victims in a sealed room or his vault along with a bowl of this mixture. A footprint found inside the vault's door was presumably made by one victim struggling to get out as she suffocated.

The Torture Chamber

Even Edgar Allen Poe could not have dreamed of the horror that awaited victims in Holmes's subterranean lair. The cavernous basement was a brick-lined torture chamber with a dissecting table under which was found a number of women's skeletons. Nearby were his box of surgical instruments for "more delicate work," a crematorium fitted with a cast-iron door and a grate that slid in and out on rollers, and a large zinc tank filled with acid. Eventually, Holmes would add an "elasticity determinator," similar to a medieval rack, that he claimed could stretch his victims to twice their normal length. In his mind, he could thereby produce a race of human giants.

In a basement storeroom, police found a bloody noose and a workbench stained with blood. Beneath the floor, they found two brick-lined vaults, each about six feet long, containing quicklime and human bones, including those of children. Presumably, the vaults were used to dispose of any bodies not cremated. Police also found piles of bones (most human) scattered and buried throughout the basement. Elsewhere in the basement, they found bloodied women's underwear. As police uncovered these horrors, a Chicago journalist began writing about the "multi-murderer" in their midst, nearly a century before the term "serial killer" was coined.

Holmes needed a skilled mechanic to modify his oven so that it would produce sufficient heat to act as a crematory. When questioned, he claimed that he planned to start a glass bending business. Although the oven was clearly too small to hold a large sheet of glass, the workman was able to climb into the 3-foot-high, 3-foot-wide, 8-foot-long firebrick-lined structure. He installed a new burner attached to a large oil tank in the alley. This allowed the oven to reach 3,000°F—more than needed to rapidly cremate an adult's body. As the technician later noted:

> In fact, the general plan of the furnace was not unlike that of a crematory for dead bodies, and with the provision already described there would be absolutely no odor from the furnace ... A dumb elevator ran from his office to the basement, and nothing would be easier than to lower a body by it to the basement and shove it into the furnace, in which

there was ample room for it and in which it would be consumed in a very brief time, leaving only an handful of ashes.

Unfortunately, the oven was removed for safety reasons (by order of the building inspector) before the police found reason to investigate it.

Most of the above information was gathered by police who, along with a building inspector, investigated the Castle after the bodies of some of Holmes's victims had been found. As their pretext for entering the building, they said they were searching for evidence in the disappearance of other women who had been in Holmes's company and then vanished.

The Victims

Holmes had a virtual harem in his Castle during the Columbian Exposition, as C. E. Davis, who ran the jewelry section of the Castle's pharmacy, noted:

> Holmes liked to have young women for clerks. And while he assumed to keep them on the jewelry side of the store, they used sometimes to have to cross the floor to the drug counter, where he was, for change or something. Mrs. Holmes noticed this and probably said something about it. After that he rigged up an electric bell in connection with a loose board near the top of the stairs leading from his flat overhead to the store, so he might be early apprised of his spouse's coming down. It was noticeable that when that bell rang he was the busiest man in Englewood.

Since he completely destroyed the bodies of most of his victims, exactly how many he raped, tortured, abused, robbed, and murdered will never be known. The best guess is that between 100 and 150 young women, as well as an additional number of men and children, were murdered. About 50 of his victims were pretty girls, most single and alone in Chicago, who came to town for the Fair. He would wine and dine them if they chose to stay at his boarding house; many never left. Up to 100 others were young female stenographers (known then as "typewriters") who answered his continual string of newspaper ads. Either before or during their employment, he put them in a special bedroom to be gassed—and then took them to his basement laboratory.

Using his master key to open their rooms, Holmes sedated some of his victims with chloroform-soaked rags before sliding their bodies into the basement via the greased chute. He would then experiment on them, extending their lives as he had those of the animals he experimented on in his youth.

Once he was through with his victims, Holmes usually cremated their bodies and dissolved any residue in his acid vat. A few, especially those with whom he had had a special relationship, ended up as articulated skeletons and were sold to medical schools. Their personal effects were also burned or dissolved unless Holmes could profit from them. Eerily, Holmes's two favorite topics of discussion with the manager of his jewelry shop were how to best use corrosive chemicals and how to disintegrate human tissues with chemicals.

Holmes once asked Mrs. Strowers, one of the washerwomen who worked for him, if she would take out an insurance policy for $10,000 naming him as beneficiary. Holmes said he would immediately pay her $6,000 for her trouble. Although she was tempted, friends dissuaded her—and so she lived.

Holmes later said of himself, "Like the man-eating tigers of the tropical jungle whose appetites for blood have once been aroused, I roamed about this world seeking whom I could destroy." A few of Holmes's best-known victims are described below.

Julia Smythe Conner and Pearl

Julia Smythe was an 18-year-old "Gibson girl" from Davenport, Iowa, who was variously described as being "sharp as a tack," "pretty as a picture," and "a shameless flirt." Standing nearly six feet tall, she was a buxom beauty with many suitors. She married Icilius T. Conner (known as Ned), a jeweler and watchmaker, in the summer of 1880. He suffered repeated business failures, and their relationship became stormy and degenerated into violent, sometimes public, quarrels. After their daughter Pearl was born in 1887, they decided to give their business, and their relationship, one more try in Chicago.

Ned applied for the position as manager of Holmes's jewelry shop. In November 1890, he began working at the store and, as part of his agreement with Holmes, lived on the Castle's third floor with Julia and Pearl. When Ned's 18-year-old sister, Gertrude, arrived for a visit from Muscatine, Iowa, Holmes quickly declared his love for her and asked her to marry him. Shocked, she fled back home to Iowa. Before she left, Holmes slipped poison into her medication bottle and, one month later, she died after taking a dose.

Shortly thereafter, Holmes made his move on Julia. By March 1891, they had become lovers. Holmes installed her as his drugstore's cashier, and their public flirtations left no doubt in customers' minds that they were a couple. Although he was loathe to jeopardize his position as jewelry store manager,

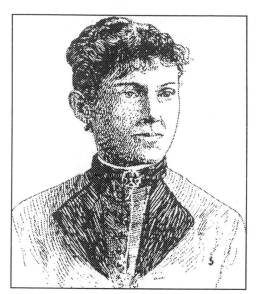

Julia Smythe Conner. (From *Chicago Daily Tribune*, July 26, 1895)

Ned eventually had to admit that his wife and Holmes were having an affair. Confronting Julia, he demanded that she cease her liaisons with Holmes; Julia refused. Ned moved out and got a new job. After a few months, he filed for divorce and left Chicago.

Julia increasingly demanded that Holmes allow her more involvement in the business. By the fall of 1891, Holmes had become tired of Julia's insistence and of her catfights and tantrums after she discovered him in bed with other women. Finally, he had had enough when, in November, she announced that she was pregnant and expected Holmes to marry her. He agreed to marry her and adopt Pearl, but he demanded that she have an abortion first—which Holmes, being a medical doctor, would perform. Procrastinating, they agreed to do it in the Castle on Christmas Eve. After putting Pearl to sleep, permanently, Holmes led Julia down a hidden staircase into the basement torture chamber. She never returned. When asked about Julia's sudden departure, Holmes replied that she had gone to join her husband.

In January 1892, Holmes learned that Charles M. Chappell, a machinist he employed, knew how to mount human skeletons. (He had learned this when he worked in the building that also housed the Bennett Medical College.) Holmes said he had a job for him and took him to the second-floor dissecting room. There, Chappell saw a woman's corpse that looked "like a jackrabbit that had been skinned by splitting the skin down the face and rolling it back off the entire body . . . In some places, considerable flesh had been taken off."

Holmes offered to pay Chappell $36 to strip off the remaining flesh and to articulate the skeleton so it could be displayed. Chappell agreed and, that night, Ben Pitezel (Holmes's assistant) hauled a steamer trunk with the body to Chappell's house. A week later, Holmes had his skeleton, which he quickly sold to Hahnemann Medical College in Philadelphia for $200. After only a few months, a surgeon, Dr. Pauling, appropriated it. The doctor displayed it in his home office, occasionally mentioning that he had never before seen a female skeleton that stood nearly six feet tall.

Emeline Cigrand

Emeline Cigrand was drawn into Holmes's web by unusual circumstances. She worked as a stenographer at Dr. Leslie Enraught Keeley's institute in Dwight, Illinois. The Institute provided treatment for alcoholics based on the quack Keeley (or Gold) Cure. Among the nearly half a million Americans who tried the remedy, which was probably made of gold salts and vegetable compounds, was Ben Pitezel, who actually went to the Institute for his treatments. While there, he was struck by the 24-year-old Emeline's beauty and tried to impress her by talking about his rich and famous employer, Dr. Holmes. When Pitezel returned and described the naïve, shapely blond, Holmes immediately wrote to offer her a position as his private secretary at a salary of $18 a week, considerably more than she was making at the Institute. She arrived in Chicago in May 1892, and took a room a block away from the Castle.

Holmes lavishly wooed Emeline with flowers, sightseeing excursions, fashionable dinners, and shopping trips. He even bought her a bicycle. By mid-summer, she had become Holmes's mistress and, in early fall, she wrote to acquaintances that she expected to marry him. Perhaps because he had two other wives, he asked Emeline to refer to him as Robert E. Phelps. He also told her that he was the son of an English lord and that they would honeymoon in Europe.

When Emeline's cousins, Dr. and Mrs. B. J. Cigrand, visited Chicago in October, they were not impressed with Holmes or the Castle. Dr. Cigrand decried its poor construction, especially the winding staircase and the inferior wood that had been used in the entire structure. Emeline paid no attention. The city building inspector later confirmed Dr. Cigrand's opinion, saying, "The structural parts inside are all weak and dangerous. Built of the poorest and cheapest kind of material."

Before their wedding, planned for December 7, 1892, Holmes asked Emeline to address a dozen envelopes to her closest relatives and friends, explaining that he would enclose the printed marriage announcements and mail them. On December 6, Holmes asked Emeline to get a document from the walk-in vault next to his office. As she searched for it, he slammed the steel door shut and engaged the lock. Seated in a chair next to the safe, Holmes pressed his ear to the door and listened as Emeline, realizing her situation, screamed in terror. He became so excited that he masturbated multiple times into his handkerchief over the next several hours while she used up the safe's oxygen supply.

The next day, Holmes and Pat Quinlan, the Castle's caretaker and another accomplice to Holmes's insurance scams, carried a heavy trunk out of his office and into an express wagon. Holmes then disappeared for two days. On December 17, Emeline's family and friends received her marriage announcement. Not long after that, Dr. Holmes sold a female skeleton to LaSalle Medical School. When he wrote his confession, Holmes claimed that he killed Emeline because she was about to leave him for someone else—a patent lie.

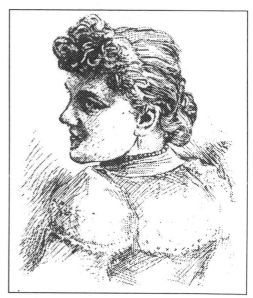

Emeline Cigrand. (Sketch circa 1895)

Minnie and Nannie Williams

Minnie Williams and her sister Nannie disappeared nearly without a trace. Holmes, ever the liar, could not even keep his own lies straight. He admitted first meeting Minnie Williams when he was in New York City in 1888 under the alias Edward Hatch, in Boston a year later, during a business trip to Mississippi in 1886 while traveling under the alias Harry Gordon, and when she replied to his ad for a stenographer.

However, and whenever, they originally met, by March 1893, Minnie was employed as Holmes's private secretary and some weeks thereafter she became his mistress. She was a plain, short-legged, plump woman with light brown ringlets framing her baby face. While she was not as beautiful as Holmes's prior mistresses, she had one hidden quality—she was heiress to property in Fort Worth, Texas, that was worth more than $40,000 ($594,000 in 2002).

Smooth-talking Holmes had Minnie, described as "naïve," sign the property over to him, her "handsome, wealthy, and intelligent" boyfriend "Harry." Since Minnie regularly corresponded with her younger and not-quite-as-naïve sister Nannie, Holmes recognized that there was a potential problem. If he killed Minnie, Nannie would ask embarrassing questions. Therefore, he told Minnie to invite Nannie to join them in Chicago to see the World's Fair. The three got along famously, and Nannie soon referred to Holmes as "Brother Harry."

On July 3, 1893, all three spent the day at the Fair. The next day he got Nannie to write a letter home describing her wonderful experience. He then took her on a tour of his Castle and showed her the vault—it was the last thing she ever saw. (Police later found what Holmes said was Nannie's naked footprint on the inside of the vault, evidence that she had struggled to break out.) A short time later, Holmes picked up Minnie at her apartment. Saying that they were going to meet Nannie, Holmes took Minnie on her last ride. Holmes later admitted that he took her to a house about eight miles east of Momence, Illinois, where he poisoned her and then buried her body in the basement.

Other Victims

After his conviction for murdering Benjamin Pitezel, Holmes confessed to 27 murders and 6 attempted murders in an article paid for by newspaper mogul William Randolph Hearst. How many of these admissions were true, and how many were amalgams of several murders, descriptions of his techniques, or complete fiction cannot be known.

Holmes claimed that his first murder victim was a Dr. Robert Leacock of New Baltimore, Michigan, who was a friend and former schoolmate. Holmes allegedly killed him in 1886 to collect his $40,000 life insurance policy. According to Holmes, he next killed a Castle tenant, Dr. Russell, over a rent dispute. After braining his colleague with a heavy chair, he tidily disposed of the corpse by dissolving the flesh in his basement acid bath, producing a salable skeleton. He wrote that this was the first skeleton he sold to a Chicago medical college; they usually paid between $25 and $45 for each one. Because producing anatomical skeletons proved to be too time consuming, he later contracted out the work—after the face and other identifying marks had been removed, of course.

After killing Julia Smythe Conner and her daughter, Holmes claimed to have killed a fishing buddy for his money. This was followed by the murder of a land speculator, supposedly with an accomplice who crushed the man's skull so thoroughly that the skeleton was of no use to the medical schools. His next murder was more pragmatic. He suffocated Lizzie, one of his maids and Pat Quinlan's mistress, in the vault both to guarantee that Quinlan would not leave his employ to follow her and to solve the inconvenient problem of her pregnancy.

Holmes claimed that his next victims were killed to protect himself from discovery. Mrs. Sarah Cook, a pregnant stenographer who worked for Holmes, burst in on him as he was preparing Lizzie's body for shipment. He quickly stuffed Mrs. Cook and her niece into the vault, thus guaranteeing their silence. He next killed Emeline Cigrand. Then, imitating the infamous body snatchers Burke and Hare, Holmes tried to simultaneously kill three waitresses who worked in his restaurant so that he could sell their bodies to a medical school. Using chloroform, he attempted to suffocate them in their beds, but the three fought back and escaped in their nightgowns.

Beautiful Rosine Van Jassand was his next victim. Holmes persuaded her, first, to work with him and, then, to become his mistress. He killed her using potassium ferrocyanide and buried her body in the basement.

Holmes's janitor, Robert Latimer, discovered the insurance schemes and tried to blackmail Holmes. According to Holmes, he confined him within one of the secret rooms to starve him to death, but his pleadings and a need to use the room for another purpose finally led Holmes simply to kill him. Latimer's escape attempts supposedly resulted in the partial destruction of a wall, which the police found when they finally investigated.

Varying his methods, Holmes next killed Miss Anna Betts by purposely putting poison, instead of medicine, in the prescription he filled for her. He killed Julia Conner's sister, Gertrude, the same way. His next victim was lured to the Castle from Omaha, Nebraska, with a promise that he would purchase her valuable Chicago real estate. Holmes gave her the money and got the deed; she died in the vault and he got his money back.

Once his basement crematory was operational, Holmes was eager to use it. He claimed that the first cremation was Mr. Warner of the Warner Glass Bending Company. Holmes wrote, "I closed the door and turned on both the oil and steam to their full extent. In a short time not even the bones of my victim remained." With an accomplice, he then enticed a wealthy Wisconsin banker named Rodgers into the Castle's secret room. There they alternately starved him and used gas to nauseate him to induce him to sign bank drafts totalling $70,000. Once his money was gone, they murdered him using chloroform and disposed of his body via the very convenient and obliging medical schools.

A woman tenant, a male fair-goer, and the Williams sisters came next. Holmes then traveled to Leadville, Colorado, and shot Millie Williams's brother "in self defense" to collect the insurance. Aside from the Pitezels, this was the last murder that Holmes admitted committing.

Ever the consummate liar, Holmes not only omitted scores of brutal murders, but also confessed to least three that he didn't commit. After his syndicated confession appeared throughout the United States and much of the Western world, both "the late" Mr. Warner and Holmes's "deceased" former employee, Robert Lattimer, appeared—alive and well. Another of Holmes's "victims" was known to have died in a train wreck rather than at the hands of this prolific murderer. Undoubtedly, other unnamed victims died in the manner that Holmes vividly described for Warner and Lattimer. As Philadelphia's district attorney, George Graham, said after prosecuting him, "The confession is a mixture of truth and falsehood. Holmes never could help lying."

Georgiana Yoke — An Unwitting Accomplice

Holmes married three women. Although he was a bigamist, he apparently took these vows seriously, at least enough so that all three "wives" survived him. In 1894, although he hadn't divorced either of his first two wives, he married again; this new wife was Georgiana Yoke.

Holmes met the petite, 23-year-old blond in March 1893, while she worked as a salesclerk at Chicago's Schlesinger & Meyer's department store, but he was involved with the Williams sisters and could not pursue the relationship. As soon as the sisters had been dealt with, he turned his attention to Miss Yoke. Neighbors from her small hometown of Franklin, Indiana, described her as having a lively intelligence, a gay smile, a sharp nose and chin, and amazingly large blue eyes. She soon became smitten with Holmes or, at least, with the bogus persona she saw.

Holmes told Georgiana that he was an orphan and was changing his name to that of his mother's bachelor brother, Henry Mansfield Howard, to ensure that his uncle would bequeath his property to him. Holmes had no such uncle, but he did change his name to avoid recognition as a bigamist, and possibly also to avoid his creditors, who were finally closing in on him. By November 1893, Georgiana and "Howard" were engaged.

By this time, Holmes knew that he would have to leave Chicago, but, before going, he tried to perpetrate one last scam. After he had taken out nearly $21,000 of fire insurance on the Castle and its contents with four different companies, the building's roof suddenly burst into flames. Holmes was not there at the time, but Pat Quinlan was. The entire top floor burned, although the rest of the building remained intact. Holmes's dubious reputation, combined with evidence that the fire had started simultaneously in several locations and that Holmes, rather than the fictitious owner named on the policy, had tried to collect the money, raised the insurance investigators' suspicions. The companies refused to pay, although they never filed criminal charges against him.

The fire spurred on his creditors. By late November, they threatened to have Holmes arrested if he did not immediately pay the nearly $50,000 he owed them. Holmes and Ben Pitezel quickly left Chicago. Holmes sporadically reappeared over the next year to visit Myrta and their daughter Lucy in Wilmette. Pitezel never returned.

In January 1894, Holmes, using the name Henry Mansfield Howard, married Georgiana in Denver, Colorado. They honeymooned in Fort Worth, Texas, while Holmes tried to wrest as much money as he could out of the parcel of land he had acquired from the late Minnie Williams. Checking into the city's fanciest hotel under yet another alias, H. M. Pratt, and posing as a wealthy investor, Holmes built a large three-story office building on his land. As before, he acquired the materials, labor, and furnishings using credit and fraudulent notes. Within two months, he had defrauded local businessmen (and at least one prominent lawyer) of more than $20,000. In March, Holmes stole a freight car of thoroughbred horses and shipped them to Chicago. Texas lawmen, never kind to horse thieves, came after him and he was forced to flee in the middle of the night.

Holmes and Georgiana then traveled to St. Louis, where they met up with Ben Pitezel. On June 15, 1894, Holmes (under the alias Howard) again attempted one of his favorite scams. Buying a little pharmacy with a small down payment, he fully stocked it on credit. After selling the merchandise, he falsified a sale of the business to a third party, actually Pitezel, to whom he referred creditors. Although he had successfully used such scams before, this time he was playing with the wrong crowd. On July 19, the Merrill Drug Company had him arrested for attempted fraud.

While jailed in St. Louis, Holmes shared a cell with the infamous train robber Marion C. Hedgepeth, known as "The Handsome Bandit." This association would be Holmes's downfall. Hedgepeth, a cattle rustler, bank and train robber, and cold-blooded killer, was known as the fastest gun in the Southwest. By age 20, he was being pursued by lawmen from Wyoming, Colorado, and Montana. A tall man with black wavy hair and dark eyes, he normally wore a blue suit, striped cravat, brown derby, and spit-polished shoes. During his nationally publicized trial in St. Louis, hundreds of women surrounded the courthouse each morning to catch a glimpse of him and sent flower baskets to his cell each afternoon. Nevertheless, he was sentenced to 25 years in the Missouri state penitentiary.

In an attempt to demonstrate that he was Hedgepeth's equal in crime, Holmes revealed the details of an insurance scam he was planning with Pitezel. In return for the promise of $500 from the insurance money, Hedgepeth gave Holmes the one thing he lacked: the name of a cooperative lawyer, Jeptha D. Howe, who "had underworld connections." For Hedgepeth, this exchange provided information he could trade to the authorities; for Holmes, it was a mistake. But Hedgepeth received only a letter of gratitude for the information that he later supplied to authorities, and he remained in jail for nine years. He later died in a shoot-out while attempting to rob a Chicago saloon.

Holmes was released on bail on July 28, but the authorities had second thoughts and rearrested him the next day. Georgiana bailed him out again on July 31. He left St. Louis for New York and then traveled to Philadelphia, where the couple reunited on August 5, 1894. They had what seemed like an ideal, although frenetic, life and Holmes appeared to be the wealthy husband she had been seeking. Georgiana was shocked when he was later arrested in Boston.

The Pitezel Scam

During the Chicago days, only one person knew of all Holmes's activities— his weak-willed, but strong-bodied, assistant, Benjamin F. Pitezel. He was known to his family by his middle name, Freelon; however, during his time with Holmes, he also used the aliases of B. F. Perry, Benton T. Lyman, L. T. Benton, H. S. Campbell, Robert Jones, and Robert E. Phelps. The last insurance scheme he worked out with Holmes ultimately killed them both.

Pitezel was a big man who stood 6'2" tall and weighed about 190 pounds. He had a laborer's muscles and hands, thick black hair, and a neatly trimmed mustache. His handsome visage was marred by a warty growth on the back of his neck and a broken nose and several missing teeth resulting from alcoholism's ravages and the bar fights it produced. He briefly worked at numerous jobs, including circus roustabout, janitor, railroad itinerant, and lumber mill hand. He had also been jailed for petty larceny, forgery, and horse stealing.

In 1887, Pitezel impregnated Carrie Canning, a Methodist minister's daughter. After a hasty wedding, Dessie was born. Their second child, Etta Alice, was born less than two years later, followed ultimately by four more children, one of whom died of diphtheria.

In November 1889, Pitezel answered Holmes's ad for carpenters to build his Castle, thus meeting the man who would employ him for the rest of his foreshortened life. Hired as a construction worker, Pitezel soon began doing Holmes's bidding on other, more questionable projects.

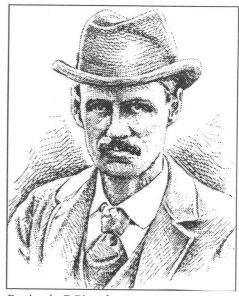

Benjamin F. Pitezel. (Sketch circa 1895)

By the end of 1893, despite his best efforts, Holmes was going broke. On November 9, 1893, Holmes took out a $10,000 life insurance policy on Pitezel with the Fidelity Mutual Life Association of Philadelphia. He planned to fake Pitezel's death by having him "disappear" to Philadelphia; Holmes would then substitute a disfigured corpse and collect the money from Mrs. Pitezel, the beneficiary. The two planned this scam for more than a year, but almost lost their chance when Pitezel, increasingly addicted to alcohol and short of funds, didn't pay the $157.50 premium. Sending a telegraphic money order, they got the payment to the insurance company's office with only a few hours to spare.

Carrie Pitezel only grudgingly went along with the scheme. She had no fondness for Holmes and distrusted the plan, but agreed to participate to improve their family's desperate financial straits. (Holmes had kept most of the proceeds from their prior scams—supposedly to reinvest for Pitezel.) Dessie also learned the plan's big picture when a drunken Pitezel told her, "Just remember—if you see it in the paper that I'm dead, don't you believe it. It's a fraud. That's all I can say."

On July 29, 1894, Pitezel caught the train for Philadelphia. Georgiana Yoke had bailed Holmes out of the St. Louis jail only the day before, outraged that her husband had been, as he characterized it, victimized by unscrupulous competitors. Eventually, all three ended up in Philadelphia, the site of the insurance company's main offices, which Holmes thought assured a more rapid pay out.

Meanwhile, on August 9, Pitezel, under the name B. F. Perry, rented a small house on Callowhill Street and set himself up as a patent dealer. The dingy brick row house was separated from the city morgue by only a narrow alley. A sign across Pitezel's storefront read "B. F. Perry—Patents Bought and Sold." With little to do in his shop, Pitezel quickly became a fixture at the local tavern.

On Sunday, September 2, as Pitezel lay in a drunken stupor, Holmes stole into his room and killed him with chloroform. According to Holmes's publicized account:

> It was necessary for me to kill him in such a manner that no struggle or movement of his body should occur, otherwise his clothing being in any way displaced it would have been impossible to again put them in a normal condition. I overcame this difficulty by first binding him hand and foot and having done this I proceeded to burn him alive by saturating his clothing and his face with benzine and igniting it with a match. So horrible was this torture that in writing of it I have been tempted to attribute his death to some more humane means—not with a wish to spare myself, but because I fear that it will not be believed that one could be so heartless and depraved . . .
>
> The least I can do is to spare my reader a recital of the victim's cries for mercy, his prayers and finally, his plea for a more speedy termination of his sufferings, all of which upon me had no effect. Finally, when he was dead I removed the straps and ropes that had bound him and extinguished the flames and a little later poured into his stomach one and one-half ounces of chloroform . . . I placed it there so that at the time of the post mortem examination, which I knew would be held, the coroner's physician would be warranted in reporting that the death was accidental.

The body was found two days later lying in a peaceful position. The upper half was badly decomposed because it had been positioned so that the sun would strike it throughout the day. William J. Scott, the first physician on the scene, described the corpse:

> His tongue was swollen and stuck out of his mouth, and red fluid issued from his mouth. Any little pressure on the stomach or over the chest would cause this fluid to flow more rapidly, and to raise the head a little would cause it to flow more rapidly. His mustache was singed, just as though a flame had flashed over and singed it a little bit, and also the eyebrow and the side of his head or hair.

The police believed that there had been an explosion, but the physicians weren't so sure and sent the body across the alley to the morgue for an autopsy. They found chloroform in the stomach and declared the cause of death to be "congestion of the lungs, caused by inhalation of flame, or of chloroform, or other poisonous drug." The body, according to custom, was put in the cold-house for 11 days awaiting someone to claim it. No one did, and Pitezel was buried in Potter's Field, the city burial ground. Holmes later wrote:

> I intended to kill him, and all my subsequent care of him and his, as well as my apparent trust in him by placing in his name large amounts of property, were steps taken to gain his confidence and that of his family so when the time was ripe they would the more readily fall into my hands.

Now Holmes had to collect the money. The insurance company initially balked at paying the claim, rightly thinking that it was a scam. So, accompanied by the lawyer Jeptha Howe, and with Pitezel's 15-year-old daughter Alice to represent the family and identify the body, they met with the insurance company's representative. Not one to let any opportunity go astray, Holmes forced Alice to have sex with him before their more gruesome task. He continued using her until he killed her some months later. (Confirming that, he later wrote, "Her [Alice's] death was the least of the wrongs suffered at my hands.")

At the cemetery, where the now completely putrid body had been disinterred and placed in a tool shed until their arrival, Alice (innocent to the shenanigans) became distraught. She waited outside the shed as the deputy coroner, the coroner's physician, Howe, Holmes, and insurance company representatives searched for four identifying marks: a deformed thumbnail, the warty growth on the neck, a scar on one leg, and some peculiarities of Pitezel's teeth. The coroner's physician could not find the marks. According to Detective Geyer:

> At this moment, Holmes pulled off his coat, rolled up his sleeves, took a surgeon's knife from his pocket, put on the rubber gloves, turned the body over, cut away the garments, washed off the skin at the back of the neck, and pointed out the wart, which he removed. He also showed the cut on the leg and the bruised nail of the thumb, which he also removed and handing them to the coroner's physician, he requested that he preserve them in alcohol.

"After all portions of the body had been covered up, save the mouth," Alice was led, sobbing, to the table to identify her father's teeth, which she did.

She later signed an affidavit for the insurance company stating that she "fully recognized the body as that of my father by his teeth. I am fully satisfied that it is he."

The next day, Howe, representing the widowed Carrie Pitezel, was given a check for $9,715.85—the policy amount minus the company's costs to investigate the claim. Howe charged Mrs. Pitezel $2,500 for his services. Holmes scammed all but $500 of the balance for himself by pretending to pay a mortgage Ben Pitezel owed the bank and giving her a worthless receipt. Holmes neglected to pay the one person who was angry enough and had sufficient information to be his undoing—Marion Hedgepeth. It was a fatal mistake.

For some time, Hedgepeth had scanned the newspapers for evidence that Holmes had initiated his insurance con. Since Pitezel's body was not identified at first, most national papers carried a story attempting to locate relatives. Hedgepeth recognized Holmes's handiwork and waited for his payment. When it wasn't forthcoming, he wrote a letter detailing Holmes's involvement to the St. Louis police chief. He later repeated the information in a sworn statement to the insurance company's investigators. Since this was information only the perpetrators, or one of their confidants, could know, he was taken seriously. Police, insurance detectives, and Pinkerton agents (whose insignia inspired the term *private eye*) were soon on the case.

Holmes was on the run. He spurted from city to city across the Midwest, East Coast, and Canada accompanied by Georgiana, Mrs. Pitezel, and the children. By convincing Mrs. Pitezel that her husband was hiding in a nearby city—always one beyond their present location—he persuaded her to accompany him with two of her children. (He told her that he had found a temporary home for the other children. Actually, he had them with him.) Mrs. Pitezel, traveling with her oldest daughter Dessie and her baby, never knew that she and Holmes were often on the same train and in the same city as her other three children. Georgiana didn't know about any of the Pitezels, even though she, too, often shared the same trains and stayed in the same cities. As Harold Schechter wrote:

> Holmes was performing a feat worthy of a master marionetteer: maneuvering three sets of human puppets—his wife [Miss Yoke]; Carrie [Mrs. Pitezel] and two of her children; and Alice and Nellie [Pitezel]—from one city to the next and lodging them within a short distance of each other, while keeping them completely unaware of each other's presence.

Moving the entire group to Burlington, Vermont, Holmes thought that he could "clean up the job, by removing Mrs. Pitezel and her youngest and eldest child," according to Detective Geyer. Mrs. Pitezel, however, finally suspected treachery and refused to accompany Holmes any longer. Holmes left town to think about his next step.

On October 31, detectives caught up with him in Gilmanton, New Hampshire, his hometown, where he had miraculously appeared to visit his parents. Since they thought him long dead, he explained that he had suffered a head injury while being robbed, lost his memory for more than a decade, and only recently regained remembrances of his family. This was classic Holmes—and his mother believed it. He also visited his legal-but-abandoned wife, Clara Lovering Mudgett, and their 13-year-old son.

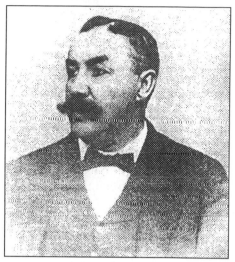

Detective Frank P. Geyer, whose tireless efforts finally led to the arrest and conviction of Mudgett/Holmes. (From *The Holmes-Pitezel Case*, F. P. Geyer, 1896)

The detectives tailed him to Boston where, fearing that he would flee to Europe, they tried to arrest him on the Philadelphia coroner's warrant for fraud. Boston police did not believe that the charge was sufficient to hold him, however, so the detectives obtained a copy of the Fort Worth, Texas, warrant for "larceny of one horse." They incarcerated Holmes on November 17. Deciding that he disliked Texas prisons more than Philadelphia jails, Holmes confessed to defrauding the insurance company. He then helped the Pinkertons lure Mrs. Pitezel to Boston, whereupon she, too, was arrested.

From his incarceration on November 17, 1894, until his execution on May 7, 1896, Holmes made a number of widely differing confessions, wrote a book explaining his actions, and testified in court. None of these descriptions match each other or the available information about his activities. As Frank Geyer, the primary Philadelphia police detective on the case, later said:

> Holmes is greatly given to lying with a sort of florid ornamentation, and all of his stories are decorated with flamboyant draperies, intended by him to strengthen the plausibility of his statements. In talking, he has the

appearance of candor, becomes pathetic at times when pathos will serve him best, uttering his words with a quaver in his voice, often accompanied by a moistened eye, then turning quickly with a determined and forceful method of speech, as if indignation or resolution had sprung out of tender memories that had touched his heart.

As for Mrs. Pitezel, police found her to be an impoverished, unpretentious woman living with her two remaining children. She was released on June 19, 1894.

The Pitezel Children

Of the Pitezels' five children, Holmes chose 15-year-old Alice, the second-oldest daughter, to help identify her father's body because Carrie Pitezel would have discovered her husband's murder. After returning from Philadelphia, Holmes convinced Mrs. Pitezel to allow him to take two more of her children, Nellie and Howard, with him so that Alice would have some company and Carrie wouldn't be noticed as she traveled to "meet her husband." Holmes, however, had no interest in traveling with the children, so he decided to kill them.

When Holmes was arrested, detectives found a tin box containing a dozen letters from Alice and Nellie to their mother and grandparents that Holmes was supposed to mail, but didn't. These gave detectives a clue about where to search for the bodies.

Howard Pitezel had been annoying Holmes by complaining about the cramped hotel rooms Holmes rented for the children, and he was the first child Holmes disposed of. On October 3, Holmes, accompanied by Howard, brought two cases of his surgical instruments—scalpels, knives, and saws—to

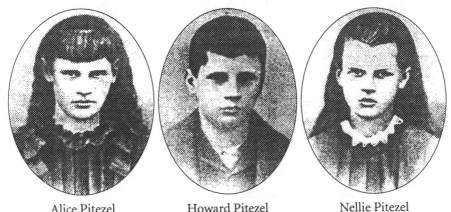

Alice Pitezel   Howard Pitezel   Nellie Pitezel
(From *The Holmes-Pitezel Case* by F. P. Geyer, 1986)

a local repairman to be sharpened. He then took Howard "on a trip," telling his sisters that Howard would be staying with his cousin in Terre Haute. Holmes rented a small wood-frame cottage in the Indianapolis suburb of Irvington, retrieved his tools on October 8, and went with little Howard in tow, to the house. Two days later, Holmes said that he called the boy into the house,

> and insisted that he go to bed at once, first giving him the fatal dose of medicine. As soon as he had ceased to breathe I cut his body into pieces that would pass through the door of the stove and by the combined use of gas and corncobs proceeded to burn it with as little feeling as tho' it had been some inanimate object.

When they searched the house months later, detectives found parts of his femur, pelvis, and skull and charred remnants of his stomach, liver, and spleen. They also found a few of Howard's belongings in the house.

On October 25, Holmes took the girls to Toronto. Renting a home on St. Vincent Street, Holmes said:

> [I] compelled them to both get within the large trunk, through the cover of which I made a small opening. Here I left them until I could return and at my leisure kill them. At 5:00 P.M. I borrowed a spade of a neighbor and at the same time called on Mrs. Pitezel at her hotel. I then returned to my hotel and ate dinner, and at 7:00 P.M. went again to Mrs. Pitezel's hotel, and aided her in leaving Toronto for Ogdensburg, N.Y.
>
> Later than 8:00 P.M., I again returned to the house where the children were imprisoned, and ended their lives by connecting the gas with the trunk. Then came the opening of the trunk and the viewing of their little blackened and distorted faces, then the digging of their shallow graves in the basement of the house, the ruthless stripping off of their clothing, and the burial without a particle of covering save the cold earth, which I heaped upon them with fiendish delight.

Detectives discovered the bodies months later, as the lead detective, Frank Geyer, recalled:

> Alice was found lying on her side with her face to the west. Nellie was found lying on her face, with her head to the south, her plaited hair hanging neatly down her back . . . As Nellie's limbs were found resting on Alice's, we first began with her. We lifted her as gently as possible, but owing to the decomposed state of the body, the weight of her plaited hair hanging down her back, pulled the scalp from off her head. A sheet had been spread in which to lay the remains, and after we succeeded in getting it out of the hole, it was placed in the sheet, taken upstairs, and

deposited in the coffin. Again we returned to the cellar and gently lifting what remained of poor Alice, we placed her in another sheet, took her upstairs, and placed her in a coffin by the side of her sister.

Investigators also found some of the children's partially burned clothes. Mrs. Pitezel went to Toronto to identify the bodies. At the "dead house," Detective Geyer related, the coroner

had removed the putrid flesh from the skull of Alice; the teeth had been nicely cleaned and the bodies covered with canvas. The head of Alice was covered with paper, and a hole sufficiently large had been cut in it, so that Mrs. Pitezel could see the teeth. The hair of both children had been carefully washed and laid on the canvas sheet which was covering Alice . . . In an instant she recognized the teeth and hair as those of her daughter, Alice. Then turning to me she said, "Where is Nellie?" About this time she noticed the long black plait of hair belonging to Nellie lying in the canvas. She could stand it no longer, and the shrieks of that poor forlorn creature are still ringing in my ears.

Toronto authorities buried the girls in St. James' Cemetery.

Trial and Punishment

Holmes was first put on trial for defrauding the insurance company, a crime to which he had already confessed. Believing that, under Pennsylvania law, the maximum sentence would be two years and that he might get off with a less severe sentence if he pleaded guilty, he agreed to do so. The judge postponed sentencing and Holmes appeared content. Investigators, though, believed that there was more to uncover, and proceeded to do so.

On July 20, 1895, Chicago detectives unearthed damning evidence when they began searching what came to be called "Murder Castle" or "Nightmare Castle." The press began screaming that police had ensnared an archfiend, a monster, and a demon. As the hysteria over Holmes intensified, pundits began blaming him for every crime that had occurred during the prior decade—a situation that the *Chicago Daily Tribune* began lampooning in its editorial cartoons. Philadelphia's Dime Museum erected a "sensational display" about his exploits. Dozens of instant books appeared, revealing the "true" but usually bizarrely inaccurate story, with lurid titles such as *Holmes, The Arch Fiend*, *A Carnival of Crime*, *The Holmes Castle*, and *Sold to Satan*. Some of them were translated for European audiences.

During the summer of 1895, in an attempt to sway public opinion, Holmes penned *Holmes' Own Story*, supposedly a detailed account of his life and misdeeds. While it certainly provides insight into the fiend's mind, much of what he wrote was simply self-serving lies—which he later recanted. For example, he related a particularly gruesome, hysterically bizarre, and unbelievable account of his attempt to acquire and transport a body to defraud an insurance company. In the tale, Holmes performs feats that any fictional hero would envy: defeating greedy assistants, detectives, and the Secret Service while overcoming numerous obstacles, including a train wreck. Finally caught, he bribes his way out of danger, but ultimately succeeds with the deception and collects $20,000. As one person later wrote, "what *Holmes' Own Story* lacked in facts, it more than made up for with melodrama . . . Holmes missed his calling when he chose medicine as career rather than the writing of dime novels."

Appended to his book, in a calculated attempt to generate sympathy, was Holmes's prison diary, in which he describes his cell:

> A thoroughly clean, whitewashed room, about 9x14 feet in size, lighted by one very narrow grated window. The entrance of the room is closed by a small latticed iron door, beyond which is still another solid door of wood, which, when closed, excludes nearly all sound, and thus renders the room practically a place of solitary confinement.

After complaining that he was permitted to send only one letter a week, was becoming accustomed to his "bed of straw," and had lost 20 pounds in jail, he wrote that "the great humiliation of feeling that I am a prisoner is killing me far more than any other discomforts I have to endure."

On September 23, 1895, Holmes was arraigned in Philadelphia's jam-packed Court of Oyer and Terminar for killing Benjamin Pitezel. Other jurisdictions had wanted to try Holmes: Toronto for Alice and Nellie Pitezel's murders, Indianapolis for Howard Pitezel's murder, and Chicago for all the murders he had committed there. But possession is nine-tenths of the law—Philadelphia had him, as well as a strong case against him.

Holmes, represented by two lawyers but already labeled by the public as the "Monster of 63rd Street," pleaded "not guilty" to the murder charge. As was the custom, after the plea, the court clerk intoned, "May God send you a safe deliverance." It seemed to foretell the final outcome. When he returned to his cell, he received a letter from his mother saying, "Herman, tell the truth whatever it may be. Remember the teachings of your mother and the influences which surrounded you in your home when you were a boy." Holmes remembered only too well and responded with his typical mendacity.

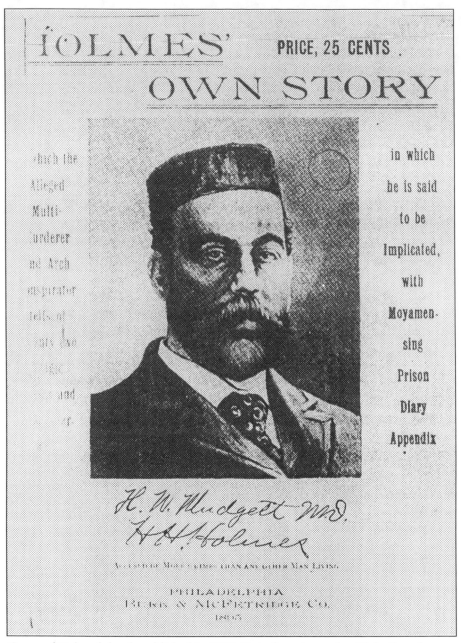

Cover of Holmes's book published in 1895. Note the autograph with both real name and alias.

On October 28, 1895, Holmes's trial began in confusion when his lawyers refused to proceed after they were denied a two-month continuance to better prepare his defense. Judge Michael Arnold threatened them with disbarment if they attempted to withdraw from the case, but Holmes countered by saying that he intended to discharge them and seek new counsel. Judge Arnold refused to allow this and demanded that the lawyers remain in court. One walked out anyway. In a bizarre turn that has been imitated by other murderers in recent years, Holmes proceeded to act as his own lawyer and interrogated the prospective jurors. Observers thought the intelligent and deceitful showman did as admirable a job as would any good lawyer.

Although the prosecutors wanted to include evidence about the gruesome murders of the three Pitezel children, Judge Arnold ruled that that evidence could be presented in a subsequent trial, depending upon the outcome of the present court case. Nevertheless, throughout the trial, the 12-man jury stared at large portraits of both the dead Benjamin Pitezel and his raped and murdered daughter, Alice.

As the trial began, the prosecutors presented so much damning evidence that even Holmes was at a loss. On October 30, he recalled his lawyers, but there was still little the defense could do. The prosecutors clearly demonstrated that the dead body was that of Ben Pitezel, that he had died of chloroform poisoning rather than from an explosion or the superficial burns, that it was murder and not suicide, that Holmes was familiar with and had visited Pitezel's Philadelphia shop and residence, and that Holmes had multiple reasons to want Pitezel dead, including the profit he made from the insurance money. The prosecution even brought in a phrenologist, who described Holmes:

> A man with a keen but intensely repulsive face: a face shaped like a hatchet, like one of those old-fashioned hatchets ... He is made on a very delicate mold. To be a great murderer he needed all his cunning and trickery, for nature gave him neither the physical strength nor the animal brutality needed for violent killing. He has killed his friends, killed, cut up, and burned little children, and murdered women whom he pretended to love. But he probably never looked one of them in the face to murder him openly.

No evidence was presented in Holmes's defense. According to Holmes, presenting defense arguments "would have been but a waste of my counsel's energies, and of my own, to have tried to convince the most impartial juries that it was a case of suicide and not a murder." Closing arguments were heard by a packed courtroom. The district attorney summarized the bizarre case:

> That was a strange story, gentlemen; if you and I had read it in fiction, we would say, perhaps, that the novelist had overdrawn or overstated the facts; that he had overdrawn the story, and made it stronger than our imagination or fancy could tolerate ... Now this strange trial is drawing rapidly to a close ... [but] there is no middle ground in this case. it is the highest crime known to the law under the circumstances surrounding the deceased, for he was poisoned to death, and the poisoning itself indicates a clear intent to kill.

Holmes's young lawyer delivered the defense's closing (and only) remarks, but it was a hopeless effort. Judge Arnold, in giving his instructions to the jury, said, "Truth is stranger than fiction, and if Mrs. Pitezels' story is true, it is the most wonderful exhibition of the power of mind over mind I have ever seen, and stranger than any novel I have ever read."

The jury was then sent to a room to deliberate. Not a person stirred from their seat in the courtroom. Three hours later, the jury returned and Holmes was brought back into the courtroom. The clerk intoned: "Jurors, look upon the prisoner; prisoner, look upon the jurors. How say you, gentlemen of the jury? Do you find the prisoner at the bar, Herman W. Mudgett, alias H. H. Holmes, guilty of the murder of Benjamin F. Pitezel or not guilty?"

"Guilty of murder in the first degree," the foreman replied. Each jury member then repeated the phrase as they were individually polled. Actually, they had agreed on the verdict before their jury room door closed, but had found it unseemly to condemn a man to death that quickly. They had waited until after their dinner to return to the courtroom. On November 18, Holmes's lawyers moved for a retrial based on 13 supposed errors Judge Arnold had made. The Pennsylvania Supreme Court turned down this request on November 30, 1895, and affirmed the verdict. Holmes was sentenced to hang.

On April 9, 1896, Holmes signed a lengthy confession in which he claimed to have killed 27 people and attempted to kill 6 others. How much of this was true is questionable, since the evidence contradicted some of the confession's "facts." Yet, undoubtedly, his confession portrays at least some of his methods and murders. Revealing something of his personality, Holmes wrote:

> To-day I have every attribute of a degenerate—a moral idiot. Is it possible that the crimes, instead of being the result of these abnormal

conditions, are in themselves the occasion of the degeneracy? . . . I committed this and other crimes for the pleasure of killing my fellow beings, to hear their cries for mercy and pleas to be allowed even sufficient time to pray and prepare for death—all this is now too horrible for even me, hardened criminal that I am, to again live over without a shudder.

True to his avaricious precepts to the end, Holmes wrote his confession for the $7,500 that William Randolph Hearst paid to reprint it in his papers. In a desperate scam to save his own life, Holmes wrote to both Mrs. Pitezel and Detective Geyer during the week before his death, trying to entice them into advocating a commutation of his sentence. To Mrs. Pitezel, he offered remuneration of the funds he had stolen; to Geyer, he offered supposed accomplices in some of his killings. Neither took the bait.

On May 7, 1896, Holmes ate a substantial breakfast at Philadelphia's Moyamensing Prison. Then he gave instructions for disposition of his estate (Myrta had already acquired everything of value) and wrote letters to his various wives, relatives, and even friends of some of his victims. He climbed the steps to the gallows, accompanied by the prison warden and city sheriff. Catholic priests from his newfound religion followed. Holmes then coolly addressed the 51 assembled onlookers, including Detective Geyer and the president of Fidelity Mutual, whom he had swindled. Confounding everyone, he recanted his prior detailed confessions:

> The extent of the wrongdoing I am guilty of in taking human life is the killing of two women. They died by my hands as the results of criminal operations. I wish also to state, so that no chance of misunderstanding may exist hereafter, that I am not guilty of taking the lives of any of the Pitezel family, either the three children or the father, Benjamin F. Pitezel, for whose death I am now to be hanged. I have never committed murder. That is all I have to say.

After he finished his speech, he bowed to his audience and briefly embraced his lawyer, who fled the gallows in tears. After kneeling to receive Last Rites, he stepped onto the trapdoor and held his hands behind him to be handcuffed, as the executioner lowered a black satin hood over his head. Holmes was heard to say, "Take your time. You know I am in no hurry." But the noose was swiftly placed over his neck and the trapdoor immediately sprung.

The rope went taut and Holmes's body began twitching as the rope slowly twisted, rotating his body. They let it hang for another 20 minutes before he was finally pronounced dead and his body was tossed, "like a bag of potatoes," into a waiting cart. Holmes's distorted and discolored face made even the physicians in attendance squirm and avert their eyes.

Herman William Mudgett, aka H. H. Holmes et al., was dead at age 35. His secrets would be buried with him.

The Aftermath

Like many graverobbing anatomists of his time, Holmes was petrified of the idea that his body would be dissected or his brain removed for examination. He had reason to worry, since at least one medical school anatomist had offered his lawyer $5,000 for Holmes's corpse.

Holmes left specific instructions for burial, which were followed. His body was placed in a pine box filled with cement; it weighed more than a ton and took two dozen men to move. The coffin was then taken to Holy Cross Cemetery in Delaware County where, after a brief Roman Catholic service, it was buried in a 10-foot-deep hole within a double plot and covered with a 2-foot-thick layer of cement. (Called "cementation," this method was eventually used to keep Abraham Lincoln's body safe from body snatchers.)

During his incarceration and trial, Holmes's public image went from the "prince of insurance swindlers" to the "king of fabrication" and, finally, to the "versatile butcher." As the *Chicago Times-Herald* wrote:

> to parallel such a career one must go back to past ages and to the time of the Borgias or Brinvilliers, and even these were not such human monsters as Holmes seems to have been. He is a prodigy of wickedness, a human demon, a being so unthinkable to the mind that no novelist would dare to invent such a character.

Following his execution, the *Chicago Journal* was just as blunt:

> The nerve, the calculation and the audacity of the man were unparalleled. Murder was his natural bent. Sometimes, he killed from sheer greed of gain; oftener, as he himself confessed, to gratify an inhuman thirst for blood. Not one of his crimes was the outcome of a sudden burst of fury—"hot blood," as the codes say. All were deliberate; planned and concluded with consummate skill.

Even the liberal *New York Times* agreed, "It takes a very convinced opponent of capital punishment to maintain that any better disposition could have been made of the wretch Holmes."

We will never know the exact number of Holmes's victims, since he refused to divulge information about them. Obsessively, he had destroyed all evidence of most of these unfortunates in his basement acid bath and crematorium. As America's first—and most prolific—serial killer, he had solved a key problem: how to safely and completely dispose of the victims' bodies.

On August 19, 1895, after Chicago police had completed their initial investigation but before additional Castle secrets could be exposed (and shortly before it was to go on display as a tourist attraction called "The Murder Museum"), Holmes's building mysteriously burned to the ground.

In describing "the Monster of 63rd Street," an early edition of *The Guinness Book of World Records* lists Mudgett/Holmes as "the most prolific murderer known in recent criminal history." In *A Criminal History of Mankind*, Colin Wilson wrote, "Like the Ripper, Holmes is a kind of grim landmark in social history. But his sadism was far more cold and calculating."

And Herbert Webster Mudgett was a physician.

World's Columbian Exposition of 1893

Timing is everything in life—and in death. The lantern that drew the moths to Dr. Holmes's flame and to his nightmarish castle was the World's Columbian Exposition of 1893, held to celebrate the 400th anniversary of Columbus' first voyage to the New World. Chicago, the *nouveau riche* "hog butcher to the world," narrowly won the honor of hosting the fair over New York, Washington, D.C., and St. Louis when the U.S. House of Representatives approved their bid on February 24, 1890, and President Benjamin Harrison agreed in December of that year.

The extravaganza was built on a 633-acre stretch of boggy Jackson Park shoreline, seven miles south of central Chicago. In February 1891, 7,000 of what would eventually become 40,000 laborers began preparing the land so they could finish the buildings by the October 21, 1892, deadline. Chicagoans would be amazed and proud as this utopian mini-city of intricate waterways and lagoons fed by Lake Michigan and buildings gleaming like alabaster marble arose out of swampland. It was a huge construction project, ultimately devouring 75 million board-feet of lumber, 18,000 tons of iron and steel, 120,000 incandescent lights, and 30,000 tons of "staff" (off-white Plaster of Paris molded around fibrous jute cloth to create a marble effect). It was so amazing that more than 3,000 people a week first paid 25 cents and, later, 50 cents just to watch the construction.

Although the project was not quite complete, 80,000 people cheered the 10-mile-long parade that passed through the city to open the fair site. The Exposition itself opened six months later on May 1, 1893, and 200,000 people attended the opening ceremonies. When opened, the site contained 200 buildings, including 14 Beaux-Arts-facaded "great" buildings with 63 million square feet of floor space. The 11-acre Manufacture and Liberal Arts Building, as officials were quick to boast, was bigger than the U.S. Capitol, Winchester Cathedral, Madison Square Garden, and the Great Pyramid of Giza combined.

Called the "New Jerusalem" and "The White City" (because of the buildings' color), the exposition featured George W. Ferris's first wheel, Little Egypt's lewd dancing, a 2,500-foot-long formal lagoon, and a mile-long sideshow called the Midway Plaisance (with "probably the greatest collection of 'fakes' the world has ever seen," said *The Century* magazine). Among the Midway's attractions were the Sliding Railway (10¢ admission), the Ferris Wheel (50¢), the Turkish Village ($1), the Street in Cairo ($1.10), and the Balloon Ascension ($2). Bringing in a camera cost an extra $2 a day!

continued . . .

World's Columbian Exposition of 1893, continued

Among foodstuffs that made their first appearance at the Exposition were the hamburger, the hot dog bun, caramel-coated popcorn and peanuts (shortly thereafter known as Cracker Jacks), Aunt Jemima Syrup, Cream of Wheat, Shredded Wheat, Pabst Blue Ribbon Beer, Juicy Fruit chewing gum, and diet carbonated soda. There were 65,000 exhibits and restaurant seating for 7,000 people.

Fifty-four countries besides the United States exhibited, including the still-independent Hawaii. Modern marvels, such as the University of Chicago's 70-ton Yerkes telescope and the newly invented telephone, phonograph, and motion picture, were shown alongside oddities such as Canada's 22,000-pound "Monster Cheese" and two model Liberty Bells, one made of oranges and the other of wheat, oats, and rye. Buffalo Bill's Wild West Show held performances just outside the fairgrounds. It was no wonder that the entire nation yearned to attend. As novelist Hamlin Garland wrote to his parents, "Sell the cook stove and come. You *must* see the Fair."

More than 27 million people, including 25 percent of the U.S. population, did attend during its six-month run from May 1 to October 31, 1893. On "Chicago Day," October 9, over 700,000 people attended. But the fair ended with a whimper. The planned gala to commemorate its closing was scrubbed when Chicago's five-term mayor, Carter Harrison, was shot dead two days earlier by an embittered office seeker. Then, on January 8, 1894, a fire destroyed three major Exposition buildings and, six months later, fire leveled even more "staff" structures, including the magnificent Manufacture and Liberal Arts Building.

With hundreds of Columbian Guards and plainclothes detectives patrolling the grounds, the Exposition had been relatively safe. What happened when visitors left the grounds, however, was a different story. Many of these visitors needed lodging and Dr. Holmes planned to make a killing. Exactly how many people (primarily women) he lured to his Castle is uncertain, but about 150 were later cited as missing after making contact with him.

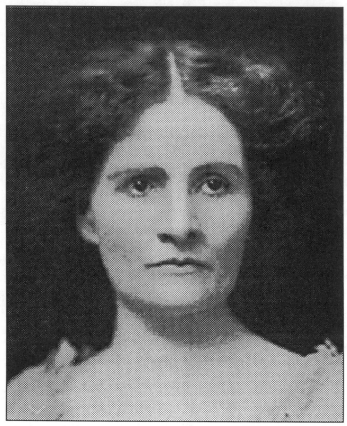

Linda Burfield Hazzard, D.O. (1868–1938).

4

The Starvation Doctor

Linda Burfield Hazzard, D.O.

The body, draped with a white sheet, seemed ready for burial. No sign of life could be detected until the eyes suddenly opened and stared. A man, shrunken almost to a skeleton, moaned and moved his hand in a vague gesture.

A woman strode up to his bed. "It's time for your therapy," she said commandingly.

"No, no, I can't do it," he replied.

"Nonsense. That's the only way for you to heal. You only have eight more days of fasting. Now for your therapy." She removed the sheet and began vigorously pounding on his forehead with her knuckles. His soft moaning could scarcely be heard over the "rap, rap, rap" on his skull.

"Turn over now, and we'll proceed on your back."

His only memories were of weeks upon weeks of scant vegetable broth, Dr. Hazzard's pounding treatments, and the enemas. For hours at a time, he would keep quarts of water in his bowels, his belly swollen beyond belief, becoming dizzy with the pain and weakness that overcame him. It was terrible, but that was the treatment. She said it would make him see again.

"Turn over, we have to continue the treatment."

He didn't stir. He would never move again. Dr. Linda Hazzard had "cured" another one.

~

The Making of A "Doctor"

Occasionally praised as one of the "many unsung heroines among women who were Hygienic professionals," Linda Burfield Hazzard is best remembered as a cold-blooded zealot who killed while administering her starvation diet cures. "Dr." Hazzard saw herself as part of the great women's emancipation movement of the early twentieth century, and she often played that card to her advantage. She denounced traditional M.D.s and D.O.s as followers of errant precepts in a male-dominated profession. Women, she claimed, knew how to cure.

With religious zeal, she promoted her own healing methods: rigid prolonged fasts, frequent enemas, and pseudo-osteopathic manipulations, in which she severely pounded her patients' backs, heads, and foreheads with her fists. These were markedly unlike the spinal manipulations practiced by her fellow osteopaths, who derided her as a quack.

Although she never graduated from a medical school or passed a licensing examination, Hazzard was granted a medical license to practice osteopathic medicine and fasting under Washington State's 1909 *Medical Practice Act*. She was "grandfathered in" after waging a legal battle to show that she had practiced medicine for at least two years. She was not averse to practicing her deadly arts without a license, however, and did so in Minnesota, California, and New Zealand using her "Dr." title.

What little medical training she did receive was part of a course of study to become an osteopathic nurse. When later questioned about her education, she said that she had studied "at two osteopathic institutions, but it would be useless to name them, for they have both ceased to exist."

Early Years

Linda Burfield was born in 1868 in Carver County, Minnesota, the eldest of seven children. Her Canadian-English mother, Susan Neal, married her American father, Montgomery Burfield, a Civil War veteran, in 1869. In 1878, the family homesteaded in Star Lake Township in Ottertail County, Minnesota. Her parents were vegetarians, a practice Linda later incorporated into her dietary system.

Linda's views on traditional medicine were soured by an itinerant doctor who visited the Burfield children annually. Probably a barely adequate practitioner, he treated the children for non-existent intestinal symptoms.

As she later remembered:

> This physician was convinced, as were the majority of his profession at that day, that all children harbored intestinal parasites, and that periodic doses of some vermifuge were essential. Therefore I, in company with my brothers and sisters, was given some blue mass pills, a strong mercurial preparation. I now allow, what of course I could not then suspect, that this powerful poison did irreparable injury to my intestines, retarding and preventing their development and growth to such degree that even to this day I am compelled to resort to the enema daily.

"Blue mass," also called calomel (mercurous chloride), was so toxic that the Union Army Medical Corps discontinued its use during the Civil War. The Burfield children suffered frequent vomiting and diarrhea, and Linda ultimately blamed her need for frequent enemas on the "medication."

In 1886, at age 18, Linda married Erwin A. Perry, who was her senior by 14 years and the son of a well-to-do pioneer family. They settled in Fergus Falls, Minnesota, and had two children: Rollin, in 1889, and Nina Floy, in 1891. But she was too ambitious to stay at home and, in April 1898, she left Erwin and sent her son and daughter to live with her mother. The divorce was finalized in the fall of 1902, and Linda assumed her maiden name of Burfield. Although her profligate son eventually came to live with her, she and her daughter never reconciled. Out of spite, Linda left Nina $1 in her will.

Minnesota

After partially completing her training as an osteopathic nurse and spending a short period of time learning "fasting" under a physician's tutelage, Linda announced that she was a "doctor of osteopathy." In 1898, she opened an office in downtown Minneapolis and advertised that "Dr. Burfield" practiced osteopathic medicine and fasting therapy. She was able to do this due to a loophole in Minnesota law. While an 1855 statute gave the University of Minnesota's faculty the "right to organize" the medical profession and an 1887 law established a medical board to register and examine physicians, it wasn't until 1927 that the board was given the right to refuse applications and revoke licenses.

With the goal of becoming a world-renowned advocate of "starvation therapy," Burfield took on hopeless cases such as patients with diabetes (before insulin was discovered), terminal kidney diseases, syphilis, and paralysis. She claimed that she could cure them all. And, until Gertrude Young died, no one examined her methods, and her practice grew.

Gertrude Young had suffered a stroke when she was only 39 years old. Due to paralysis in a foot and an arm, she had profound difficulty caring for herself. In addition, the muscle contractures caused her significant pain and she was desperate for relief. In October, 1902, Young consulted "Dr." Burfield, who started her on a 40-day fast to cure her. Instead, she quickly withered away and died.

U. G. Williams, M.D., a traditional physician who also was the Hennepin County coroner, had examined Young during her fast and had told the nurse that her patient would die if she didn't eat. After Young died, he arranged for an autopsy to be performed at the University of Minnesota. Based on the examiner's finding of death by starvation, Dr. Williams announced that Young had been the victim of "Dr." Burfield's cruel and unnecessary quackery, and pushed for an indictment against her. On November 20, 1902, a headline in the *Minneapolis Daily Times* screamed: "Coroner in Crusade Against Starvation Curists Urges Prosecution as Sequel to Woman's Death."

Investigators discovered that Young's jewelry had disappeared, but Linda claimed not to know anything about it. When reporters asked her whether she had a medical license, she replied, "Thank God, I have no license to kill!" Actually, because she was not licensed to practice medicine and there was no statute restricting quack treatments, she could not legally be held accountable for the death. "Dr." Burfield saw this loophole in Minnesota's law as a vindication of her methods.

Throughout her life, Linda Burfield doggedly pursued her dreams, ignoring any obstacles—legal or otherwise. She often proclaimed that her starvation diet had cured cancer, tuberculosis, psoriasis, heart disease, epilepsy, insanity, and toothaches. She was a dynamic speaker and promoted her gospel of health in a manner that would have made the most zealous preacher proud.

Linda Burfield's stormy career as a doctor had begun, but a tempest of another kind occurred when she fell in love with Sam Hazzard.

Sam Hazzard

Samuel Christman Hazzard was a handsome man, standing over six feet tall with a military bearing. Those who knew him well described him as a "bright, intelligent, well-educated Lothario." Born in 1869 in Pottsville, Pennsylvania, he entered the United States Military Academy at West Point on June 15, 1889. Shortly after graduating and receiving his commission, he married the vivacious and intelligent Agnes Hedley.

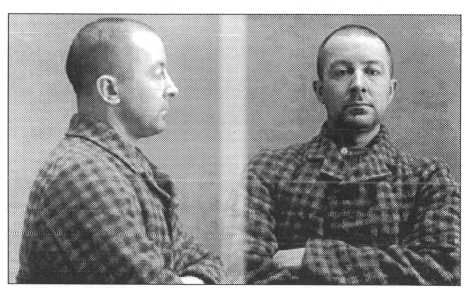

Sam Hazzard—prison photographs. (Stillwater Prison Collection, Minnesota Historical Society)

Three years later, in 1896, he was appointed instructor of modern languages at the Academy because he could fluently read and speak French, Spanish, German, and Latin. He was soon promoted to the prestigious post of military adjutant. However, everything was not as it appeared.

Sam Hazzard had taken a mistress. Thus, when he was promoted to first lieutenant of artillery in April 1899 and was scheduled to be transferred, he did everything in his power to stay with his new love. After he repeatedly sent messages to his commanding officers saying that his father was desperately ill, they reluctantly granted him extended leave. As soon as Hazzard left the base, angry creditors and people he had swindled began to notify the army about his unpaid bills. The army had to investigate the flood of complaints against him, including one that claimed he had misappropriated army funds. Hazzard resigned from the army, but they still issued orders for his arrest. So he fled, leaving both his wife and his mistress. He became Sam "Hargrave" and disappeared; at some point, he divorced Agnes.

By 1902, Sam Hazzard was working as an insurance salesman for American Credit Indemnity out of Chicago. He was still using the last name "Hargrave" to keep the U.S. government from locating him. There he met Viva Estelle Fitchpatrick, the twice-divorced flighty daughter of an Iowa state senator. They became "an item" and, when Sam's employer moved him to Minneapolis in February 1903, Viva followed in March. Sam met Viva the day she arrived and, almost as an afterthought, hurried her into the court commissioner's office to get married, telling his cohorts at work only that he needed to take a few hours off. This offhand wedding was a harbinger of things to come.

Exactly how Linda Burfield and Sam Hazzard met is unclear, but when Linda decided to wed Sam, the "man of her dreams," it didn't matter to her that he was already married. On November 11, 1903, a minister married Sam and Linda in her medical office. Sam spent the next few nights with Viva, but he soon announced that she was not his legal wife and that he was now married to "Dr." Burfield. He then quit his job to manage Linda's career.

But Sam and Linda had misjudged their adversary. With her father's support, Viva got the Hennepin County attorney to file bigamy charges against Sam Hargrave, alias Hazzard. The case became the sensation of Minneapolis. Viva's father also contacted Elihu Root, the U.S. secretary of war, about his son-in-law the deserter. Root sent Secret Service officers to arrest Hazzard for forgery and cashing government vouchers for personal use. But Sam was already in jail, so they let him be.

Linda continued to publically proclaim that she was Sam's legal wife, but they fought a losing legal battle that ended with her public humiliation and Sam Hazzard's two-year incarceration in the state penitentiary for bigamy. Linda visited him in prison, but pressure from Viva and her powerful family led Sam to announce his intention to return to Viva.

Linda and her strong will eventually triumphed. Sam was released from prison on October 30, 1905 and, rather than reuniting with Viva as expected, he headed directly to Linda Burfield to resume their complex relationship. While Sam had been in jail, Linda's practice had grown, and she needed Sam's help as her business manager and promoter. They never remarried to legalize their relationship and the social pressures in Minneapolis eventually became too much for Linda. By 1907, they had moved to Seattle, where she felt that she could call herself "Linda Burfield Hazzard" without facing any embarrassing questions. Sam drank heavily and had frequent dalliances throughout their marriage, despite Linda's loud and sometimes physically abusive protestations.

Seattle/Olalla

As the twentieth century dawned, Seattle had 300,000 residents and was the largest and fastest-growing city in the Pacific Northwest. The city was crisscrossed with broad brick-paved streets traversed by electric streetcars. Already populated by liberal thinkers, it was an ideal place for the Hazzards to begin their new life. Linda initially established her office downtown and commuted by ferry from her home in Olalla.

Olalla was a small, rain-soaked village, the only inhabited site on the western side of Colvos Passage off Puget Sound. Populated primarily by Finnish and Swedish homesteaders, it still had no electricity as late as 1911. Located in Kitsap County, Olalla could claim only a boardwalk built after an agonizing fundraising process, rich clam and oyster beds, and the wild strawberries that entangled the hillsides.

The residents of Olalla found Linda Hazzard an elegant and refined lady who was always dressed in the latest fashions. She was often seen walking to the ferry landing with her cocker spaniel in tow. Linda, at 43, was more handsome than beautiful; her angular jaw, and no-nonsense approach to life made her stand out. Her professional attire usually consisted of a white dress similar to those worn by nurses.

A white wooden archway over the Hazzards' circular drive, off Orchard Avenue, announced that visitors had arrived at "Wilderness Heights." The 40-acre plot, densely covered with huge Douglas firs, was accessed by a long, rutted, and usually muddy road. Blackened areas and enormous tree trunks attested to attempts to clear this gloomy tract for buildings. For the rest of her life, even during her time in prison and in New Zealand, Linda and Sam would call Olalla home, and repeatedly return.

Linda's ultimate dream was to build a majestic sanitarium on the site. The initial "healing center," however, consisted of five tiny cabins for patients, a sturdy little barn, and the cedar-shingled bungalow that was the Hazzards' home. To generate income and advertise her methods, she wrote a book, titled *Fasting for the Cure of Disease,* that was first published in 1908 and eventually went into five editions. The name of the book changed twice, first to *Diet in Disease and Systemic Cleansing* in 1917 and then to *Scientific Fasting: The Ancient and Modern Key to Health* in 1927. She also wrote a book called *The Perfect Man,* which was less successful.

The Starvation Diet

The starvation diet was actually the idea of Dr. Henry S. Tanner (1831–1919). Born in England, Tanner was a traditional Minnesota physician who came upon the idea as a result of suicidal frustration when he did not quickly recover from what he called "low gastric fever." As he described in a letter to Hazzard:

> I really believe that I am entitled to be called the father of therapeutic fasting in this country, for away back in 1877 I had given up hopes of ever regaining what might be called normal health. I was then in Minneapolis in the practice of my profession, and, after a strenuous time with a patient critically ill, I virtually collapsed. I was at such a low ebb physically and mentally at the time that I did not care whether I lived or died, and I determined that, since my drugs gave me no relief, I would starve myself to death ere I again would suffer the physical misery that had been mine for months preceding. I accordingly told Dr. Moyer, my consulting companion, that I would not again eat food until I was dead or recovered in health.

Dr. Tanner's symptoms resolved in about ten days, but, for whatever reason, he continued his fast, while drinking large amounts of water, for 42 days. Eventually, as Dr. Moyer wrote in *Forty Days Without Food*:

> The case continued until I became alarmed, and I strenuously urged Dr. Tanner to allay his gastric irritation by taking milk, which he finally consented to do. The next forenoon—that of the forty-second day of fasting—he ate a cracker and drank some lemonade, but this his stomach rejected.

After a trip to the city, Dr. Tanner returned and told Moyer, "Well, Doctor, I think I have finished affairs for good. I not only have taken a pint of milk, but have eaten five pears and half a good-sized watermelon." In her book, Linda Hazzard praised Dr. Tanner, but also castigated him for fasting without taking frequent enemas, a point on which they continued to disagree.

When members of the medical community learned about Tanner's fast, they did not believe him. As Hazzard later wrote, "Medical men especially, almost to a man, when questioned upon the subject, stated that such a fast was a physical impossibility, and medical journals published such statements as scientific facts." Nevertheless, Tanner began using fasting as the basis for his medical practice, decrying the use of drugs to treat patients. To quell persistent critics, Tanner repeated his fast in 1880, but with significant advance publicity. He later wrote to Dr. Hazzard:

> My second fast, publicly given, was called the "Great American Sensation," and its novel incidents were wired to the ends of the telegraphic world . . . My object was not money, but to relieve myself of the odium unjustly heaped upon me by the medical enemies of all righteousness . . . Every prediction of failure was nullified, and I came off conqueror and more than conqueror, in spite of the medical Goliaths arrayed against truth.

Dr. Edward Hooker Dewey (1839–1904) was the other major promoter of fasting for health. A native of Wayland, Pennsylvania, he began his medical career in a pharmacy. That experience led him to believe that "as an adaptation of means to an end, the administration of drugs for the cure of disease is one of the most unscientific of human vocations." Nevertheless, Dewey graduated from the University of Michigan College of Medicine and Surgery in 1864, just in time to become an assistant surgeon in the Union Army. After the war, he practiced traditional medicine in Meadville, Pennsylvania, a city of 10,000 people. He discovered the benefits of fasting accidentally while treating a patient. As he said in his book, *True Science of Living*:

> On a hot day in July, 1877, I entered a home to assume charge of a case of typhoid fever that was to arouse every possible faculty as by an electric charge . . . I was a very surprised physician, for, even without food, I found the tongue clean and a manifest gain in both mental and physical strength that became even marked at the time, when, to my continued surprise, food might be borne. I, however, determined to let nature continue to have her way, and from the end of the third week I watched, without trying enforced feeding, until the thirty-fourth day, when my patient, with natural hunger in evidence, began to eat and to rebuild with ultimate return to normal vigor.

Dewey went on to write his popular book, *The No-Breakfast Plan,* in 1900, and later he wrote *The Gospel of Health*. He coined the term "physiatrics" for his discipline—a term that now means physiotherapy. (Unfortunately, it also sounds almost exactly like the name of the medical specialty physiatry, or rehabilitative medicine.) Dewey's colleagues called him eccentric and even crazy. The local medical society eventually asked for his resignation.

It was from Dewey that Linda first learned of the fasting technique, and she studied with him for "one term." Although he acted as Linda's mentor, Dr. Dewey strongly disagreed with the need for enemas during treatment. Linda noted that he paid little attention to what foods he ate: "As to diet in health, the doctor exhibited the common failing of the medical profession, which then as now seems to consider food merely as fuel for the body, with but little regard for its digestibility or its nutritive content."

Dr. Hazzard's Starvation Regimen

The usual dietary regimen Linda Hazzard prescribed restricted the patient to two meals a day for a week and then to one meal a day. The diet included no meat; Linda believed that meat eaters were "foolish, disgusting, and suicidal."

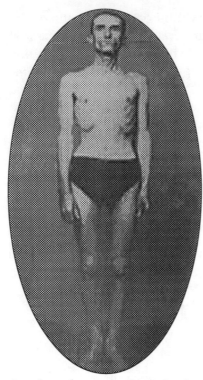

A patient who survived a 50-day fast administered by Dr. Linda Hazzard. (From *Fasting for the Cure of Disease*, 1908)

After a few more days, the only solid food allowed was a little fruit. Finally, patients were given only broth made from a few vegetables, particularly tomatoes and asparagus. Canned vegetables were often used, although patients were always told that the ingredients were fresh.

Hazzard frequently diagnosed her patients as having "digestive organs of infantile size," a ridiculous claim for healthy adults. Her treatment was to "rest" the bowels and expunge the impurities, and included frequent and prolonged enemas of "no less than three quarts."

There is an old German saying: "The illness that cannot be cured by fasting, cannot be cured by anything else." This is no doubt true if one counts death as a cure. In an otherwise healthy person who takes adequate liquids, total starvation is fatal in 8 to 12 weeks (40 to 60 days). Adults who fast for 30 to 40 days lose 25 percent of their initial weight and have an increased metabolic rate. More prolonged starvation causes weight loss of up to 50 percent in adults, and possibly more in children.

During fasting, the body tries to conserve energy and takes calories from stored fat. Eventually, the body must cannibalize its own tissues so that the person can survive, a process that Hazzard denied as "absurd." Among the organs, the liver and intestine lose the most weight, the heart and kidneys a moderate amount, and the nervous system the least. The results of starvation are most evident where prominent fat deposits normally exist; muscle mass shrinks, bones protrude, and the skin becomes thin, dry, inelastic, pale, and cold. Hazzard, however, interpreted the weight loss as being due to "removal of waste" accumulated through improper digestion; the "healthy tissue" that remained was "then ready for the process of rebuilding upon normal lines."

Starving people have a slowed pulse and decreased blood pressure because of their smaller heart and the reduced amount of blood being pumped.

Their temperature falls, and they have compromised immunity and wound healing and increased weakness—in part, because the muscles break down. Men and women lose their libido, men's testicles shrink, and women become amenorrheic. While the mind remains clear until near death, the person becomes very irritable.

Hazzard wrote in *Fasting for the Cure of Disease* that "in a scientifically conducted fast, death from starvation cannot take place when organic disease is absent . . . the life of the patient is extended through abstinence from food, since organic effort is thereby greatly reduced." She did warn that "it requires great skill to fast an individual properly, but any tyro can starve a man to death." In a statement ripe for Freudian analysis, she elaborated on the "law of hunger":

> Hunger is at all times to be distinguished from appetite. Hunger is discriminative and preserves the body. Appetite is abnormal desire and ultimately destroys. Hunger is primarily indicated in the mouth, and, if not relieved, it becomes an organic craving that can be satisfied only by digestible food; but appetite cannot be so silenced; it continually searches for this or for that; it is never satisfied.

Hazzard's justification for her patients' deaths was to say it was "inevitable."

In her books, Hazzard enclosed brochures with extravagant claims, such as her ability to cure "blindness, chronic constipation, diabetes, Bright's disease [kidney disease], and syphilis to paralysis." Sam Hazzard, much better educated than Linda, polished her writing.

Apparently, Linda Hazzard's strong personality helped convince patients to continue their fasts. A claim was made that she used hypnosis, although the line between a "magnetic personality" and hypnosis may, at times, be thin. Dorothea Williamson, Hazzard's former patient and chief nemesis, experienced the starvation doctor's powers of persuasion:

> During the time we were fasting I wanted food oh so much, but she kept on saying just wait a little bit. Finally I got into such a condition I did not care for food and really believed against my will that I did not need any.

The Victims

Whether due to Linda Hazzard's forceful personality, the fame she received from her books, or Kitsap County's lack of money to prosecute her effectively, authorities turned a blind eye to the deaths from starvation that occurred with regularity among her patients. Moreover, as many of her patients had traveled long distances for treatment, their deaths were often unnoticed—and unreported. However, the number of known deaths are more than sufficient to label Linda Hazzard a serial killer.

The first known fatality in Washington State was Daisy Maud Haglund. She died of starvation on February 8, 1908, 50 days into a fast supervised by "Dr." Hazzard. On September 26, 1908, Ida Wilcox followed her to the grave after fasting 47 days. Both were supposedly autopsied by Linda Hazzard, who listed bizarre causes of death in their records.

On March 24, 1909, after Viola Heaton died in a similar fashion, traditional physicians trained in anatomy and pathology performed the autopsy and determined that she had died of starvation. "Dr." Hazzard's actions were finally a matter of public record. Physicians who autopsied Blanche B. Tindall after her death on June 18, 1909, following a 28-day fast prescribed by Hazzard, found that she, too, had died from starvation.

Somewhere along the line, Linda and Sam apparently began to use her "cure" to murder patients for money. In 1909, Eugene Stanley Wakelin, the 26-year-old son of aristocrats, arrived from New Zealand to take "Dr. Hazzard's fast cure." The Hazzards welcomed him warmly, presuming that he had a large fortune. While there, Wakelin died under mysterious circumstances; his body was found near the Hazzard property in a badly decomposed state. Whether he died from starvation or from gunshot wounds, as is listed on the death certificate, is unknown. What is clear is that Linda Hazzard had appointed herself the administrator of Wakelin's (relatively small, as it turned out) estate. Upset that so little money was in Wakelin's account, she wired New Zealand after his death claiming that Wakelin's debts to her had not been paid.

Earl Edward Erdman died next. Otherwise healthy, the 24-year-old civil engineer suffered from frequent bouts of indigestion. After three weeks of starvation therapy, daily enemas, and osteopathic treatments under Hazzard's supervision, Erdman was rushed to Seattle's City Hospital. The once-robust young man was so emaciated that his ribs could be counted while he lay covered with a sheet; he died soon after his arrival. At autopsy, the cause of death was found to be "starvation." Despite this finding, the coroner reaffirmed that Washington State had no law under which they could prosecute Linda Hazzard. On March 29, 1910, a headline in the *Seattle Daily Times* read: "Woman 'M.D.' Kills Another Patient."

In an ironic twist, the next day's headline read: "Dr. Hazzard Gets License." Along with 28 chiropractors, other osteopaths, and individuals who practiced hot-air therapy, mechanotherapy, and electrotherapy, the Washington State Supreme Court ordered the state board of medical examiners to grant Linda Hazzard a medical license, based on her claim that she had practiced as a "doctor" for more than two years (as the law required) before the state's medical practice act went into effect.

The newly licensed doctor then killed some more patients. Maude Whitney died on July 20, 1910. Once again, Hazzard performed the autopsy herself and diagnosed "chonic pancreatis" [sic]. Frank Southard, a somewhat overweight and well-regarded principle in a large law firm, died on March 29, 1911. He quickly lost 77 of his 230 pounds under Dr. Hazzard's supervision and then went into kidney failure. Unfortunately, he also went to Dr. Hazzard for treatment of that condition and died soon thereafter. About the same time, C. A. Harrison, the publisher of *Alaska-Yukon Magazine*, became another victim.

John "Ivan" Flux, another of Hazzard's victims, had come to America from Gloucester, England, with the goal of buying a ranch. According to his father, Flux had several hundred dollars when he left home. The Hazzards, however, claimed that he had only $70 when he died on February 10, 1911, after a 53-day fast. Again, Linda Hazzard performed the autopsy; she stated that the unfortunate lad had died of pneumonia.

Although Linda claimed that she had supervised Flux's treatments, in reality, he had been left alone for more than two weeks before he died. After questions were raised about his death, a letter mysteriously appeared from a "J. F. Gallagher" who claimed to be another patient. He wrote that he had witnessed Flux's last hours and that his symptoms were consistent with pneumonia. "Gallagher" was never found. On August 21, a *Tacoma Daily News* headline asked: "Did Dr. Hazzard Invent Gallagher?"

The known death toll was rising rapidly, and rumors abounded that many more needless deaths were occurring among Dr. Hazzard's patients. The authorities, therefore, tried to intervene when they heard of another pending death in May 1911.

Lewis E. Rader, a publisher and state legislator, was dying from Dr. Hazzard's starvation therapy. Health inspectors tried to move him to a site where his health could be restored, but he refused to go. Before anything else could be done, Linda moved him to an undisclosed location. Rader died on May 11, 1911, leaving behind a wife and four sons. This once-robust man, who stood 5'11", weighed less than 100 pounds at death. Dr. Hazzard's autopsy report listed a number of vague causes of death, including "prolapsis" of the stomach.

The body was cremated at the funeral home she always used when her patients died.

There may have been collusion involved in Rader's death. He had a troubled relationship with his wife and, in an article written after his death, the *Seattle Daily Times* noted a curious coincidence: the Raders had transferred the title to "Wilderness Heights" to the Hazzards. The story ended suggestively, stating, "Rader's widow now lives near Dr. Hazzard's place and is on friendly terms with the starvationist."

Once again, the coroner exclaimed, "I am helpless in this matter." But, in the 1912 edition of *Fasting for the Cure of Disease*, Hazzard noted that of 2,500 patients, 18 had died while under her care—a death rate of just "seven-tenths of one percent." Dr. Hazzard performed autopsies on these patients and reported that the findings proved that the presence of organic disease made those deaths "inevitable."

Dorothea and Claire Williamson

Officials in Seattle had had enough. They were finally ready to stop what they saw as Dr. Hazzard's killing spree, and the case of the Williamson sisters seemed to offer the opportunity. It helped that the women were wealthy British citizens. After the story broke, state and county officials were pressured to act by Lucian Agassiz, the British vice consul in Tacoma, Washington.

Dorothea (Dora) and Claire Williamson, both in their early thirties, were the orphaned daughters of a well-to-do British Army medical service officer. Dorothea was born in Trichinopoli, India, and Claire in London. They had been educated in Switzerland, England, and France. Their father was injured in India and died at age 39, two months after Claire's birth. Their mother died when Claire was 14, and Dora, who was just four years older, acted as guardian for her sister. Both sisters were described as having perfect porcelain skin, blue-green eyes, delicate hands, and a manner befitting the upper class. They disdained corsets, a convention Linda Hazzard also decried. The two were extremely close, and neither had yet found a man for whom she would leave her sister.

With a fortune of over $1 million inherited from their grandfather (more than $18 million in 2002) and real estate holdings in Canada, the United States, England, and Australia, the sisters traveled around the world in comfort, with 14 trunks of elegant belongings. Their travels in 1910 and early 1911 had taken them from Liverpool in England to Quebec, and then to Toronto.

From there, they crossed Canada, visiting distant relatives at each stop, until they arrived at Vancouver Island, where they stayed at the elegant Empress Hotel. Claire planned to return to London in May 1911 to begin training as a kindergarten teacher. Dora intended to travel to Australia to visit more relatives before she returned to London.

Despite their obvious good health, the sisters were convinced that they were chronically ill. They visited clinics wherever they traveled in search of the latest "magic cures." A London osteopath had told Claire that her uterus had dropped back onto her spine and that her ovaries were inflamed. Dora suffered from "acute rheumatic pains in her knees." They both had considered visiting Dr. Kellogg's (of corn flakes fame) well-known sanitarium in Michigan, but decided that it would be too arduous a journey.

On September 2, 1910, Claire spotted an advertisement in a Seattle newspaper for *Fasting for the Cure of Disease* written by Dr. Linda Burfield Hazzard, and she sent for it. At a cost of $1.25 (and, eventually, her life), it was the worst investment she ever made. Five days later, the book and a brochure for Dr. Hazzard's sanitarium arrived.

After reading the book, the sisters wrote to Dr. Hazzard telling her that they had decided to travel to Seattle to take her cure. Linda wrote back that the sanitarium was not yet completed. She sent a regimen for them to follow, including instructions for a local woman osteopath to do "internal massage" on Claire's uterus and then pack her vagina with boric acid- and glycerin-soaked cotton batting. They were also to begin daily enemas. The correspondence continued and Dr. Hazzard suggested more therapeutic changes: The sisters were to continue the enemas and to begin eating only vegetable broth and cornbread. Although they were lifelong vegetarians, the sisters found the regimen difficult to tolerate. (They were charged $5 for this advice.)

In January 1911, Dr. Hazzard wrote that she could treat the sisters in Seattle and transfer them to the sanitarium in Olalla once the building was ready. The cost to each sister would be $60 per month for daily office visits. If "additional consultations" were required, there were more fees. Hazzard could arrange for them to rent a furnished apartment near her office in the Northern Bank and Trust Building.

Since their relatives scoffed at their pseudo-medical treatments, Dora and Claire said simply that they were going to Canada "on business." They arrived at Hazzard's office on February 27, 1911, where they immediately began the starvation diet without a physical examination or answering any questions about their medical history. Given that the women had already decreased their

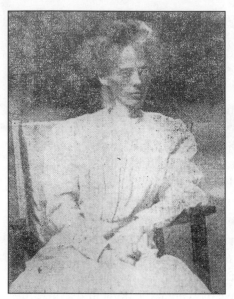

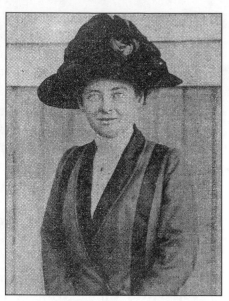

Dora Williamson when rescued from Olalla; she weighed 50 pounds. (Courtesy of Tacoma Public Library)

Dora Williamson recovered; during the 1912 murder trial. (Courtesy of Tacoma Public Library)

diet, the doctor immediately started them on twice-daily vegetable broth meals and several vigorous walks a day. They also were given "internal baths"—enemas of up to six quarts of warm water at a time given over a two- to three-hour period—to "eliminate the poisons."

Although they had never fainted before, it became commonplace within the first week of their new dietary regimen. Dora became semiconscious, while Claire seemed to perpetually sleep. A neighbor in their apartment complex later testified that the few times she saw them, their bodies had wasted away to skin and bones, and that she often heard the two women moaning loudly at night in obvious agony. A homeopathic-trained nurse, Nellie Sherman, was hired to help with the sisters' treatments. Even with Ms. Sherman's help, Claire became so weak that she could not walk out to her apartment's sun deck.

Forty years old when the Williamson sisters first encountered her, Nellie Sherman had become a rigid Dr. Hazzard devotee, and even perjured herself during the subsequent trial. Yet, at one point, Nellie did consult another physician when the sisters seemed near death. Dr. Augusta Brewer was known as a reputable osteopathic physician who thought little of Dr. Hazzard or her methods. He advised Nellie to immediately give the sisters more food if they were to survive. She didn't.

On April 21, 1911, the Williamson sisters, wrapped in dark blue wool blankets, were carried to two ambulances and then on board the sternwheeler *Virginia*, which took them to Olalla. In the ambulance, the Hazzards' lawyer put a letter in front of the almost incoherent Claire for her to sign. It turned out to be a codicil to her will giving her jewels and money to Dr. Hazzard. Those who saw the women were aghast at their emaciated appearance, although Linda arranged to have them off-loaded at an isolated landing.

The women were lodged in the Hazzards' unfinished attic, since the "sanitarium" was still many years away from being built. Linda insisted that the women remain apart and walled off areas of the attic for each one. Once the sisters were completely debilitated, Dr. Hazzard began pressing them for information about their estate and their relatives. As they were too weak to write on their own, she arranged for a secretary from her attorney's office to write letters and legal documents for them, including periodic transfers of money. She also coaxed them into allowing her to store their jewelry, land deeds, and other valuables in her office safe.

Claire died on May 18. When her uncle and her lifelong nanny and friend, Miss Conway, viewed her body at the funeral home, neither could identify it as that of Claire. The body was hastily cremated and no one could verify the rumors that Hazzard, or the funeral home on her behalf, had switched bodies at the viewing to prevent Claire's terrible condition from being publicized. After Claire's death, Dora was placed in a tiny cabin that had a window without glass and a rickety plank door; witnesses later described it as a henhouse.

A lawyer hired by Miss Conway finally wrested Dora from Wilderness Heights 93 days after she had arrived. She had lost at least half her body weight and had almost lost her sanity as well. The Hazzards presented Dora with a bill for the sum of $2,000 (about $36,000 in 2002), of which she supposedly still owed $700. The bill—almost a ransom—was paid on the condition that Linda would return the valuables she had taken from Dora and Claire.

Months after her recovery, Dora was shown a forged bank draft transferring $583 to Sam Hazzard. She was shocked when she learned that Linda had had herself appointed as Dora's legal guardian for both her medical and personal affairs. It was then less of a surprise when she found that a check to Linda Hazzard for $1,005 had been drawn on Claire's account. The Hazzards had also taken $110 of Dora's pension and $540 from her savings account. Eventually, the court overturned both the guardianship and the exorbitant charges, and made the Hazzards return all but $597 to Dora.

The Trial

On August 4, 1911, a Seattle paper printed an article claiming that Linda Hazzard "is planning to flee. She's going to New York and Hong Kong . . . she's going to teach her methods to the royal family!" With the public announcement that she was a flight risk, Kitsap County's attorney finally agreed to prosecute Dr. Hazzard for Claire's murder, but only if Dora Williamson would pay the costs for the witnesses. She agreed, and a warrant was issued for Linda Hazzard's arrest. (The British vice consul had asked the British government to pay some of the costs for prosecuting the bogus physician who had killed three British subjects—Claire, Flux, and Wakelin—but they declined.)

On the afternoon of August 5, 1911, Deputy Sheriff George Posse arrived at Wilderness Heights with the warrant to arrest Linda Hazzard for first-degree murder. Since Kitsap County was too poor to maintain its own jail, Linda was taken to spend a few days at "Deputy" Mrs. W. O. Breed's home until she either posted bail or was sent elsewhere for incarceration. She had no intention of going to jail, so her supporters scrambled to find $10,000 for her bond. Finally, Pacific Coast Casualty Company paid the money, and she was freed.

On August 7, 1911, the banner headline in the *Tacoma Daily News* read: "Officials Expect to Expose Starvation Atrocities. Dr. Hazzard Pictured as Fiend." Seattle's *Patriarch* ran a story under the headline "Here is Another 'Superwoman'":

> What's in a name?—"Hazzard."
>
> Linda Burfield Hazzard "tortures her victims to death." Let us see; is this not the same "Hazzardous" outfit that got away with "L.E. Rader" by the "starving process" some few months since? . . .
>
> To think that "systematic murder" can be conducted right under our very nose by a notorious cold-blooded woman with a "doctor's diploma," is not only a blast upon our morality but it is a challenge of our sanity. This "Hazzardous" murderous systematic "Lucretia Borgia" is fortunate that she is not in the country from whence "her victims came," or she would in less than four weeks be lying side by side with the late "Dr. Crippen" instead of being subjected to a bond of a paltry $10,000 . . .
>
> We have got this wicked "Superwoman" with a "doctor's diploma" in our grasp. Shall we do her justice? Or shall we do ourselves an injustice and make a "heroine" of her? The "prohibitionists" should place her upon a pinnacle of fame for she is a rigid abstainer. [For information on the deadly Dr. Crippen, see Chapter 7, *The Minor Players*.]

Relatives of her victims thought that it was about time Dr. Hazzard was prosecuted for her greed and quackery, foremost among them Dora Williamson. She filed a $25,000 civil suit against Hazzard and her too-friendly funeral home for her anguish over Claire's unauthorized autopsy and the removal of her organs at the funeral home. Among the evidence never presented in court was that Hazzard had sold Claire Williamson's teeth for a few dollars after she died. Although the civil suit was dismissed, the judge did force Hazzard to return her "outrageous and unreasonable" fees.

Linda pleaded "not guilty" to the murder charge and began a series of legal maneuvers to delay the trial. Although the publicity actually helped generate more patients for her practice, the Hazzards rapidly drained their financial resources. Standing outside the Kitsap County courthouse, Linda announced that her "sanitarium" would be closed until she was exonerated, which she expected to happen soon.

The murder trial began on January 15, 1912. During the trial, Hazzard eschewed the starched white uniform she normally wore for a brown velvet gown and a hat decorated with ostrich feathers. She was distressed when only men were selected for her jury. (Rather than the conspiracy she claimed it to be, the jury was selected from voter rolls. Since women in Washington had just received state voting rights in 1910, no women had voted in the prior election.)

More than 100 witnesses testified during the trial, including 11 doctors for the prosecution and 4 for the defense. Typical of the prosecution physicians, local practitioner Dr. T. J. Baldwin said that Hazzard's starvation treatment demonstrated a "gross ignorance of the healing art . . . a gross disregard on [her] part of ordinary and usual care and knowledge of the human body." The past president of the Medical Licensing Board, called by the defense, testified that they had had no choice but to grant a license to Linda Hazzard.

Linda Hazzard saw the trial as a battle between traditional medicine and the proponents of natural cures. Her lawyers argued that Hazzard was a healer and that the problem actually lay with her patients—especially the Williamson sisters. The lawyers, however, had little to say when handwriting experts showed that Claire's diary entry bequeathing her diamonds to Dr. Hazzard and her staff had been written by the doctor herself.

Unfortunately, the trial did not attempt to answer many of the questions the grisly situation raised. The regional United Press Leased Wire Service sent out just such a list:

- Did Mrs. Hazzard hold autopsies over, dissect and cremate all the patients who died at her establishment?
- If she did, what became of the corpses?
- Did she cremate the remains to cover up the cases?

- What was in the coffins buried, supposedly containing bodies of her patients?

Linda Burfield Hazzard was found guilty only of manslaughter. As the *Town Crier* proclaimed:

> It is interesting to note that not one of the jurors who tried Mrs. Hazzard believed her innocent. The sole question was on the degree of guilt, and there is no doubt that her sex alone saved her from the verdict of murder.

On February 7, 1912, the judge sentenced Dr. Linda Burfield Hazzard to serve from 2 to 20 years of hard labor at the penitentiary in Walla Walla, Washington.

While released again on bond during her appeal, Hazzard gave numerous speeches advancing her cause. Although she supposedly had suspended her practice during this period, she supervised a protégé who starved one infant to death and then tried to repeat the process on a second infant and her mother. The mother, who was known to have received "osteopathic treatments" from Hazzard, died of starvation, but the infant was rescued. Simultaneously, another emaciated person was found dead at Wilderness Heights.

The Washington State Board of Medical Examiners waited until July 1, 1912, to revoke Linda Hazzard's medical license. The revocation seemed to have little effect: Mary Bailey died in mid-March 1913, while undergoing treatment at Wilderness Heights. A coroner's inquest found that she had died of starvation, but, since authorities knew Hazzard would shortly be incarcerated, they didn't pursue the case. Fred Ebbeson also died during this period after a 49-day fast administered by a Hazzard disciple. (He had been unable to afford treatment from the "doctor" herself.)

Just before Thanksgiving in 1913, the Washington Supreme Court rejected Hazzard's appeal. But, rather than wait to be escorted to the prison, Linda Hazzard simply arrived with a suitcase after Christmas. This was a first, and no one knew what to do. They did, however, check that the new inmate's photograph matched that of Dr. Hazzard to ensure that her fanatical followers had not arranged to have someone take her place. In a letter written to help the warden understand his unusual wife, Sam Hazzard wrote:

> [Linda] has not been conducive to patience in her disposition. She may say things that will tend to make your matron think that she would like to overturn all penological rules, but these remarks should be taken as that outcome of her reform spirit, and not as criticism upon the present management or surroundings.

The Deadly Aftermath

The Washington State Parole Board released Linda Hazzard after she had spent only two years in prison. However, they denied her request to move to California. Six months later, Governor Ernest Lister granted her a pardon on the condition that she fulfill a prior promise and leave the United States. She agreed, although she was upset that the pardon did not restore her medical license. She and Sam sailed to New Zealand, where she set up a lucrative practice under the various titles of "physician," "dietitian," and "osteopath."

In *Scientific Fasting: The Ancient and Modern Key to Health*, Hazzard wrote of her trial, incarceration, and release. As usual, she glossed over or altered many of the details:

> Called to the Pacific Coast in 1906, I decided there to remain, and in the summer of that year I opened offices in Seattle. Soon after this I began to encounter organized persecution from medical sources, aided by newspapers controlled by the profession. Such deaths as occurred under my care received the widest publicity, and the accounts written concerning them were distorted and filled with implication, innuendo, and threat. These articles eventually accomplished the end sought by their authors, for in 1912 I was brought to trial charged with having willfully caused the death of an English woman patient through starvation.
>
> A jury divided amongst itself, but urged to decision by a prejudiced judge and by public sentiment inflamed by a public press, determined that my crime was that of manslaughter, and I was thereupon sentenced to a minimum term of two years in the penitentiary. I served these years day by day in anguish of body and of mind, until finally the then Governor of Washington became convinced of my innocence and of the monstrous injustice that had been done, and he granted to me an unconditional pardon, restoring all of the rights and privileges which by reason of my conviction I had forfeited.

By 1920, she had returned to Olalla with enough money to begin building her grand sanitarium. When finally erected, the building was impressive. The white, wood-framed structure had dormer windows extending over a porch that ran the full length of the building. A grand foyer dominated the interior and a dark oak staircase led up to two floors. There was also a basement where Hazzard performed autopsies on her patients; they continued to die under her ministrations. How many is uncertain, since they were often buried without formalities or records.

Linda called her sanitarium the "Wilderness Heights Institute of Natural Therapeutics," and referred to it as a "school of health." Others called it "Hazzard's Lodge" and, eventually, it became known as "Starvation Heights." She continued to refer to herself as "Dr. Hazzard," despite her lack of a medical license, and soon regained her local prestige. When she tried to supervise a case in California in April 1922, however, authorities arrested her for violating that state's Medical Practice Act. In 1923, she was arrested on the same charge in Washington (finally!) when Leonard Ritter died after an 84-day fast. Although a jury found her guilty, she received only a $100 fine and no jail time.

In May 1935, the sanitarium burned down. Linda thought it was due to a conspiracy, but the fire actually started in Sam's room. Whether the fire was intentional was unclear, but Sam tried to interfere with efforts to save the sanitarium equipment, noting that "everything is insured."

Epilogue

Linda Burfield Hazzard died in 1938. Sam Hazzard continued to reside at "Starvation Heights" in an alcoholic stupor until his death eight years later. Linda's estranged daughter returned only to sell the property.

In the end, the prosecutor at Hazzard's trial was wrong when he said, "This case will, I believe, be a death blow to quack medical and healing individuals and institutions throughout the country." It wasn't. Natural healing bookstores, among others, still sell Linda Hazzard's books, and fasting remains a part of naturopathic curricula.

As always, *caveat emptor*—because Linda Burfield Hazzard was, for the deadliest part of her career, a licensed physician.

Unorthodox Medical Practices

Orthodox medicine took millennia to finally reach the point where a sick person stood a better than 50-50 chance of recovery after seeing a physician. For a long time, people who saw the negative results of medical treatments knew that, whenever possible, it was best to avoid a physician's care.

During the 1800s, traditional medicine advanced slowly. Many of the medications dispensed and the therapies prescribed caused much more harm than good. Physicians could provide patients only with narcotics to ease pain, a few disease-specific remedies such as digitalis and quinine, immunizations, and general anesthesia. One of America's leading physicians, Oliver Wendell Holmes, Sr. admitted, "If the whole *materia medica* [list of available drugs] as now used could be sunk to the bottom of the sea, it would be all the better for mankind—and all the worse for the fishes."

It was against this backdrop that many people turned to other medical systems. The number of alternative practitioners increased; by the late 1800s, they comprised about 15 percent of U.S. physicians.

Thomsonians

Samuel Thomson (1769–1843) was the leader of the *Thomsonians*, the first American movement that presented an alternative to traditional physicians. A combination zealot and con man with no formal education, he railed against the special privileges (licenses) of the medical establishment. He denounced bloodletting and calomel (mercurous chloride) in favor of his own patented system of botanical medicines.

His medicines induced sweating and vomiting to cure disease. He sold the right to use them to families for $20. Thomson organized these families into "friendly societies" to lobby state legislatures to repeal or emasculate their existing medical licensing laws. This proved to be successful: By the 1840s, almost all state laws that had once limited the practice of medicine to trained practitioners were revoked. Many states would not have strong enough laws to prevent unnecessary deaths from quack practitioners until the early twentieth century. In most cases, though, traditional physicians have been the ones who developed pseudo-medical systems.

Homeopathy

After graduating from a prestigious German medical school, Samuel Hahnemann (1755–1843) began experimenting on himself with various medicinal compounds. When he tried cinchona bark, the raw form of quinine that was used to treat malaria, he seemed to get malarial symptoms; experiments with other medications produced similar results. He developed these findings into *homeopathy*. Its practitioners still believe that minute amounts of a substance

continued . . .

Unorthodox Medical Practices, continued

that produces symptoms of a disease in a healthy person can alleviate those symptoms in a patient. Hahnemann called his concept "the law of similars," or likes are to be cured by likes (*similia similibus curantur*). While homeopaths are still licensed in some states, today it is naturopaths who most often use this approach, as well as many of the remedies discussed below.

Homeopaths left two lasting impressions on the English language. First, they began to use "allopath" as a derogatory term for any doctor who used medications that would cause the opposite symptoms from those of the disease in healthy people. When most of these practitioners disappeared with the advent of modern scientific medicine, "allopath" came to denote M.D. physicians. Second, the term "homeopathic dose" now means such a minuscule amount of a medication that it will have no effect.

A clear benefit of homeopathy was its rejection of bloodletting, an often-lethal practice that was common in the United States up until the Civil War. Prior to the Civil War, most homeopaths were physicians who had trained in regular medical schools. After the war, homeopaths were evicted from the standard medical associations, so they formed their own medical schools, hospitals, and societies. Except for the medications they used, most homeopathic colleges and hospitals had training almost identical to that of traditional medical schools.

Eclectics
The rise of homeopathy split the Thomsonians; the more educated went on to join yet another branch of medicine, the *eclectics*, begun by Wooster Beach (1794–1868). Their substandard medical schools imitated traditional medical education, except that they promoted the use of drugs of mineral origin and substituted resinous drugs for the more common alkaloids.

Popular Health Movement
Declining to use any medications at all, Sylvester Graham (1794–1851) began the *popular health movement*. He advocated many of the lifestyle changes that physicians now encourage—regular bathing (a rarity at the time), fresh air, exercise, proper diet—and railed against gluttony, sexual permissiveness, tight clothing, and medications.

The diet he proposed was strictly vegetarian, and it eliminated coffee, tea, and pastries in favor of his still-popular Graham cracker. Graham's "drugless practitioners" felt that by following these precepts, physicians would become irrelevant. Critics claimed his "sublimated Puritanism" took the joy out of both the kitchen and the bedroom.

continued . . .

Unorthodox Medical Practices, continued

Hydropathy

Made popular by Austrian peasant Victor Priessnitz, *hydropathy* was purported to cure chronic diseases, such as arthritis and gout, with water, either by drinking it or bathing in it. Initially making a "splash" in Europe, the system was imported into the United States in the 1840s, and two medical schools based on this theory were established. By the mid-1850s, hydropathy was practiced in at least 27 medicinal spas in the East and Midwest. Healing spas still exist, but are most popular in Europe.

Magnetic Healing

Also known as "animal magnetism" and "mesmerism," *magnetic healing* was the product of Dr. Franz Mesmer (1734–1815), an Austrian physician who believed that a magnetic fluid flowed through the body. Imbalances in the flow, in a concept akin to the Chinese *yin-yang*, caused diseases, particularly those of the nervous system. (Magnetism does exist in the body, and is the basis for magnetic resonance imaging (MRI).) Mesmer began treating patients in Germany, and then in France, with what would now be called hypnotism, and developed almost a stage show in which patients would faint when he waved his hands.

One of his French disciples, Charles Poyen (d. 1844), brought the technique to the United States in 1837. He trained hundreds of "magnetizers," wrote a book, and began a journal, *The Psychodinamist*. Poyen's activities stirred massive resistance among the clergy, the scientific community, and traditional physicians, and forced his return to France. Nevertheless, magnetic healing continued to be popular in the United States throughout the 1800s, and it is still a favorite folk remedy. Hypnotism is also used by a variety of practitioners, including traditional physicians.

Osteopathy

All the methods mentioned above influenced Andrew Taylor Still, the founder of *osteopathy*, one of the practices that Linda Burfield Hazzard claimed to use. Born August 6, 1828, in Jonesville, Virginia, Still was the third of nine children. His father had been a Methodist preacher, but, when Andrew was born, he was supporting his family by farming and practicing medicine. He returned to the ministry nine years later. Andrew received a diverse education as he traveled with his missionary family. In 1853, married and with two children, he gave up farming and apprenticed himself to his father in medicine—a common method of medical education, especially in the American West.

When the Civil War erupted, Andrew enlisted in the 9th Kansas (U.S.) Calvary as a hospital steward. In April 1862, he returned home, organized his own unit,

continued . . .

Unorthodox Medical Practices, continued

and was commissioned a captain. He was later promoted to major. Of his war experience, he later wrote,

> During the hottest period of the fight, a musketball passed through the lapels of my vest . . . another minie-ball passed through the back of my coat, just above the buttons, making an entry and an exit almost six inches apart. Had the rebels known how close they were to shooting osteopathy, perhaps they would not have been so careless.

Still returned home to resume his career as a traditional physician. Despite his military experience, his strong Methodist upbringing influenced him to abstain from alcohol. This in turn led him to question the role of medications, many of which were alcohol-based "tinctures" or laced with opiates or cocaine. A zealot, he began thinking of traditional physicians not only as the purveyors of these poisons, but also as their victims. In June 1874, he disassociated himself from traditional medicine.

His departure from medicine, in favor of "laying on of hands," had dire consequences. His neighbors, church, friends, and relatives turned against him, and he ended up in Kirksville, Missouri. There, with no local opposition, he opened a small practice as a "magnetic healer." Eventually, to support his family in Kirksville, he traveled the countryside as an itinerant healer.

In the late 1870s, Still added "bonesetting" to his armamentarium. The traditional English practice of bonesetting had existed in America since colonial times, the most famous practitioners being the Sweet family of New England. As did other bonesetters, Still used his abilities not only to set fractures and reduce dislocations, but also to manipulate joints, including the spine, in the belief that pain was due to a "bone out of place," a claim ridiculed by traditional physicians.

Still advertised that he was the "lightning bonesetter" through the 1880s. Around 1880, he began manipulating the spine and adjacent ribs to cure not only orthopedic problems, but also asthma, headache, heart disease, extremity paralysis, varicose veins, and a host of other diseases. Dressed in a rumpled suit and a slouch hat, and with his pants stuffed in his boots, he traveled with his sons around Missouri, plastering hundreds of flyers in each town and then giving a show. According to eyewitnesses, "with his intuitive insight, he would pick out a cripple, or someone with a severe headache or some disease that he could cure quickly, and demonstrate before the anxious crowds."

By 1889, his much-improved reputation allowed him to stay in Kirksville and run an extremely successful infirmary. He decided to call his brand of medicine

continued . . .

Unorthodox Medical Practices, continued

"osteopathy," based on the Latin word for "bone" combined with the stem of "pathology." In 1892, in conjunction with the European-trained Dr. William Smith (1862–1912), he opened the American School of Osteopathy at Kirksville.

Contemporary doctors of osteopathy, D.O.s, now embrace the same pharmaceutical and surgical therapies as do their M.D. counterparts. Both M.D. and D.O. medical schools have essentially the same requirements and curricula, but the latter also offer courses in osteopathic manipulation medicine, reflecting their initial link with spinal manipulation. About half of all osteopathic medical school graduates do their specialty training at M.D. institutions, and osteopaths practice at most hospitals in the United States.

Chiropractic

Chiropractic and *naturopathy* began about the same time as osteopathy. In September 1895, Daniel David Palmer (1845–1913), a Canadian-born magnetic healer, performed his first "adjustment." He claimed to have cured a patient's deafness by realigning her spine. Shortly afterward, Palmer relieved a patient's heart trouble by adjusting her vertebra. These experiences led him to believe that all diseases could be treated by relieving pressure on nerves as they exit the spinal canal. And so chiropractic was born. During the early period of chiropractic, Palmer was accused of stealing Still's methods, and he was successfully prosecuted for practicing medicine without a license.

Nevertheless, he and his son, Bartlett Joshua Palmer, persevered and started the first of many chiropractic colleges (graduates earn a D.C. degree). To further confuse matters, adherents with similar views, who called themselves "naprapaths" and "neuropaths," began practicing—they were even licensed in a few states. Through World War II, chiropractors were on many hospital staffs (especially in obstetrics) and practiced psychiatry as well as general medicine. Today, chiropractors have returned primarily to performing spinal treatments.

Naturopathy

Sent to the United States to introduce hydrotherapy, Benedict Lust, M.D., D.O., added the use of natural and folk therapies to create *naturopathy* in 1896. Dr. Lust started the first naturopathic medical school in the United States as a two-year post-graduate program. It quickly evolved into a four-year program, with educational standards typical of most of that era's medical colleges.

While many of the early unorthodox medical fields have disappeared, naturopathy, also known as "natureopathy," "naturopathic medicine," and "naturopathic health care," endures and has incorporated many of their methods.

continued . . .

Unorthodox Medical Practices, continued

Practices vary by region of the country, the local laws, and the practitioner, but can include mechanotherapy (also called Swedish movements), reflexology, lymph-drainage, massage, physiotherapy, electrotherapy, phototherapy, psychotherapy, suggestotherapy, heliotherapy (using the sun), spondylotherapy, botanic medicine, and folk medicine. Practitioners also employ clinical nutrition, detoxification, hydrotherapy, homeopathy, herbs, "Chinese medicine" (including acupuncture), natural childbirth, manipulation similar to that of chiropractic, and stress counseling.

In Washington State (Dr. Hazzard's home base), which has the most expansive licensing laws for naturopaths, these practitioners are permitted to dispense some medications. Oregon allows them to do minor surgery. There are three accredited naturopathic schools in the United States, but a substantial number of practitioners receive their N.D. degrees from mail-order schools.

Mechanotherapy
Mechanotherapists advocate treating all diseases by mechanical methods, such as massage, traction, passive motion, compression, and pressure. This is similar to modern physical therapists. The system is based on the work of Dr. Gustaf Zander's Mechanico-Therapeutic Institute in Stockholm in the late 1800s. Mechanotherapists can still be licensed in Ohio.

Unfortunately, quackery, be it folk medicine, voodoo, or the newest fad of injecting or ingesting unusual substances, still has a place in our lives. Whether it is the need to believe in miracles, or because of limitations—despite astonishing advances—in medicine, people continue to search for magic cures.

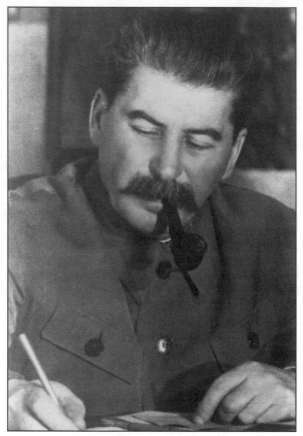

Joseph Stalin, circa 1935. (© ArchivePhotos/PictureQuest)

5
Big Lies

The Russian Doctors' Plots

In the 1930s and 1950s, there were notorious conspiracies involving two groups of prominent Russian physicians who were put on public trial for plotting to kill government officials by the "deliberate application of improper medical treatment." The Russian press called them the "Doctors' Plots." Confessions were heard in open court, medical experts agreed with the findings, and Soviet documents and news sources recorded the exploits of these "foul murderers and traitors hiding behind the masks of doctors" who were found guilty of treason against the Stalinist regime.

But did a cadre of influential physicians actually conspire to kill Soviet politicians through "bad medicine"—twice? Even today, the true story of these alleged doctor-conspirators is shrouded by innuendo, coerced confessions, and perjured testimony. Experts in Russian history are, in general, only vaguely aware of both trials. But, thanks in part to the opening of once-secret Soviet records, the story of two groups of doctors who suffered the destruction of their professional reputations, imprisonment, torture, and, in some cases, death because they supposedly plotted to kill high-ranking Soviet leaders can finally be told.

The "Doctors' Plots" were set against the background of fear and distrust that permeated Stalinist Russia. People disappeared at random—plucked off the street on their way to work, dragged from their homes in the middle of the night, or snatched out of classrooms as they taught. Rewards went to the co-worker who named names, the child who denounced her parents, and the student who dutifully copied any of the professor's statements that could be construed as anti-Soviet.

Millions of people vanished into the Gulag, a system of prison labor camps that stretched into the far reaches of Siberia. Some of these individuals had, for one reason or another, fallen out of favor with the prevailing political hierarchy. Others were seen as enemies in the paranoid delusions of an all-powerful leader—Joseph Stalin.

In reality, the "victims" of the physician conspiracies of the 1930s, one of whom was the famous writer Maxim Gorky, all died of natural causes. The "plots," their "discovery," and the public show trials that followed were actually staged events, all part of Stalin's plan to justify his great purges, which caused the deaths of 40 million Soviet citizens. By late 1938, 8 million people were in the Gulag; over the next 15 years, 12 million died in these prison camps.

And, in 1953, the aging and increasingly paranoid dictator was ready to initiate another wave of witch hunts and vicious purges. A second group of doctors—mostly Jewish—was accused of practicing bad medicine, once again igniting public fears and tapping into longstanding anti-Semitic feelings. Only Stalin's death prevented another catastrophic purge of talented doctors (and others) caught in the wrong place and the wrong time in history.

[NB: Because the Russian names have been translated from the Cyrillic alphabet, multiple spellings exist. The spellings used here are the most common, although not necessarily the most phonetically correct.]

~

Joseph Stalin — The Real "Serial Killer"

Russia has a long history of paranoid tyrannical rulers. Joseph Stalin was just the latest, but he exceeded his czarist predecessors in both his tyranny and the number of people killed due to his capricious dictates. Born Iosif Vissarionovich Dzhugashvili in Gori, in Russian Georgia, on December 6, 1878 (his birthdate is often incorrectly cited as 1879), he was either of Georgian or Ossetian descent. Stalin's legal father was an abusive drunken shoemaker, although rumors persist that Stalin may have been the product of an illicit liaison.

Stalin's upbringing resulted in what psychoanalyst Daniel Rancour-Laferriere called his overt

> paranoia, megalomania, sadism, power hunger, vindictiveness, and self-control . . . Stalin's mother adored him, his father hated him. Even as a positive, elevated self-image was being built in little Soso [his nickname] by his mother, that self-image was being undermined by an abusive father whose love he desperately craved . . . Consequently, in adulthood, Stalin had to live with two affective extremes: he worshiped himself and he hated himself. The first he externalized by promoting a narcissistic cult of personality. The second he dealt with by instituting a reign of terror, by turning the hatred outward.

At his mother's urging, young Iosif entered Tiflis Seminary, the region's equivalent of a university, where he studied for the priesthood. A friend from his seminary days later described Stalin as seeing "only the negative, the bad side ... [He] had no faith at all in men's idealistic motives and attributes."

Stalin quit his studies in May 1899 to work with anti-Czarist Georgian- nationalist revolutionaries, adopting the code name "Koba," the same as that of a fictitious Georgian freedom fighter. Although he had a bond with Georgia by birth, Stalin would be instrumental in ruthlessly sup-

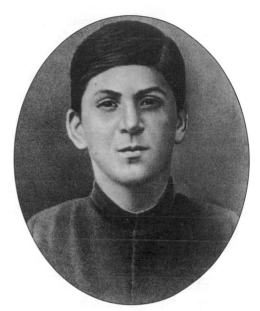

Young Stalin, 1893.

pressing Georgian autonomy after the Bolshevik Revolution and in incorporating the region into the Soviet Union. He later dropped his obviously Georgian name to better fit in with his Bolshevik Party comrades—and so it would be easier to remember.

Stalin's revolutionary activities eventually forced him into exile, where he met Vladimir Lenin. Neither thought much of the other—Stalin didn't seem to impress very many people during that period. A British diplomat who met Stalin at a meeting of the new Bolshevik government's Central Executive Committee in 1918 later said that Stalin "did not seem of sufficient importance" to be worthy of much notice. "If he had been announced then to the assembled Party as the successor to Lenin, the delegates would have roared with laughter."

Like Napoleon and Hitler, Stalin was short—only 5'4"—and tried hard to blend in with his country's main ethnic group, the Russians. He had thick black hair and a mustache that poet Osip Mandelstam described as "cockroach whiskers." Yugoslav diplomat Milovan Djilas described Stalin as "ungainly ... His torso was short and narrow, while his legs and arms were too long." Boris Pasternak, one of the few Jewish literary giants that Stalin did not exterminate, said of his first encounter with the dictator:

> A man looking like a crab advanced on me out of the semi-darkness. The whole of his face was yellow and it was pitted all over with pock-marks [from childhood smallpox]. His mustache bristled. He was

dwarfish—disproportionately broad and apparently no taller than a 12-year-old boy, but with an old-looking face.

A childhood accident left Stalin with an atrophied left hand and a weak left arm that would not bend at the elbow or rotate at the shoulder. As a result, he often wore a glove or, Napoleon-like, kept his hand tucked inside his jacket. He was also self-conscious about his crooked teeth so he rarely smiled. When young, he was known to be slovenly and unkempt; eventually, however, he adopted a uniform as his usual dress and became vain about his appearance.

Leon Trotsky, Stalin's comrade and, later, chief nemesis, described him as "an outstanding mediocrity." He also called Stalin the "Super-Borgia in the Kremlin," which referred to his supposed poisoning of political enemies, and "the gravedigger of the revolution." This comment was insightful, since Stalin greatly admired his ruthless and bloodthirsty predecessor, Czar Ivan the Terrible, and saw him as a role model. But Stalin thought that Ivan's mistake was not liquidating enough of his enemies; he would not make the same mistake. While Ivan's *Oprichnina* killed 4,000 boyars, Stalin executed over 7 million people between 1935 and 1940 alone. Indeed, Stalin executed more "revolutionaries" than had all the Czars combined. The "Doctors' Plots" of 1938 and 1953 were but two of the many schemes he hatched to justify his mass killings.

So, how did this slovenly, forgettable non-Russian come to reign over the Soviet Empire for nearly a quarter century? As historian Helen Rappaport wrote, it was:

> a combination of natural guile and intelligence, a flair for duplicity, and a disregard for human suffering that got Stalin to the top. In so doing he proved that a political leader did not necessarily have to be a great military man or a great theoretician to achieve power and stay there. He was happy to leave the intellectualizing to the likes of Lenin.

As historian James Abbe noted, "there is nothing of the fanatic about Stalin: he is just a deliberate, persistent, calculating person whose faculties coordinate." He also had a politician's tremendous recall ability; he never forgot a face. In Stalin's case, however, he immediately labeled individuals, remembering them for later punishment.

Stalin assumed the role of Gensek (General Secretary) of the Communist Party in April 1922 and held that position until 1952. He transformed that position into the pinnacle of power within the Communist Party and, thus, within the Soviet Union. In a 1923 letter sent to the Party hierarchy, Lenin expressed concern about what Stalin would do with this position:

> Comrade Stalin, having become General Secretary, has concentrated enormous power in his hands; and I am not sure that he always knows how to use that power with sufficient caution ... Stalin is too rude, and this fault, entirely supportable in relations among us communists, becomes insupportable in the office of General Secretary. Therefore, I propose to the comrades to find a way to remove Stalin from that position and appoint to it another man who in all respects differs from Stalin on one superiority—namely, that he be more tolerant, more loyal, more polite, and more considerate to comrades, less capricious, etc.

In his "Secret Speech" to the Twentieth Party Congress in 1956, Khrushchev later spoke about Stalin's excesses:

> Stalin acted not through persuasion, explanation, and patient cooperation with people, but by imposing his concepts and demanding absolute submission to his opinion. Whoever opposed this concept or tried to prove his viewpoint, and correctness of his position, was doomed to removal ... and to subsequent moral and physical annihilation ...

Yet, both in public and in private, Stalin exuded an aura of calm, rational self-control. In negotiations, he was skilled at gamesmanship, often permitting long periods of extended silence to both impress and intimidate others. When answering a question, his voice was low, guttural, and often unintelligible. This slow and methodical speech was intentional, and used partly to hide his Georgian accent.

Once he assumed power, Stalin systematically rewrote Bolshevik and Soviet history to emphasize his role, diminish his shortcomings, and lay the blame for errors on others. He had no qualms about manipulating historical facts and commented that "paper will put up with anything that is written on it." Indeed, schoolbooks with Stalin's version of Soviet history were used in the country's schools until the mid-1980s, when historians wrote more accurate versions. Photographs were also altered to erase the images of those who had fallen from his good graces. Leon Trotsky's image, for example, virtually disappeared from all photographs.

During his life, Stalin consciously developed a "cult of personality." He encouraged the masses to refer to him as *batyushka*, or "little father," a religious appellation previously applied to the czars. In a characteristically grandiloquent phrase, Party chief Sergey Kirov wrote in 1934 that Stalin was "the greatest man of all times, of all epochs, and peoples." Yet nowhere was this contrived adoration better seen than in various titles that the Soviet media bestowed upon him during his life: Generalissimo, Genius of Mankind, Grand

Strategist of the Revolution, Great Friend of the Children, Great Helmsman, Great Internationalist, Great Leader, Great Master of Daring Revolutionary Decisions and Abrupt Turns, Greatest Genius of All Times and Peoples, Honorary Pioneer, Leader of the World Proletariat, Leading Light of Science, Standard-Bearer of Communism, Supreme Military Leader, and Transformer of Nature.

To promote pervasive distrust and fear throughout the country, Stalin developed a web of secret police and informants, rewarding those who informed on others. Stalin's own increasing paranoia was evident to those around him. According to Nikita Khrushchev, a close colleague who later assumed Stalin's position:

> Stalin was a very distrustful man, sickly suspicious; we knew this from our work with him. He could look at a man and say: "Why are your eyes so shifty today," or "Why are you turning so much today and avoiding to look me directly in the eyes?" The sickly suspicion created in him a general distrust even toward eminent Party workers whom he had known for years. Everywhere and in everything he saw "enemies," "two-facers" and "spies."

Isaac Babel, a famous Yiddish writer who later died in prison, said of those times: "A man talks frankly only with his wife, at night, with the blanket over his head."

The Gulag and "The Great Terror" (1936–1938)

During Stalin's 25-year tenure as Soviet dictator, he periodically instituted purges, called *chistki* or "cleansing," including the two-year period in the 1930s that historian Robert Conquest termed "The Great Terror," implying a parallel with France's eighteenth-century Reign of Terror. Political parallels aside, only 17,000 people died in France—not even one day's death toll when Stalin was at his most ruthless. Historian Helen Rappaport estimates that, including executions, the deaths of those sent to the Gulag, and deaths from forced farm collectivization and famine, Stalin directly caused the deaths of around *40 million* Soviet citizens!

Stalin's murderous policies actually began with the 1929–1930 drive to collectivize peasant farms. This resulted in the 1932–1933 famine, which, compounded by Stalin's refusal to send assistance and to appeal for foreign aid, resulted in the deaths of 7 million people. In the early 1930s, 70 percent of the prisoners in the labor camps known as the Gulag were peasants displaced from their land in the mass-collectivization program. During the purges of 1936–1938, large numbers of the intelligentsia and professionals were added.

Stalin had greatly expanded the Gulag, a vast network of corrective labor camps, detention centers, and prisons set up in Siberia by the Czars and then added to by Lenin's *Cheka* (*Chrezvychainaya kommissiya*, Extraordinary Commission for Combating Counterrevolution and Espionage, 1917–1923), or secret police, in 1919. The Gulag, an acronym for *Glavnoe upravlenie ispravitelno-trudovykh lagerey* (Chief Administration of Corrective Labor Camps), eventually stretched from Moscow's environs for 6,000 miles to the Siberian Far East in Kolyma. Most of the 35 major camp clusters, themselves comprised of 200 or more individual camps with up to 2,000 prisoners each, were located in Siberia. By 1930, they were controlled by the secret police.

Both criminals and political prisoners ended up in the Gulag; the hardened criminals generally fared better in the survivalist environment. In August 1932, a new Soviet law allowed children as young as 12 years old to be sent to the labor camps. By the end of 1939, it has been estimated that almost 12 million prisoners were being held in the Gulag. Many died while crammed into boxcars or the holds of ships on their way to the camps. More died because of the camps' horrific conditions and minimal rations. During World War II (WWII), the Gulag was enlarged when Stalin's NKVD (secret police) forcefully deported the minority population of Chechens, Crimean Tartars, and Volga Germans. German and Japanese prisoners of war were also sent to the Gulag.

Stalin used prison labor extensively; without it, he could not have industrialized the Soviet Union in such a short time. The most common work was construction, which was often performed without tools. Prisoners also commonly worked in gold, coal, and uranium mines without any safety precaution, and in logging. This work was all performed in the most extreme weather conditions. One woman prisoner described digging the building foundations at Norilsk, some as deep as 40 feet, with her bare hands:

> When you had finished you would get into the bucket for the earth, like in a well, and they would pull you out. More than once the rope broke. And that was that. The bodies were left at the bottom. Norilsk is built on bones.

Life expectancy in the camps was less than 10 years. Estimates are that half of all prisoners died within 3 years; prisoners assigned to uranium mining usually survived only 3 months. Between 1928 and 1953, between 40 and 50 million people were sent to the camps and, at the time of Stalin's death in 1953, as many as 12 million prisoners were still there. No one knows how many died before the Gulag was finally disbanded in 1956.

Stalin's purges began in the late 1920s with public trials of engineers from heavy industry and the railroads, who were charged with being "wreckers" and "enemies." Stalin found the excuse he needed to begin his mass killings when Leonid Nikolaev sneaked into Leningrad's Communist Party headquarters on December 1, 1934, and discovered the Party chief, Sergey Mironovich Kirov, *in flagrante delicto* with Nikolaev's wife. Being prone to violence and emotionally unstable, he shot Kirov dead. Kirov, a well-liked moderate, instantly became a hero and martyr, thus influencing his country's political future in death more than he could ever have expected to in life.

Stalin's first step was to issue special instructions to follow "in dealing with terrorist acts against officials of the Soviet regime," the infamous "Lessons of the Events Connected with the Evil Murder of Comrade Kirov." Condemning the forces that were supposedly arrayed against the country, the "Lessons" set the stage for military court trials with no rights to legal defense or appeal, a time limit of ten days, and execution of the accused. This rule remained in effect through the three famous "Purge Trials," or "Show Trials," of the late 1930s.

August 1936 saw the first of the show trials in which major Party figures admitted their "treachery" before being shot. The terror escalated when, shortly thereafter, Stalin appointed Nikolai Ivanovich Yezhov, "the bloodthirsty dwarf," as head of the secret police. The second show trial was held in January 1937, and the third, which included those involved in the "Doctors' Plot," was in March 1938. According to one Western observer, handpicked Soviet citizens witnessed these trials while "sitting there like schoolchildren out for a treat, in their neat blue suits and tidy dresses . . . men and women who could be counted on to place the correct interpretation on what they saw and heard, to benefit from the lessons and, for that matter, the warnings which it might contain."

Dimitri Volkognonov, a politician-writer, explained the purpose of the trials:

> A feature of the trials was Stalin's desire not merely to destroy his opponents, real and imagined, but first to drag them through the mud of amorality, betrayal and treason. All the trials are an unprecedented example of self-abasement, self-slander, self-condemnation. This often took on a ludicrous appearance, as the accused insistently claimed to be traitors, spies and murderers.

Although he instituted and directed them, Stalin so distanced himself from the mass killings that the Russian word describing the worst period, between 1936 and 1938, is *Yezhovshchina* (the time of Yezhov), implying that the secret police chief, rather than the dictator himself, was responsible for the brutalities. The two were of like mind: where Stalin once said, "One death is a

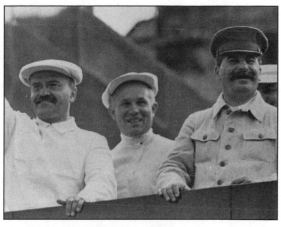

Vyacheslav Molotov, Nikita Khrushchev, and Joseph Stalin, 1936. (© Sovfoto/Eastfoto/PictureQuest)

tragedy—a million is a statistic," Yezhov quoted a Russian proverb, "Better that ten innocent people should suffer than one spy get away. When you cut down the forest, wood chips fly." During this period, one of every eight Soviet citizens became a "wood chip"—and was either executed or sent to the Gulag.

Proportionately, the Communist Party leadership suffered the most casualties. For example, of the 139 elected representatives attending the Seventeenth Party Congress in 1934, 98 had been executed by 1938. One million regular Party members, 5 First Secretaries of the Komosomol, and 6 Politburo members were also executed.

Unbelievably, Stalin nearly destroyed the Red Army's leadership prior to WWII. Among those who received "eight grams of lead" via an automatic pistol to the back of the head were: 3 of the Soviet Union's 5 Marshals (the highest rank), including the army's chief of staff; half of the generals, including 13 of the 15 army commanders; 8 of the 9 fleet admirals and admirals grade I, including the navy's commander-in-chief; 50 of 57 corps commanders; and 15,000 officers and other army personnel.

The worst excesses were stopped in early 1938, when Stalin removed Yezhov from his position and replaced him with Lavrenty Pavlovich Beria. Beria immediately shot 150 of Yezhov's followers within the secret police. Yezhov himself was arrested on April 10, 1939, and he was secretly shot on February 4, 1940. Stalin thought that the secrets, including those of the "Doctors' Plot," would disappear with Yezhov's death—and, for many years, they did.

The 1938 "Doctors' Plot"

The 1938 "Doctors' Plot" was Stalin's calculated scheme to entrap his political challengers, remove perceived enemies, and mobilize the populace to solidify his power. The alleged conspiracy made international news, stimulated a new wave of Soviet anti-Semitism, and resulted in the torture and death of innocent physicians.

This third public trial, generally known as the "Bukharin Show Trial," took place in Moscow in March 1938. It had two purposes. The first was to disgrace Bukharin, an eloquent and charismatic economist and potential rival to Stalin, whom Lenin had described as "the darling of the Party."

The second was to answer foreign criticism of the two prior purge trials. The question had been asked: How could only one death [Kirov's] have resulted from the dozens of well-organized terrorist groups that the prosecution claimed were operating in the Soviet Union? Stalin decided to answer these criticisms by showing that other important Soviet personages had been killed by a Bolshevik conspiracy—even though their deaths had previously been described as "natural" in news releases. Alexander Orlov, the former Soviet counter-intelligence chief, explained:

> Stalin was obliged to give the names of the leaders who had been murdered. But there were none to be found: during the last twenty years the Soviet people had heard of only that one terroristic act ... Between 1934 and 1936 in the Soviet Union several prominent political figures died of natural causes. The best known of them were Kuibyshev, a member of the Politbureau, and Menzhinsky, the chairman of the OGPU [secret police]. Besides those two men, during the same period of time the famous author Maxim Gorky died and also his son Peshkov. Stalin made up his mind to use the names of these four men. But to carry out such a plan was not an easy task even for a falsifier invested with dictatorial power.

So Stalin's government released a story stating that killer doctors, directed by their political allies—chief among them Party strategist Nikolai Ivanovich Bukharin and secret police chief Genrikh Yagoda—had conspired to stage a "palace coup." Their "plan" was to eliminate high-level officials; this would cause civil unrest and thus provide encouragement for the Soviet Union's enemies, particularly Germany and Japan, to intervene and overthrow the Communist regime. The government claimed that the accused physicians murdered the "victims"—their patients—by intentionally practicing bad medicine. No one claimed that the doctors would directly benefit from their misdeeds; rather, their supposed intention was to advance their co-conspirators' political aspirations.

Stalin knew that the public was primed to believe this story. Tales of doctor-killers had pervaded Russia from at least the Middle Ages. In fact, based on persistent rumors, Boris Andreyevich Pil'nyak penned *Tale of the Unextinguished Moon (Povest' Nepogashennoj Luny)*, a supposedly fictionalized account of Stalin arranging the 1925 death of military hero Mikhail Vasil'evich Frunze in the operating room. This may have hit too close to the mark: The author was executed in 1937 on the trumped-up charge of spying for Japan. Yet the fear of medically engineered political murders persisted.

The "Victims"

Stalin claimed that the doctors had murdered four people in succession: Vyacheslav Menzhinsky, Maxim Peshkov, Valerian Kuibyshev, and Maxim Gorky. All supposed victims were well-known among the populace, and details of their natural deaths had been published in papers throughout the country. Therefore, Stalin had to change the facts to justify arresting the doctors.

Vyacheslav Menzhinsky

The first "victim" was Vyacheslav Rudolfovich Menzhinsky, Genrikh Yagoda's boss and the chairman of the OGPU (*Otdelenie gosudarstvennoi politicheskoi upravi*, Unified State Political Directorate, 1923–1934), the dreaded secret police. The fabricated story alleged that Yagoda wanted the top spot, so he arranged (by threatening him) to have Dr. Lev Grigorievich Levin of the Kremlin Medical Service "do something about" Menzhinsky, who was one of his longtime patients.

In reality, Menzhinsky had been in poor health since 1926, when he suffered either a heart attack or a severe and persistent case of angina pectoris. Since standard medical therapy had not helped him, he tried several miracle cures. In 1932, it seemed as if Dr. Kazakov's lysate therapy was actually working. This positive outcome supposedly displeased Yagoda, who instructed Dr. Levin to advise Menzhinsky to take a "rest period" from the lysate therapy. Menzhinsky did and, in early 1933, he suffered a heart attack. He resumed lysate therapy and again improved.

On November 5, Menzhinsky was again under Dr. Levin's care when he suffered a severe case of asthma or congestive heart failure. Dr. Kazakov was summoned and got Menzhinsky through the episode. The next day, however, Yagoda supposedly summoned Kazakov to his office and threatened him with severe punishment if he did not cooperate with Dr. Levin "to bring about a quick end to Menzhinsky's useless life, which was in the way of many people." According to the concocted story, Kazakov understood both the threat and what Yagoda could do for him if he became the secret police chief, so, since he had many grudges to settle, Kazakov joined the conspiracy.

In December 1933, Drs. Levin and Kazakov allegedly injected Menzhinsky with lysates that were all potent stimulants, such as epinephrine, causing his angina to worsen. They then withdrew all treatments, but gave him large doses of digitalis, despite knowing that Menzhinsky was very susceptible to this drug's toxic effects. Menzhensky's condition rapidly deteriorated, and he died on May 10, 1934. According to Levin's coerced testimony presented at the show trial, Yagoda told him at Menzhensky's funeral:

> Well, now that you have committed these crimes, you are entirely in my hands and you must agree to what I shall now propose . . . something much more serious and important . . . A change of Party leadership is inevitable, predetermined, and unavoidable . . . The movement against the Party leaders is headed by Bukharin, Rykov, and Yenukidze. And since this is inevitable, since it will happen all the same, then the sooner it takes place the better. In order . . . to facilitate this process, we have to remove certain members of the Political Bureau and Alexie Maximovich Gorky. This is a historical necessity . . . You must help us with the means at your disposal.

Maxim Peshkov

Maxim Gorky's ne'er-do-well son, Maxim Peshkov, was at the fringes of society, tolerated primarily because of his father's fame. Already in poor health due to his chronic alcoholism, Peshkov's demise was supposedly precipitated by the doctor-conspirators who allegedly arranged for an assistant to supply him with alcohol. According to the story, this continued until, on a chilly May 2, 1934, the assistant left him lying half naked on a bench along the Moscow River. The next day, Peshkov's temperature was 102.5°F. Yet, instead of calling a doctor, the assistant supposedly gave him more alcohol.

When Dr. Levin arrived the next morning, the story went, he said that Peshkov had "light grippe." Dr. Bodmayev, a Gorky friend, disagreed and said he had an obvious case of lobar pneumonia. Dr. Levin returned with Dr. Vinogradov and began treatment. Two days later, Peshkov had improved.

Levin and Vinogradov supposedly were displeased at this turn of events and ordered large amounts of champagne for Peshkov. More realistically, Peshkov probably began drinking again on his own. Predictably, Peshkov's abdomen began to swell and his fever increased. Dr. Vinogradov was said to have administered a strong purgative "to relieve distention," aggravating his patient's condition. At that point, Gorky called in two other physicians, Professors Speransky and Pletnev, but they disagreed about what could be done to help Peshkov, whose skin was now turning blue from a lack of oxygen in the tissues (cyanosis). He died the next day, May 11, 1934.

Valerian Kuibyshev

At the time of his death, the third "victim," Valerian Vladimirovich Kuibyshev, was an important member of the Politburo, the Communist Party's policy-making committee. Since he had died of coronary artery disease, as evidenced by his anginal attacks, he easily fit into Stalin's tale of doctor-induced murders.

The story presented at the trial was that although Kuibyshev did well with small doses of digitalis, Dr. Levin began treating him with much higher doses, which can be lethal. Kuibyshev began experiencing the symptoms of digitalis toxicity, as well as more frequent anginal attacks, when the doctor purportedly began injecting him with the stimulant epinephrine. A much weakened Kuibyshev developed a peritonsillar abscess while on vacation and returned to Moscow in a debilitated condition. Dr. Levin supposedly pronounced Kuibyshev fit to resume his normal strenuous duties, but left secret orders with Kuibyshev's secretary not to call for medical help if his boss should suffer another attack. When Kuibyshev had the expected attack in early 1935, his secretary allegedly urged him to walk down the stairs, the several blocks to his home, and up the three flights of stairs to his apartment. He arrived home in critical condition. The secretary then supposedly delayed calling Dr. Levin; Kuibyshev was dead when the doctor arrived.

Maxim Gorky

Maxim Gorky (pseudonym of Aleksey Maksimovich Peshkov), who was a short-story writer and novelist, may seem like a strange target for this political conspiracy. But Stalin had few prestigious names to use as victims for his invented "plot" and, in the 1930s, Gorky was dean of the Soviet intelligentsia and the first president of the Soviet Writer's Union, with a wide and devoted international following. An ardent Stalinist, he fully supported the Communist Party and could rally the masses whenever either was attacked. He also had a close relationship with Lenin, which Stalin dearly wanted to emulate.

Gorky had tuberculosis as a child and suffered frequent relapses. Subsequently, he developed bronchiectasis with secondary emphysema. He also had episodes of angina. To escape the harsh winter weather, the 56-year-old Gorky left Russia for Italy in 1924. Eventually, Stalin lured Gorky back to Russia with an amazing array of blandishments, including honors, money, an entourage of servants, a fine home, two *dachas* (country homes), and the renaming of streets, cities, factories, and schools in his name.

As described at the trial, Dr. Levin and Professor Dmitri Pletnev, who had treated Gorky on several occasions, supposedly plotted to kill Gorky with the help of his secretary. (Pletnev was said to be a reluctant participant until he met with Yagoda, who threatened to kill his entire family.) The "plan" consisted of encouraging Gorky to take long walks and do manual labor, both of which he loved, in order to place him under stress. After his health deteriorated, Gorky went to the Crimea to recuperate, but he didn't stay long. An influenza epidemic had struck Moscow and his beloved granddaughter was sick, so he hurried back. Not surprisingly, a few days after he returned, he contracted influenza and, then, bronchopneumonia.

In June 1936, Drs. Levin and Pletnev treated Gorky. The medical records were altered to show that they had given him massive intravenous infusions of glucose and extraordinary doses of medications. For example, in only one day, they supposedly administered 40 camphor injections, 4 caffeine injections, and 2 injections each of strychnine and digalen (digitalis). In reality, given his poor state of health, it was not surprising that Gorky died on June 14. After his death, he had a grand funeral and his ashes were buried in the Kremlin Wall.

The "Conspirators"

Genrikh Yagoda

Genrikh Grigorievich Yagoda (1891–1938) was born Heinrich Yehuda in Lodz (now in Poland), which was part of the Russian Empire's Jewish Pale of Settlement. One of Stalin's closest colleagues, he arranged, under Stalin's direct orders, the murder of many of the dictator's political opponents, possibly including Kirov. Although he was guilty of many atrocities, ironically, he was innocent of the one for which he was tried and executed: masterminding the fictitious "Doctors' Plot."

Yagoda joined *Cheka* in 1920 and worked his way up the ranks. As deputy head of the secret police, he oversaw the construction of the Moscow-Volga Canal. He also organized the notorious 20-month-long building of the White Sea-Baltic Sea Canal, during which more than 60,000 of the prisoner-construction workers died. Yagoda received the Order of Lenin for his work. Subsequently, Stalin named him vice-chairman of the OGPU, the successor to the *Cheka*. Yagoda was also in charge of a secret laboratory that developed poisons, and was later accused of using these concoctions to poison various enemies.

Stalin signaled Yagoda's demise when, in 1936, he sent a telegram saying that "Yagoda has definitely proved himself incapable of unmasking the Trotskyite-Zinovievite bloc. The OGPU is four years behind in this matter." He then concocted a story that would implicate Yagoda as the person who not only assembled the doctor-killer group, but also directed their actions and then concealed information on them when they were about to be exposed.

According to the story, Yagoda first enlisted Dr. Lev Levin into the plot by using favors and threats. Yagoda knew Levin: the doctor had successfully treated him and his wife in 1930 during a severe illness. He had lavishly thanked the doctor with flowers, French wine, and a *dacha* near Moscow. He had also arranged for Levin's baggage to be exempt from inspection when he returned from his many foreign visits, enabling him to bring in duty-free items. While these gifts were not unusual, they were used to prove that Yagoda planned to enmesh Levin in the "conspiracy."

Once Dr. Levin was indebted to him, Yagoda supposedly informed Dr. Levin that Maxim Gorky was being influenced by his dissolute son, Maxim Peshkov. Yagoda then explained that the government wanted Levin, who was Gorky's family physician, to help eliminate both Gorky and Peshkov.

Yagoda was accused and tried in a "show" trial. During his trial, and perhaps knowing that Stalin secretly watched from behind a hidden screen, Yagoda shouted, "I appeal to you! For you I built two great canals!" Yagoda was shot in Lubyanka Prison on March 15, 1938. He has never been posthumously rehabilitated.

Dr. Dmitri Dmitrievich Pletnev

Dr. Dmitri Pletnev was an obvious choice for those hatching the fictitious doctors' conspiracy. A well-known Moscow physician since before the Revolution and Russia's leading cardiologist, he was a vocal opponent of the Soviet regime and longed openly for the "good old days." During the Revolution, he had been an active Constitutional Democrat (called "Kadets" after the acronym for their party's name), and advocated a limited constitutional monarchy.

After the Revolution, Professor Pletnev continued to support the cause of the Kadets (although they no longer existed), but, because of his reputation, the government left him alone. He became the editor of a leading Moscow medical journal and was a member of the Soviet medical mission to Berlin in 1932. In 1934, already in his mid-sixties, he was a delegate to the International Congress on Rheumatism.

The doctor had foolishly written in his private papers that he believed Stalin to be a paranoid megalomaniac. (Stalin had psychologist Vladimir Bekhterev poisoned in 1927 for making a similar observation.) As early as December 1936, the secret police had identified him as a potential member of their invented doctors' cabal. Pletnev knew this, but hoped that his medical reputation and his powerful patients, including Vyacheslav M. Molotov, Stalin's second-in-command, would protect him. That hope vanished with his arrest on March 5, 1937.

Pletnev's manuscript condemning Stalin was produced at the trial, as was the scurrilous accusation that the doctor sexually molested his patients. The prosecutor had arranged for a secret police provocateur, a woman often used to ensnare foreigners, to see Pletnev as a patient. After two visits, she accused the elderly doctor of assaulting her and began bothering his family at home. He called the police, but, on instructions from the secret police, they sided with the woman and released her statement to the newspaper. *Pravda* published it under the headline "Professor-Rapist, Sadist." The statement accused Pletnev of throwing himself on his patient, biting her severely on the breast and doing permanent injury, and then trying to cure the lesion. They also published a letter she supposedly had sent Pletnev:

> Be accursed, criminal violator of my body! Be accursed, sadist, practicing your foul perversions on my body! Let shame and disgrace fall on you, let terror and sorrow, weeping and anguish be yours as they have been mine, ever since, criminal professor, you made me the victim of your sexual corruption and criminal perversions. I curse you.

To demonstrate the absurdity of this charge, Dr. Yakov Rapoport later wrote:

> I knew this woman. She was a reporter for a Moscow newspaper (*Trud*, I believe) and, in my capacity as assistant rector for research and instruction of the Second Medical Institute, I had been obliged to receive her when she sought information for an article. Her appearance was far from glamorous, and it is hard to imagine her arousing any sexual passion. She was about forty, dowdy and unattractive ... The only emotion she aroused in me was the desire to be rid of her as soon as possible. And suddenly we were told that she had been the virgin victim of the "lustful" professor, a violator and sadist. I said then that one would only be moved to bite the woman in self-defense, for lack of any other means of protection.

The next day, *Pravda* published a list of national and local medical organizations holding meetings to vilify Dr. Pletnev. The following day, the paper was filled with letters from medical groups denouncing him. Ironically, among those attacking Pletnev were physicians who, 15 years later, would themselves be accused in a "doctors' plot."

For this supposed infraction, the judge—actually a senior secret police operative—sentenced the 66-year-old Pletnev to two years in Lubyanka Prison. There, secret police could work on the professor at their leisure to obtain his "confession" for killing his supposed victims.

Dr. Lev Grigorievich Levin

Born in 1870 to a lower-class Jewish family, Dr. Lev Levin graduated from the Faculty of Natural Sciences in Odessa and the Medical Faculty of Moscow. Before the Bolshevik Revolution, he had worked in various hospitals and as the physician for several industrial plants. After the Revolution, he associated himself with the People's Commissariat of Health, and worked at the Health Resort Selection hospital until he was called to serve in the Red Army.

In 1920, he began working in the Kremlin's Polyclinic, where he treated many senior Soviet government officials, including Lenin, Stalin, and Politburo members and their families. He also served on the staff of the secret police's medical service under three different directors: Dzerzhinsky, Menzhinsky, and Yagoda. He was not a member of the Communist Party and demonstrated little interest in politics. Yet Levin was later appointed consulting physician to the Medical Service of the People's Commissariat of Internal Affairs. No one (prosecution or defense) would dare to claim that his participation in the fictitious plot resulted from his political convictions.

Dr. Levin, painted in the trial as naïve, supposedly joined the plot believing that he would gain recognition by helping the conspirators (unnecessary, since he was already famous) and that Kryuchkov, Gorky's secretary, and Dr. A. I. Vinogradov, the Gorky household's consulting physician, were willing to assist him.

His important patients gave Dr. Levin an enviable position of privilege within the Soviet hierarchy. Yet, when he was entrapped in this web of deceit, no one attempted to help him. The "conspirators" supposedly considered Dr. Levin cowardly, timid, and naïve about the politics in which he was embroiled. The last claim seemed to be true. At the time of his arrest on December 2, 1937, Dr. Levin was 68 years old and had several sons and many grandchildren. The secret police gained his cooperation by threatening all their lives.

Dr. Ignaty Nikolaievich Kazakov

Dr. Ignaty Kazakov was arrested on December 16, 1937. The youngest member of the fictional physician cabal, he was only 16 years old at the time of the

Revolution. Although he never joined the Communist Party, his self-promotion and politically connected patients had gotten him appointed as head of a large and well-equipped investigative, clinical, and promotional organization, the Institute for Research in Lysate Therapy. It is believed that Kazakov was targeted, in part, because he knew too many secrets about his well-connected patients.

As with other medical zealots, Kazakov grossly overstated the value of lysate therapy, or lysatotherapy, which used modified extracts of animal glands, organs, and other body structures. He boldly claimed that lysate therapy could cure *all* human illnesses by correcting disorders of the endocrine glands—such as the thyroid, pancreas, adrenal, and pituitary—that send hormones directly into the bloodstream. He asserted that the therapy was especially effective against ailments related to aging and impotence, a great concern to many in the Soviet hierarchy.

Kazakov's future "co-conspirators" had little to do with him professionally: Professor Pletnev did not interact with him and Dr. Levin thought him a charlatan. In fact, most physicians considered him a quack and blocked him from publishing his papers and books at reputable scientific presses. As one person remarked, Kazakov used "very intricate drugs that were not only unknown to medicine, but not very well known to Kazakov himself."

Two Dead "Doctor-Killers"
Two of the accused physicians mysteriously died before going to trial.

Dr. A. I. Vinogradov, like Dr. Levin, worked in the Kremlin Medical Service. He died while in secret police custody, presumably under torture. According to the OGPU, the proceedings against him were "terminated owing to his death."

Dr. I. Khodorovsky, head of the Kremlin Medical Administration until 1938, also died while in secret police custody. Although he was named as a co-conspirator, there was no official discussion of what his role in the "plot" might have been.

The Trial and Its Aftermath
To ensure that the rigged trials ran smoothly, there was a long preparation time, during which the doctors were expected to learn their parts. As politician-writer Dmitri Volkognonov explained:

> Several months were spent in trying to break the accused. The investigators had a wide range of means to obtain the desired confession which, contrary to legal norms, would serve as the main evidence of guilt. Some

witnesses lasted as long as three months, others only a few days. Then would come the humiliating rehearsals. Once broken, the accused were forced to learn the proper version, to make prepared statements "unmasking" named people. After countless repeats of this shameful pretense, the "directors" would be informed that this or that "actor" was ready for his "premiere" . . . [Generally] the trial went smoothly. The accused agreed with the procurator, accepted the monstrous charges in a friendly spirit, readily adding a detail here and there to their own evil deeds.

Whether the doctors were tortured to obtain their confessions is unclear, although two of them did die in secret police custody, and torture was definitely employed during the 1953 "Doctors' Plot" investigation. Deputy People's Commissar Finsovsky of the secret police authorized such cruel treatment with the memo: "I authorize transfer to the Lefortovo [prison]. Beating permitted." In his "Secret Speech," Nikita Khrushchev admitted:

> Many thousands of honest and innocent Communists have died as a result of this monstrous falsification of such "cases," as a result of the fact that all kinds of slanderous "confessions" were accepted, and as a result of the practice of forcing accusations against oneself and others... The vicious practice was condoned of having the NKVD prepare lists of persons whose cases were under the jurisdiction of the Military Collegium and whose sentences were prepared in advance. Yezhov would send these lists to Stalin personally for his approval of the proposed punishment . . . Suffice it to say that from 1954 to the present time [1956] the Military Collegium of the Supreme Court has rehabilitated 7,679 persons, many of whom were rehabilitated posthumously.

The trial court appointed a Commission of Medical Experts made up of five prominent internists to review the care given the "victims." All five would later be accused in the 1953 "Doctors' Plot." In each case, this Commission was asked: "Can it be granted that properly qualified physicians could have adopted such a wrong method of treatment without malicious intent?" The Commission members uniformly answered, "No."

Similar to the "hired guns" used in today's malpractice cases, Commission members claimed that Drs. Levin and Vinogradov had not given Peshkov appropriate treatment. Of Dr. Kazakov's lysate therapy, the physicians alleged that "such a combination of methods of treatment could not but lead to the exhaustion of the heart muscles of the patient V. R. Menzhinsky, and thereby to the acceleration of his death." Nikita Khrushchev later wrote about such perjured testimony:

In our day we had people lifting up their voices in court, vouching for the truth of accusations, beating their breasts, and swearing that the accused were enemies of the people—all without any real knowledge about what had happened. A witness would endorse the verdict and raise his hand, voting for the elimination of the accused without really knowing about the facts of the alleged crime, much less the role of the alleged criminal.

Stalin's chief prosecutor for all the major show trials of 1936–1938, including that of the doctors, was Andrei Yanuarevich Vyshinsky. He had a large team, but usually took the spotlight in the courtroom, where he tried to invoke drama by routinely hurling such epithets as "vermin" and "mad dogs" at the accused. Vyshinsky, a lawyer, had taught at Moscow State University before becoming prosecutor for the Russian Soviet Federated Socialist Republic in 1931. He had originally supported the provisional Kerensky government and condemned Lenin as a traitor and a spy; however, he quickly changed sides when the Bolsheviks won, currying favor with Stalin.

After the trials, he retired as a prosecutor, was elected to the Soviet Academy, and, in 1939, became a member of the Central Committee of the Communist Party. Vyshinsky was then named deputy commissar of foreign affairs and, in 1949, replaced Molotov as minister of foreign affairs. On Stalin's death, he was appointed chief Soviet delegate to the United Nations, effectively removing him from national politics. He died in New York a year later.

Vyshinsky knew he was prosecuting innocent men, but, he wrote, "one has to remember comrade Stalin's instructions, that there are sometimes periods, moments in the life of a society and in our life in particular, when the laws prove obsolete and have to be set aside."

After prolonged incarceration, interrogation, and possibly torture, the three surviving physicians pled guilty. Dr. Levin needed no prompting in court; he had learned his part in the farce very well. He admitted that he had organized the plot with Yagoda and had ordered Kazakov to poison Menzhinsky so that Yagoda could assume control of the secret police. He also admitted killing Peshkov with Drs. Vinogradov and Pletnov by instigating his pneumonia and then treating him inappropriately. And he again confessed to purposeful malpractice in the case of Kuibyshev.

Dr. Levin said that he also arranged to have an already ill Maxim Gorky put in circumstances, such as repeatedly moving from an overheated room to the freezing cold, which resulted in his death. Levin was also accused of, but did not admit to, conspiring with the now-disgraced Nikolai Ivanovich

Bukharin in the December 1, 1934, killing of Sergei M. Kirov, and of trying to poison Yagoda's successor, Nikolai Yezhov.

Dr. Kazakov confirmed Levin's testimony and emphasized his fear of Yagoda, who allegedly told him, "If you make any attempt to disobey me, I shall find quick means of exterminating you." Dr. Pletnev also testified that Yagoda made threats against himself and his family. The physicians' prominent defense lawyers asked the court for mercy. They justified their request by downplaying their clients' role in the plot and stressing Yagoda's blackmail as the motivating factor. Levin testified about Yagoda:

> He reiterated that my refusal to carry this out would spell ruin for me and my family. I figured that I had no other way out, that I had to submit to him. Again, if you look at it retrospectively, if you look back at 1932 from today, when you consider how all-powerful Yagoda appeared to me, a non-Party person, then, of course, it was very difficult to evade his threats, his orders.

The court heard only briefly from Yagoda, formerly of the secret police. Looking cornered and desperate, he testified, "I gave Levin instructions to bring about the death of Alexei Maximovich Gorky and Kuibyshev, and that's all." He also said, "I did not bring about the death of either Menzhinsky or Max Peshkov." But, in a deposition before trial, he had said, "I summoned Kazakov and confirmed my orders . . . He did his work. Menzhinsky died." He also stated before the trial that he "had guilt for causing" Peschkov's illness.

Bulanov, Yagoda's personal assistant and a secret police veteran, dutifully perjured himself and said that there had been a plan to topple the government with the assistance of both organized subversive groups and outside governments. He also described Yagoda's laboratory, where poisons were prepared for the secret police. As to the doctors themselves, he testified:

> As far as I know, Yagoda drew Levin into, enlisted him in the affair, and in cases of poisoning generally, by taking advantage of some compromising material he had against him.

The court was not moved by the physicians' protestations of innocence. Prosecutor Vyshinsky demanded the death penalty, saying that the defendants "must be shot like dirty dogs! Our people are demanding one thing: Crush the accursed reptiles! Time will pass. The graves of the hateful traitors will grow over with weeds and thistles."

At 9:25 P.M. on March 12, 1938, the court retired to consider their verdict. Returning at 4:00 A.M., they ordered that Drs. Levin and Kazakov be shot and all their property confiscated. As an accessory rather than an active participant and "because of his old age," professor Pletnev was sentenced to 25 years in prison, confiscation of all personal property, and a loss of political rights for five additional years.

Dr. Levin and Dr. Kazakov were immediately shot in the cellars of Lubyanka Prison. Robert Conquest described the typical scene:

> The cellars of the Lubyanka were really a sort of basement divided into a number of rooms off corridors . . . The condemned handed in their clothes in one of these rooms and changed into white underclothes only. They were then taken to the death cell and shot in the back of the neck with a TT eight-shot automatic. A doctor then signed the death certificate, the last document to be put in their files, and the tarpaulin on the floor was taken away to be cleaned by a woman specially employed for that purpose. At the Lefortovo, the corpses were cremated.

Dr. Levin's son, who worked for the People's Commissariat for Foreign Affairs, was arrested and never heard from again. Dr. Pletnev was sent to Orel Prison, where he was re-sentenced to death on September 8, 1941, and killed three days later. A number of other prominent doctors were later quietly implicated in this "affair." As a group, they were called "Gorkyists" for the most noted victim, and they were sent to the Gulag to meet various fates.

Was there a conspiracy? Alexander Orlov, former Soviet counter-intelligence chief, dismissed the possibility of a "Doctors' Plot":

> That legend is so absurd that it can be discredited completely by a single question: why was it necessary for the old and highly respectable physicians to commit murder for Yagoda when they could have warned their distinguished patients that Yagoda had ordered their murder and that he directed a conspiracy against Stalin and the Soviet Government? The physicians had plenty of chances to tell about the terroristic plans of the Politbureau as well. Professor Pletnev, in particular, could have told the whole story to Molotov, whom he had treated, and Dr. Levin, who worked in the Kremlin, could have informed Stalin himself about the sinister designs of Yagoda.

Suggesting that Stalin could at least have come up with a better story, Robert Conquest wrote:

> As for the effects of the trial, once again neither the ineptitudes [sic] of the plot nor the partial denials of the accused made any difference . . . Once more, a vast network of assassins was discovered. At least eight groups were working on the destruction of Stalin [and others] . . . And, this

time, they were shown not simply to be under the protection of high officials in the Party and the Army, but actually to have been nourished and
sponsored by the NKVD [secret police] itself. Seldom can terrorists have
had such advantages as those supposedly enjoyed by the plotters . . . But
the results had been negligible. Assassinations had indeed been carried
out, but only by doctors . . . It is an unimpressive result and the conclusion—that the best way to assassinate anyone was to wait until he got
ill—was not very encouraging to anyone desiring speedy action.

In 1988, the Soviet government posthumously "rehabilitated" all those
involved in the fiasco, except for secret police chief Genrikh Yagoda.

The 1953 "Doctors' Plot"

Stalin's final "Reign of Rerror" was a series of major, although relatively
unpublicized, purges. The aging tyrant had turned 70 in 1949, and his life of
chain-smoking and 16-hour days had taken its toll. He had withdrawn from
some of his usual activities, and those who would succeed him were beginning
to assume stronger positions within the Party and the government. Yet, Stalin
felt that he needed to regain control.

In 1949 and 1950, he had about 3,000 senior Party officials from Leningrad, including members of the Politburo, arrested and tortured; many were
then shot. Stalin was now ready to begin another great purge like those of the
1930s. All he needed was a way to justify and promote his mass killings to the
public.

The linchpin he decided to use was anti-Semitism, long entrenched in
Russian culture. Since the rise of post-WWII Zionism and the establishment
of Israel in 1948, Stalin had become obsessed with Jews in Soviet society,
writing: "I can't swallow them, I can't spit them out. They are the only group
that is completely unassimilable." Khrushchev considered Stalin's anti-
Semitism:

> [to be] a major defect in his character . . . As a leader and a theoretician
> he took care never to hint at his anti-Semitism in his written works or in
> his speeches. And God forbid that anyone should quote publicly from any
> private conversations in which he made remarks that smelled sharply of
> anti-Semitism.

But a Soviet expert believes that Stalin settled on an anti-Semitic campaign
because his "Hate America" campaign wasn't energizing the population and,
thus, "darker, more archaic, aggressive instincts had to be aroused by Stalin

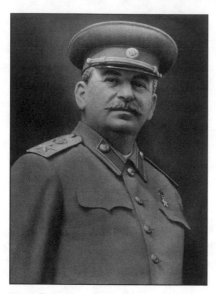

Joseph Stalin, 1948. (© Sovfoto/ Eastfoto/ PictureQuest)

inside Russia in order to deflect hatred from the regime itself."

In the late 1940s, Stalin initiated rabid official anti-Semitism with new restrictive laws and sanctioned violence against Russian Jews. He began with editorials in *Pravda* and *Kultura I zhizn* accusing the mostly Jewish literary, music, and theater critics of "ideological sabotage." In what was known as the "Anti-Cosmopolitan Campaign," editors claimed that various prominent Russian Jews were "rootless cosmopolitans" of a "nonbasic" nationality who "demolished national pride" and "fawned on the West."

In an attempt to destroy the last vestiges of Jewish culture and identity in the Soviet Union, the government dissolved the Jewish section of the Writer's Union, closed the Yiddish presses, and removed Jewish literature from bookstores and libraries. They also closed the last two Jewish schools, as well as Jewish theaters and choirs. Jews were summarily fired from leading scientific, academic, military, media, and legal positions and were also purged from the Communist Party leadership. As a joke of the time went, "Moses led the Jews out of Egypt, and Stalin led them out of the [Communist Party] Central Committee."

In what became known as the "Crimean Affair," 25 of the leading Yiddish writers were arrested in 1948 and at least 14 were secretly killed in Lubyanka prison on August 12, 1952. The remainder did not survive imprisonment. Historian Yakov Rapoport later wrote, "Jewish culture in the Soviet Union was put before the firing squad, its finest representatives physically destroyed."

At the time of Stalin's death, *Pravda* was set to publish a letter from prominent Jews called "The Jewish Statement." It had been signed under coercion, and condemned the Jewish doctors allegedly involved in the plot and requested transportation for all Jews to "the developing territories in the East (Siberia)" to protect them from the wrath of other Soviet citizens. Continuing the work of the last czar, Nicholas II, who deported Jews from the Baltic provinces during World War I, almost all Soviet Jews were to be deported to concentration camps in Siberia, Kazakhstan, and Birobidzhan.

Renowned physicist Andrei Sakharov later wrote, "After Stalin's death we heard that trains had been assembled in the beginning of March to transport Jews to Siberia and that propaganda justifying their deportation had been set in type, including a lead article for *Pravda* entitled, 'The Russian People are Rescuing the Jewish People.'" Alexander Sozhenitsyn alleged in *Gulag Archipelago* that Stalin planned to publically hang the doctors in Red Square, ensuring that anti-Jewish pogroms would ensue and allowing Stalin to "save" the Jews by resettling them in Siberia and Kazakhstan, as he had already done with several other minority groups during WWII.

The Story: The Doctor-Poisoners

Reprising the scenario of the 1930s, Stalin planned to eliminate prominent doctors who had signed death certificates for important Soviet politicians, accusing them of murder through intentional malpractice. Physicians were an obvious target of Stalin's anti-Semitic assault. In 1951, about 35,000 (16%) of 215,000 Soviet doctors were Jewish. In Stalin's mind, Jews were linked with the United States, science, and medicine. Moreover, by calling the Jewish doctors "poisoners," he fed into old anti-Semitic lies that Jewish doctors started plagues and killed non-Jewish patients.

Stalin had signaled that the accusations, the doctors' trial, and their public executions would begin a new set of purges. In prior purges of intellectuals, engineers, military officers, geologists, agronomists, and other public figures, nearly all were found guilty and quietly executed after secret trials. Since the "conspirators" in this case were so well-known that their abductions could not be hidden, and because Stalin needed to set up his "rescue" of the Jews to Siberia, the opposite tack was taken—the news was widely disseminated.

To that end, Stalin announced the discovery of nine "doctor-conspirators," some of whom were dead, who were charged with killing two prominent Soviet officials and plotting to kill others. The arrests began in November 1952, and official notice was given on January 13, 1953, by Radio Moscow, *Izvestia*, and *Pravda*, although the entire list of those accused, arrested, and, in some cases, executed would not be known for many years. *Pravda* reported the story on the front page:

> A group of saboteur-doctors, [a] terrorist group, uncovered some time ago by organs of state security, had as their goal shortening the lives of leaders of the Soviet Union by means of medical sabotage. Investigation established that participants in the terrorist group, exploiting their position as doctors and abusing the trust of their patients, deliberately and viciously

undermined their patients' health by making incorrect diagnoses, and then killed them with bad and incorrect treatments.

The headline for an accompanying editorial, also on the front page, screamed across two columns, "Vicious Spies and Killers under a Mask of Academic Physicians." *Pravda* elucidated Stalin's theory of an international conspiracy—and emphasized the involvement of Jewish physicians as poisoners:

> The majority of the participants of the terrorist group . . . were recruited by a branch office of the American secret service—the international Jewish bourgeois-nationalist organization called "Joint" [American Jewish Joint Distribution Committee]. The filthy face of this Zionist spy organization, covering up their vicious actions under the mask of kindness, is now completely revealed . . . Unmasking the gang of poisoner-doctors struck a blow against the international Jewish Zionist organization . . .
>
> The bigwigs of the USA and their English junior partners know that to achieve domination over other nations by peaceful means is impossible. Feverishly preparing for a new world war, they energetically send spies inside the USSR and the people's democratic countries: they attempt to accomplish what the Hitlerites could not do—to create in the USSR their own subversive "fifth column" . . . Exposing the gang of poisoner-doctors struck a shattering blow to the Anglo-American war mongers.

The American Jewish Joint Distribution Committee (JDC), or "Joint," was actually a philanthropic (and generally anti-Zionist) organization founded in 1914 with the cooperation of the Soviet government for the relief and rehabilitation of Jewish victims of war and persecution in 60 countries. In the 1920s, most of their efforts were within the Soviet Union, which before World War II had the world's largest Jewish population.

Over the next seven weeks, until Stalin died, Moscow's four major newspapers, *Pravda, Izvestia, Komosomol Pravda*, and *Labor*, published 49 articles concerning the "Plot" and the need to remain vigilant against the associated terrorist groups. Hundreds of Soviet publications joined in the hysteria, splashing coordinated attacks against the "traitorous Jewish doctors" and their accomplices on their front pages. On January 25, the eighteenth anniversary of Kuibyshev's death, they reminded their readers that this current episode was only a reprise of the 1938 "Doctors' Plot," when the nation had been "villainously done to death by monsters who were disguised as doctors . . . The foul hirelings of foreign imperialist intelligence agencies brought about his death."

Boris Shcharansky, father of Anatoly (the "Prisoner of Zion"), was working as a reporter for a local newspaper, *Sozialistik Donbass,* at the time. He recalled a meeting where the staff was instructed to write about "bad doctors, bad workers, takers of bribes." They were told to find and print as many explicitly Jewish names as possible. Just such an article was published on February 26, 1953, stating that city doctors (all those named were Jewish) not only lacked proper medical degrees, but also had misdiagnosed and maltreated patients (all of whom had Russian names). Afterward, the Party boss called to congratulate the staff on the "useful exposé."

The stories had the desired effect. As historian Louis Rapoport wrote, "The revelations about the grand plot electrified the ordinary Russian, who immediately began to think about his local clinic or hospital physician, wondering whether he could possibly be safe, if powerful men like Zhdanov were not." Across the Soviet Union, a witch hunt was stirred up "against doctor-poisoners, Zionist agents, spies, and wreckers, and every Jewish doctor with a Jewish-sounding name was nervous and edgy." According to Yakov Rapoport:

> One professor of medicine after another was arrested. The medical world was not simply deflated, it was crushed. Nobody knew anything for certain, but it was clear that yet another exposure of a conspiracy was in the offing—this time among the top men in the medical profession—and everyone in that group who was still at large expected arrest each night."

Not only doctors were targeted. In many of the largest cities, nearly all Jewish medical school professors who had not been arrested were dismissed. And, upon graduation, all Jewish medical students were sent to the most remote regions, such as Kamachtka, Yakutia, and Siberia.

The "Victims"

While the doctors were accused of planning to kill several unnamed Party members and military leaders, only two Soviet officials, Aleksandr Shcherbakov and Andrej Zhdanov, were named as their "victims." Both had actually died from natural causes complicated by alcoholism.

Aleksandr Shcherbakov

Aleksandr Sergeevich Shcherbakov was the head of the Soviet Army's Main Political Administration and a candidate-member of the Politburo when he died in 1945 at age 44. Zhdanov's brother-in-law, Shcherbakov had partnered with Maxim Gorky, a "victim" of the 1938 "Doctors' Plot," to lead the newly formed Soviet Writers' Union. The partnership soon deteriorated as Shcherbakov's push to stress politics over art seriously diminished the quality of new publications.

Although *Pravda* stated that "the criminals likewise cut short the life of Comrade A. S. Shcherbakov by incorrectly employing strong drugs in his treatment," Khrushchev later wrote that alcoholism killed Shcherbakov, as it had Zhdanov.

Andrej Zhdanov

Andrej Aleksandrovich Zhdanov had been a Politburo member since 1939. At the time of his death in 1948, at age 52, he was the Central Committee's secretary. A Bolshevik since 1915, Zhdanov had risen to become Leningrad's (St. Petersburg) political boss—ironically filling the position of the assassinated Sergey Kirov, whose death had sparked the 1938 "Doctors' Plot" trials. In that capacity, he led the defense against Germany's siege of the city (1941–44). For this achievement, Stalin promoted him to major general and transferred him to Moscow in 1944. He became the Soviet spokesman on the arts, and condemned famous writers, musicians, filmmakers, and even scientists for their ideological impurity.

In 1947, Zhdanov oversaw the establishment of the Soviet Union's international propaganda arm, Cominform (Communist Information Bureau). For three years, Zhdanov and Stalin were linked by marriage, when his son married Stalin's daughter, Svetlana. Zhdanov's death was followed by the notorious Leningrad Affair, during which his enemies (primarily Georgy Malenkov and Lavrenty Beria, under Stalin's orders) purged 2,000 of his associates and subordinates. In actuality, Zhdanov may have had a heart attack, but it was complicated by his uncontrollable and obviously terminal alcoholism. Nikita Khrushchev, who frequently worked with Zhdanov during this period, wrote:

> Before his death, Zhdanov had been in poor health for some time . . . [He] wasn't able to control himself when it came to drinking. He was pitiful to watch. I even remember that in the last days of Zhdanov's life, Stalin used to shout at him to stop drinking. This was an astounding thing because Stalin usually encouraged people to get drunk. But he compelled Zhdanov to drink fruit water and suffer while the rest of us were drinking wine or something stronger.

Yet, four years after his death, *Pravda* dutifully reported the Party line, writing that "taking advantage of the illness of Comrade Zhdanov, [the doctors] intentionally concealed a myocardial infarction [heart attack], prescribed inadvisable treatments for this serious illness and thus killed Comrade Zhdanov."

Agent-Provocateur — Lydia Timashuk

In August 1948, soon after Zhdanov's death, Lydia Feodosevna Timashuk, a secret informer (*sekrety sotrudnik*) for the State Security Ministry, wrote a report suggesting that he had died as a result of faulty diagnosis. Timashuk, described by a former KGB (Committee for State Security) official as a "violent anti-Semite," had the lowest level medical degree, which allowed her to work only as a technician. She had toiled for nearly two decades as an x-ray technician at Kremlin Hospital, and hated both Dr. Sophia Karpai, the head of electrocardiography, and Dr. M. B. Kogan, who had refused her request to upgrade her medical degree. Both physicians would later be arrested in connection with the "Plot."

Her report, as well as subsequent letters on the same theme, found their way to Mikhail Dmitriyevich Ryumin, who was in charge of fabricating evidence against the Kremlin doctors. Ryumin, a former SMERSH (WWII counterespionage unit) interrogator, gave Timashuk's letters to Stalin who, in mid-October 1952, read one of them to his inner circle during the Nineteenth Party Congress. It claimed that Zhdanov's death was a case of medical murder. Khrushchev was present and recalled:

> If Stalin had been a normal person, he wouldn't have given Timashuk's letter a second thought. A few such letters always turn up from people who are psychologically unbalanced or who are scheming to get rid of their enemies. But Stalin was more than receptive to this sort of literature... But how could you find even ten percent truth in a letter like Timashuk's?

Timashuk was now thrust into the limelight. On November 10, 1952, the previously unknown technician had an article published in the prestigious *Klinisheskaya Meditsina* (*Clinical Medicine*). That same issue, not coincidentally, omitted the names of Drs. Vinogradov and Vasilenko, two of the doctors accused, from the list of the journal's editorial board.

On January 20, 1953, Lydia Timashuk was awarded the Order of Lenin "for assistance rendered to the government in exposing the 'Physician-murderers.'" Describing the technician as a "doctor," articles in popular magazines praised her as the "dear daughter of our country." She was compared favorably to Joan of Arc, poems were written about her, and one article described how "a simple Soviet woman, an ordinary doctor [had caught] the venal vermin who hid a knife and poison under their snow-white frocks . . . these degenerates with serpents' stings in place of hearts."

The "Consipirators"

Solomon Mikhoels

Unlike the 1938 episode, no high-ranking politicians were accused of master-minding this "Doctors' Plot." The only non-physician officially implicated with this group of "saboteur-doctors" was the Jewish leader Solomon Mixajlovich Mikhoels, who had been murdered five years before the "Plot" was announced. This supposed ringleader was an internationally respected Yiddish actor and stage and movie director who directed the Moscow Jewish State Theater. He was so well-known that he gave private recitals for Stalin, and Albert Einstein hosted his visit to the United States. During WWII, Stalin appointed Mikhoels to head the government's Jewish Anti-fascist Committee (JAC).

A key component of the government's plan was the dissolution of the JAC and the murder of its most prominent member, Mikhoels. The JAC had been formed in April 1942 by prominent Soviet Jews. According to Khrushchev, its purpose was "to publicize the successes of the Red Army and to expose the atrocities committed by the Germans in the Ukraine." The effort was very successful, garnering massive support and millions of dollars from the West, especially the United States, to aid Russia's struggle against Nazi Germany. After WWII, the JAC became the focal point for the reemergence of a Russian Jewish identity.

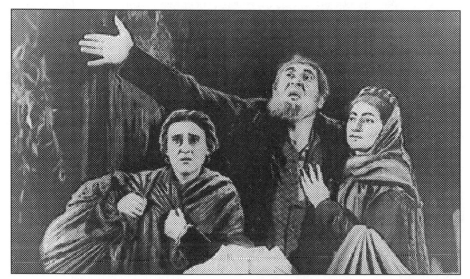

Solomon Mixajlovich Mikhoels (center) on stage in the final scene of "Tevye the Milkman" at the Lvov Jewish State Theater in 1947, just before it was closed down.

In 1948, Stalin felt that the JAC had outlived its usefulness and ordered the NKVD to kill Mikhoels. He was promptly murdered and his body was dumped on a city street in Minsk, where a truck ran over it to make it seem like an accident. According to Khrushchev, "They killed him like beasts. They killed him secretly. Then his murderers were rewarded and their victim was buried with honors." Mikhoels was given a prominent obituary in *Pravda* and a state funeral. His denunciation came much later.

The "Saboteur-Doctors"

The rest of those falsely accused were physicians. Most were well-known and associated with Kremlin Polyclinic (Hospital). Stalin had ordered all members of the Politburo, the Central Committee, the Central Executive Committee, the secret police, and the army hierarchy to receive their medical treatment from Kremlin Polyclinic. Near the end of Stalin's reign, foreign Communist Party dignitaries also received medical treatment there, among them French Party leader Maurice Thorez and Bulgarian dictator Georgi Dimitrov. From its inception, most Kremlin Polyclinic doctors were Jews. Khrushchev said:

> These doctors could only have been the best and most trusted of their profession. Only men well known and much respected in the Soviet medical world had been enlisted to work in the Kremlin hospital. But they were arrested and thrown in jail like common criminals.

The most famous doctors arrested in conjunction with the supposed plot were Vladimir Vingradov (the only one not Jewish), Miron Vovsi, Boris Kogan, Lina Shtern, Sophia Karpai, Yakov Etinger, Eliazar Gelstein, and Yakov Rapoport. Some of these physicians were actually arrested long before the "conspiracy" was publically announced. The accusations against them were bogus and often bizarre. When the "Plot" was announced, they were lumped in with the conspirators to give their arrests validity and to bolster the case against the accused.

Dr. Vladimir N. Vinogradov

Dr. Vladimir N. Vinogradov was a giant of Soviet medicine. An impeccably groomed doctor with a well-trimmed goatee, he was Joseph Stalin's personal physician and chief of Moscow Medical Institute. Widely published, primarily in the field of infectious diseases, he had received many honors, including four Orders of Lenin—one as late as February 27, 1952. Like many of the accused physicians, Vinogradov had served on the Medical Commission during the 1938 "Doctors' Plot" trial, and he had probably given false information that helped convict his colleagues.

His big mistake was telling Stalin, in 1952, that he was at risk for stroke and should have "complete rest, freedom from all work." Stalin saw this advice as part of a conspiracy to remove him from power. He angrily demanded Vinogradov's immediate arrest, screaming, "Leg irons! Put him in leg irons!" (Stalin had recognized that his health was deteriorating rapidly and, for the first time in 50 years, he quit smoking.) Dr. Vinogradov was proven correct when Stalin died of a stroke the next year.

Arrested on November 9, 1952, before the official announcement of a plot, Vinogradov was charged with deliberately administering incorrect medical treatment to Soviet Party and government officials and of being "an old agent of British Intelligence." He was later charged as being one of Zhdanov's murderers (he had signed Zhdanov's death certificate). When Stalin was asked what should be done with his non-Jewish personal physician, he replied, "So you don't know what to do? Link him to the 'Joint.' He's a weak character . . . he'll sign anything for you." In jail, the elderly Vinogradov readily endorsed every confession he was asked to sign.

Dr. Miron S. Vovsi

Dr. Miron S. Vovsi, another giant of Soviet medicine, was a large, balding, "homely" man. He had developed a new classification for angina pectoris and had authored many scientific publications. During WWII, Major General Vovsi was head of the Red Army's Medical Division and their chief internist. He was awarded the Order of Lenin "for heroic acts during the fighting for Leningrad," and had also garnered the Red Banner of Labor, the Order of the Red Star, and other high Soviet honors.

As one of Kremlin Polyclinic's senior physicians, he treated the highest Soviet leaders. He was also a professor, department chairman, and scientific director at Basmanov Hospital and at Botkin Hospital, where both Soviet citizens and foreign diplomats were treated. By 1950, he was also directing a research team at the Institute of Therapy of the USSR Academy of Medical Science. Solomon Mikhoel's first cousin, Vovsi had also served on the JAC. Like Vinogradov, he had given testimony, probably false, during the 1938 "Doctors' Plot" trial and had been extremely vocal in demanding the accused physicians' execution.

The 55-year-old professor was arrested on November 11, 1952, and taken to Lubyanka, where the interrogations began. After being kept awake by powerful lights shining in his eyes and being repeatedly beaten, he was ordered to admit that he had been an agent of Hitler's Gestapo, the U.S. Central Intelligence Agency, and the Israeli Mossad. His captors threatened, "We'll quarter you, hang you, impale you." When he said that he could invent things to stop the beatings, his interrogator told him:

> You yourself won't need to invent anything. The MGB [security service] will provide you with every sentence of your testimony. You will have to study it carefully and to remember without any lapse all the questions and answers which the court will put to you. This case will be ready in a month or two. During this time you will be preparing yourself so that you will not compromise the investigation.

He was warned that his wife had also been arrested, and that if he did not cooperate, his small son might become an orphan. Although Dr. Vovsi survived Stalin by five years, he eventually died from a sarcoma that developed in the torture scars on his leg.

Dr. Boris Borisovich Kogan

Dr. Boris Borisovich Kogan, second-in-command at Moscow Medical Institute (Kremlin Hospital), was a famous cardiologist and internist. He had more than 100 articles and books to his credit on topics such as medical history, asthma, occupational medicine, myocardial infarctions, and social hygiene. Described by a former student as "brilliant, talented, vibrant, and alive," he was the school's most popular lecturer.

Kogan was an elegant dresser, and was chauffeured around Moscow where he associated with the Communist elite. He treated Soviet leaders at Kremlin Polyclinic and was the principal physician to Dimitrov, the Bulgarian dictator who died in 1949. He had also treated Zhdanov. Like some of his colleagues, he had testified during the 1938 "Doctors' Plot" trial. Kogan was arrested in November 1952, after which the secret police searched his apartment all night, checking for poisons, secret weapons, and incriminating documents—none were found. After Stalin died, he was released and ultimately returned to his position. Kogan died of natural causes in 1967.

The recently opened KGB/FSB archive revealed a document from March 23, 1953, in which the secret police admitted: "It is now established that the statements by Kogan and Vovsi . . . were extorted through brutality and beatings."

Dr. Lina Solomonovna Shtern

Dr. Lina Solomonovna Shtern was born in Latvia and educated in Switzerland. She had been a biochemistry professor at Geneva University before moving to the Soviet Union in 1925. A top Soviet physician-researcher and a renowned physiologist, she had developed a method of obtaining hormonally active drugs, as well as a technique that cured tuberculous meningitis. She was in great demand to present at scientific meetings, and could do so in most European languages. Shtern was the only female member of the Soviet Academy of Science and had been elected to the USSR's Medical Academy. She, too, had been active in the JAC.

Seventy years old at the time of her arrest in January 1949, Dr. Shtern spent most of her imprisonment in Lubyanka Prison. She was transferred to a punishment cell at Lefortovo Prison for 20 days of "hell," during which time she was forced to remain standing, had hallucinations, and was certain that she was going mad. She was released in 1953 and her research laboratory was ultimately restored.

Dr. Sophia Karpai

Dr. Sophia Karpai, chief of Kremlin Polyclinic's electrocardiography division, had co-authored a textbook, *Electrocardiogram Analysis*, which propelled her to her position as the country's foremost electrocardiologist. When she was arrested in the summer of 1951, her colleagues described her as still a stunning beauty at age 45, as well as a talented contralto singer.

Despite the around-the-clock interrogations she periodically endured in Lubyanka Prison, over a period of two years, she was the only Kremlin Polyclinic physician who was not coerced into admitting guilt in the "Plot." However, the incarceration and constant interrogation turned her hair gray, gave her asthma, and left her seriously ill.

Dr. Yakov G. Etinger

Dr. Yakov G. Etinger was the clinic director at First Gradskaya Hospital and professor and chairman of the Department of Internal Medicine at Stalin Medical Institute (also known as the Second Moscow Medical Institute). Colleagues described him as "an extremely bright, great diagnostician and internist who was often called in to consult on the cases of the highest ranking people in the country." Unfortunately, he also had the unhealthy habit of talking too much about politics. Arrested in December 1950 with his wife, Dr. Etinger died in prison on March 2, 1951, before the list of "doctor-plotters" was published. His adopted son, a student at Moscow University, mysteriously disappeared shortly before the arrests and was never heard from again.

Other "Saboteurs"

A number of physicians were simply added to the list of those accused and then arrested after the first announcements were made. Nearly all were Jewish and well-known, and many were associated with Kremlin Polyclinic or its ancillary facilities. In some cases, they disappeared without a trace. And, while some names are known, many others have never been recorded.

Dr. Eliazar M. Gelstein was a brilliant researcher and clinician who held the post of director of the Clinic of Internal Diseases at Moscow's Second Medical Institute for more than two decades. During WWII, he was appointed chief therapist (chief medical officer) of the Leningrad front, for which he received numerous medals and was made an Honored Scientist. Ill and slandered by the reports of "his part" in the "Doctors' Plot," he resigned from his post at the Medical Institute. He was arrested in 1953 and died a broken man in 1955.

Dr. Yakov L. Rapoport was an anatomical pathologist who headed a research laboratory at the prestigious Institute of Morphology and chaired the Pathology Department of First Gradskaya Hospital, one of the oldest and largest hospitals in Moscow. A Communist Party member, he would later write a book describing this shameful episode in Soviet history from the victims' perspectives.

Arrest, Prison, and Interrogation

Boris Pasternak, one of the few Jewish writers to survive Stalin's purges, described the climate Soviet citizens endured during this period in his book, *Dr. Zhivago*:

> One day Lara went out and did not come back. She must have been arrested in the street, as so often happened in those days, and she died or vanished somewhere, forgotten as a nameless number on a list that was afterwards mislaid, in one of the innumerable mixed or women's concentration camps in the north.

At midnight on February 2, 1953, the secret police arrested Dr. Yakov Rapoport at his home. They preferred making arrests between 11 P.M. and 3 A.M. to increase their victims' terror, often hauling them away in black vans ("Black Ravens") which were labeled "meat" or "milk." Dr. Rapoport was taken to Lubyanka Prison, one of three Moscow prisons used for "politicals" (the dreaded Lefortovo and the "special section" of Butyrka were the other two), where officials performed a cavity search on the elderly professor.

The fortress-like Lubyanka, on Dzerzhinsky Square (named for *Cheka's* founder, Felix Dzerzhinsky), served simultaneously as a prison from which few ever emerged, and as the Moscow headquarters of the Soviet secret police. One hundred prisoners were often crammed into cells designed for 25. At the height of the Great Terror, up to 200 people a day were shot in its grim cellars. One person described Lubyanka as having the "atmosphere of a front-line hospital—screams, groans, broken bodies, stretchers."

Dr. Rapoport described what he saw of Lubyanka:

[I] was led by a guard through some inner corridors and staircases to my cell . . . I felt I had seen [it] before—but where? It was a square yard enclosed by four walls, four stories high. Metal netting was stretched over the yard at the level of each floor, and a gallery some two meters wide ran along the perimeter of the square on each floor. Along the edge of the gallery ran iron banisters to which the interfloor [anti-suicide] netting was attached. A multitude of doors, now closed, looked onto the gallery. They obviously led to cells . . . I had seen it in a Soviet film about a revolt in America's Sing-Sing Prison . . .

A door was opened, and I was led into a solitary cell. Its furnishings consisted on an iron bedstead covered with a thin mattress and a little table with an aluminum bowl, an enamel mug, and a spoon—standard prisoner issue. The cell was narrow—about a meter and a half wide and no more than three meters long. In the wall opposite the door, high up near the ceiling, was a small grilled window with a sloping sill cut through the thickness of the wall. To the right of the door was a radiator, also covered by a grille, which issued barely perceptible heat. And—the cell was quite posh—opposite the bed there was a trap above a tiny semi-circular sink and a cone-shaped toilet . . .

When the door of the cell closed behind me and I was alone, exhausted and driven to the limits of my endurance by the preceding events and two sleepless nights—it was the afternoon of the third day . . . [I] was immediately introduced to the meaning of "special regime." I found out I was not alone—a watchful eye followed my every movement through the peephole in the door. The eye belonged to a woman who suddenly materialized in my cell . . . She growled at me: "Get up! It's forbidden to lie down in the daytime" . . .

So I spent my first day in prison, tortured by fatigue, overwhelmed by the nightmarish events, and denied the only escape physiology dictated—protective inhibition, that is, sleep.

Dr. Rapoport's interrogation experience was milder than many of the others arrested. In political cases, prisoners generally were not told of the charges against them, but rather were encouraged to confess to anything that they considered criminal. The interrogator's first words were usually the same question used in the Spanish Inquisition: "Will you tell me the hypothesis you have formed of the reason for your arrest?"

If they were reluctant to confess after a few interviews, some prisoners were "softened up" before interrogation. For example, Jozsef Lengyel, a Hungarian writer, was taken from the ordinary cell in which 275 men lived "on, between and under 25 iron bedsteads" and placed for two weeks in a "hermetically closed space." When he returned to his original cell, his former companions did not recognize him. At Lubyanka, others were sent to the "kennel"—a heated basement cell, about 15 feet square, with no ventilation except a slit under the door—for a week or more. All inmates put in the "Black Hole" suffered from eczema, nausea, and palpitations.

After 24 hours, Dr. Rapoport was transferred to the infamous Lefortovo Prison, which was worse than Lubyanka. As he said, "I was gripped by fear. Lefortovo had a terrible reputation, the worst of all the Moscow prisons. It was believed that nobody ever left it alive, that the very fact of confinement there was tantamount to a death sentence." Indeed, prisoners who refused to sign a confession were taken to Lefortovo for further "inducements."

The nightly interrogation sessions focused on two main themes: Jewish bourgeois nationalism and his participation in terrorist acts perpetrated by the fictional organization of killer doctors. Dr. Rapoport was grilled about his writings, his speeches, and his work; the interrogator had a two-volume dossier on his subject. After repeatedly refusing to sign a confession, he was placed in handcuffs that were designed to tighten with any sudden movement. This went on for weeks, during which time he got almost no sleep.

One evening, his interrogator asked him technical medical questions related to severe illness. He was also asked who were the best specialists to treat the problems; they were all in jail as part of the "conspiracy." Later, he discovered that Drs. Miron Vovsi and Eliazar Gelstejn had been asked the same questions, obviously about Stalin's illness. After this incident, the interrogations continued, but "the investigator grew lazy, [and] was less emphatic in his questions."

On March 14, five days after Stalin's funeral, Dr. Rapoport was briefly transferred back to Lubyanka Prison. There, he met with a general who commented that "the 'professor' did not look like one at all: closely cropped hair, unshaven, a long nose on a shrunken face, dressed in a prison robe with no buttons, a crumpled jacket also without buttons, loose trousers barely held up by one remaining button." The general said to him, "Yakov Lvovich [the familiar form of his name], please forget what happened at the interrogation. You know, anything can happen during an investigation." Subsequently, prison life eased quite a bit. In retrospect, Dr. Rapoport believed that this prison time was to restore him to a semblance of his pre-incarceration appearance before his release. Nevertheless, he weighed 31 pounds less on his release than when he entered prison.

Finally, on April 3, 1953, he was again transferred to Lubyanka in his civilian clothes. He was told by another general, "Well, I had you brought here to inform you that you have been completely exonerated and will be released today." "This news was too much for me," wrote Dr. Rapoport, "and I broke into tears. All the bitterness of the past months and the shock of this unexpected finale found release in those tears."

The general continued: "I have arranged for you to be brought home by car . . . Give your family a call from the downstairs telephone to let them know you're coming." Before he left the prison, they handed him a certificate stating that the charges had been dismissed and the documents that they had seized, including his passport, doctoral diploma, war medal certificates, professor certificate, and Party card.

Torture Methods

Not everyone in secret police custody was as lucky as Dr. Rapoport. On January 29, 1936, a coded telegram from Stalin, who was fond of "physical methods," officially gave permission to the secret police to torture prisoners to obtain confessions. On January 20, 1939, the order was passed down to regional party committees. It read:

> The Party Central Committee explains that application of methods of physical pressure in NKVD practice is permissible from 1937 on, in accordance with permission of the Party Central Committee . . . It is known that all bourgeois intelligence services use methods of physical influence against the representatives of the socialist proletariat and that they use them in their most scandalous forms.
>
> The question arises as to why the socialist intelligence service should be more humanitarian against the mad agents of the bourgeoisie, against the deadly enemies of the working class and of the collective farm workers. The Party Central Committee considers that physical pressure should still be used obligatorily, as an exception applicable to known and obstinate enemies of the people, as a method both justifiable and appropriate.

The bizarre Stalinist legal code required that the accused confess to their crimes—even if they were innocent. According to Khrushchev:

> When Stalin said that one or another should be arrested, it was necessary to accept on faith that he was an "enemy of the people" . . . What proofs were offered? The confessions of the arrested, and the investigative

judges accepted these "confessions." [sic] And how is it possible that a person confesses to crimes which he has not committed? Only in one way—because of application of physical methods of pressuring him, tortures, bringing him to a state of unconsciousness, deprivation of his judgment, taking away of his human dignity. In this manner were "confessions" acquired.

Both male and female prisoners were typically beaten, often with sandbags. When the injuries were fatal, police physicians would certify that the person had died "from cancer." Another method was the *stoika*, in which a prisoner was forced to stand on tiptoe against a wall for several hours or more or was placed in a "standing cell" that only allowed that position. One or two days of this would break nearly any prisoner. More mundane was sleep deprivation, with police teams interrogating a prisoner without interruption for hours or days. A week of this treatment without food or sleep was enough to break even those who resisted physical torture.

Sometimes interrogators would combine the two methods. Prisoners, including some of the doctors, would be forced to stand for 18 hours a day, with interrogation lasting 16 of those hours. During the 6-hour "sleep period," guards pounded on the door every 10 minutes, at which time prisoners had to jump to their feet and say a specified phrase, such as "Detainee No. 1473 reports: strength one detainee, everything in order."

One prisoner wrote:

> Cold, hunger, the bright light and especially sleeplessness. The cold is not terrific. But when the victim is weakened by hunger and by sleeplessness, then the six or seven degrees above freezing point make him tremble all the time. During the night I had only one blanket . . . After two or three weeks, I was in a semi-conscious state. After fifty or sixty interrogations with cold and hunger and almost no sleep, a man becomes like an automaton—his eyes are bright, his legs swollen, his hands trembling. In this state he is often convinced he is guilty.

Interrogators tormented prisoners by feeding them salty food and depriving them of liquids. Other methods included tying them in contorted positions, ripping out nails, breaking bones, urinating on them, extinguishing cigarettes on their skin, or beating them with truncheons over their kidneys or genitals. According to historian Robert Conquest:

> Needles, pincers, and so on are sporadically reported, and more specialized implements seem to have been in use at the Lefortovo. But on the whole some appearance of spontaneity was maintained. Feet and

fingers were stamped on. Broken-off chair legs were the usual weapon for beatings, which were distinguished from "torture." But as one very experienced prisoner says, this distinction was rather absurd when a man came back after such a beating with broken ribs, urinating blood for a week, or with a permanently injured spine and unable to walk.

They also used psychological torture, such as threatening prisoners with guns, directing other prisoners to describe the horrors of physical torture, or playing recordings of others moaning—sometimes they were told it was their spouse. When physical and psychological torture was not sufficient, prisoners, including the doctors in this case, were fed meals laced with scopolamine, a sedative that causes nightmares.

To emphasize that they meant business—as if it could be doubted, given their methods—MGB guards were stationed outside the homes of family members. The doctors were warned that if they did not cooperate, their families would "suffer." Writing about the "Doctors' Plot" case, Khrushchev later recalled:

> Stalin was crazy with rage, yelling at Ignatiev and threatening him, demanding that he throw the doctors in chains, beat them to a pulp, and grind them into powder. It was no surprise when almost all the doctors confessed to their crimes. I can't blame them for slandering themselves.

Both *Pravda* and *Izvestia* reported that all the doctors had admitted their guilt in this "Plot." This is not surprising, given the methods used to get them to confess.

The Aftermath

On the last sentient evening of his life, Stalin repeatedly asked his henchmen about the case's progress—and specifically about Dr. Vinogradov, who had been his personal physician. Secret police chief Lavrenty Beria told him, "Apart from his other unfavorable qualities, the professor has a very long tongue. He has told one of the doctors in his clinic that comrade Stalin has already had several dangerous hypertensive episodes." "Right," said Stalin. "What do you propose to do now? Have the doctors confessed? Tell Ignatiev that if he doesn't get full confessions out of them, we'll reduce his height by a head." "They'll confess," Beria replied. "With the help of Timashuk and other patriots, we'll complete the investigation and come to you for permission to arrange a public trial." "Arrange it," Stalin grunted.

Later that night, on March 1, 1953, Joseph Stalin had a massive stroke; he died on March 5. This immediately aborted the doctors' trial, which was to begin the next day. Stalin's minions, including Khrushchev, quickly tried to distance themselves from the stigma of the enormous pogrom they had helped plan. Russian leaders had always tried to divert attention away from their failures by whipping up anti-Semitic hysteria; this time it failed only because of Stalin's sudden demise and the new leadership's need to jockey for power.

On April 3, 1953, agent-provocateur Timashuk's Order of Lenin was rescinded after the Presidium of the Supreme Soviet determined, "in view of the true circumstances coming to light," that it had been "incorrectly awarded." She then resumed her old job at Kremlin Polyclinic among those she had denounced, seemingly not at all disturbed by the disaster she had precipitated. Subsequently, she was awarded the Order of the Red Banner of Labor, second only to the Order of Lenin.

In an event that startled foreign observers, Beria announced on April 4, 1953, that the "Doctors' Plot" was bogus and that the erstwhile "criminals" would be released. A list naming the 15 arrested physicians was finally made public. *Pravda* reported that the case against the doctors had been reexamined and that the charges were false. It said, in part, that the physicians accused "of wrecking, espionage and terrorist activities against the active leaders of the Soviet Government [had been] unlawfully arrested by the former Minister of State Security of the USSR, without any legal basis." It went on to say that the confessions had been obtained using "unacceptable means."

Two days later, on April 6, *Pravda* went even farther, railing against the "despicable adventurers" who accused the good doctors "by means of a case they themselves had fabricated to foment in Soviet society . . . feelings of national hostility . . . [and] tried to kindle feelings of racial hatred." The paper also criticized the Medical Commission for not investigating the medical cases of the alleged victims and for simply signing "false accusations against a group of medical leaders." The same day, *Pravda's* lead editorial described the just-released doctors as "honest and esteemed figures of our State" and extolled the late Solomon Mikhoels as "that honest public figure and People's Artist of the USSR who has been shamelessly slandered."

The doctors, except for those who had died under torture, and many wives who had also been incarcerated were exonerated and freed. They were admonished to "forget everything" and to keep quiet about their experiences. Most were able to return to their prior positions, although local Party officials continued to harass many over their alleged involvement in the "Plot."

The accelerating official anti-Semitism slowed and, in 1954, Ministry of State Security official M. D. Ryumin and some police officers involved in the case were executed for fabricating evidence against the physicians. Plans to deport Russian Jews, already discussed in the Politburo, were dropped.

In his Secret Speech to the Twentieth Communist Party Congress on February 25, 1956, Khrushchev revealed that Stalin had personally ordered that the bogus cases against the doctors be developed as the beginning of a new purge. Khrushchev later wrote that "the so-called Doctors' Plot . . . was a shameful business . . . a cruel and contemptible thing." Summing up Stalin's career, Khrushchev said:

> There are those who argue that Stalin was motivated by his concern for the well-being of the people and not selfishness. This is crazy. While concerned for the interests of the people, he was exterminating the best sons of the people! . . . It's always a complicated thing to argue for the acquittal of a mass murderer.

Epilogue

The Soviet physicians accused of multiple murders were innocent of those charges—unlike the other physicians in this book. However, many people in both Russia and the West still believe that they were serial killers. As Adolf Hitler said, "The great masses of the people . . . will more easily fall victims to a big lie than to a small one."

The popular media and historical writers, swayed by misinformation and Stalinist sympathies, have perpetuated these lies. These include the 1941 book, *Mission to Moscow*, written by the former U.S. ambassador to Moscow, Joseph E. Davies, and the infamous movie of the same name. John Dewey, who led the American commission investigating the trials, said that this movie was "the first instance in our country of totalitarian propaganda—a propaganda which falsifies history through distortion, omission or pure invention of facts." Cable channels still show this movie, thus continuing to slander these doctors. Hopefully, this chapter will help to rehabilitate the memories of these leaders of their medical communities.

Stalin's Ignoble Death

By the late 1940s, Stalin's mental health had begun to deteriorate, his memory was failing, and his fear of physical debility and death had increased. Yugoslav diplomat Milovan Djilas described the aging Stalin as having "quite a large paunch, and his hair was sparse though his scalp was not completely bald. His face was white, with ruddy cheeks . . . His teeth were black and irregular, turned inward. Not even his moustache was thick or firm."

His paranoia was such that Khrushchev heard him say in 1951 that "I'm finished. I trust no one, not even myself." On January 12, 1953, the night before the new "Doctors' Plot" was announced in the media, Stalin attended a performance at the Bolshoi Theater. A member of the Polish troupe who performed described Stalin as seeming "very old and 'gaga.'" It would be his last public appearance.

After a typical late night with colleagues that lasted into the early morning of March 1, 1953, Stalin failed to emerge from his quarters. His servants were afraid to disturb him and only dared to enter Stalin's rooms late that evening. A bodyguard found the exalted leader lying on the floor, semiconscious and soaked in his own urine. Rather than immediately getting medical help, they put him on a sofa and summoned Politburo members who decided that Stalin's snoring noises meant that he was "sleeping peacefully." Actually, some believe that these politicians may have tampered with Stalin's anticoagulant medication to help cause his stroke. In any event, no doctors were summoned until the following morning.

Once involved, physicians from the Moscow Academy of Medical Sciences used extraordinary, and sometimes bizarre, methods to save his life. After Stalin was transferred to his Kuntsevo *dacha*, neurosurgeon and "reanimationist" Dr. Galina Chesnokova worked non-stop for three days using leeches, along with accepted medical methods, trying to cure him. Ironically, some of the prestigious doctors who had been arrested in the "Doctors' Plot," and were still in jail, were consulted about the case. They only learned who the patient was after their release.

Stalin never spoke again and, at 9:50 P.M. on March 5, 1953, according to his daughter, he died "a difficult and terrible death." His body was immediately embalmed at the Lenin Mausoleum and then lay in state in Moscow's Hall of Columns. For the millions of soviet citizens who had never known another leader, news of his death came as a shock. (In a tragic postscript, 500 people were crushed in the crowd trying to view his corpse.) Stalin's funeral was held on March 9 and his body was put on display in the Lenin Mausoleum.

Nikita Khrushchev succeeded his former mentor. He formally denounced Stalin on February 25, 1956. His demeaning comparisons between Stalin and Lenin during his four-hour "Secret Speech" at the Twentieth Congress of the Communist Party effectively ended official praise for the dead dictator. The final blow came in 1961, when Stalin's preserved corpse was removed from Lenin Mausoleum and buried. Removal of Stalin statues, portraits, and place names soon followed.

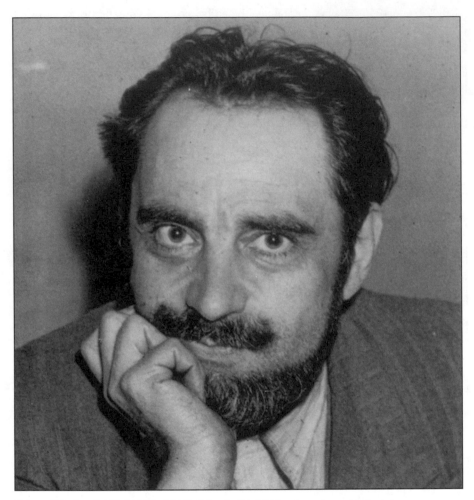

Marcel Petiot, M.D. (1897–1946), March 17, 1946. (AP/Wide World Photos)

6

French Death Trips

Marcel André Félix

"This won't hurt a bit," he said, as he plunged the
She stared plaintively at her husband and tried to be b
she needed this shot to enter Argentina. Tears welled up
realization that her family would soon be safely out of
of the German menace and able to start a new life.

She glanced at her husband, who had already had hi
well: his eyes had glazed over and he was slumping i
wrong?" she tried to ask, but the words came out garbled
ing to her? She tried to stand, but her legs wouldn't m
becoming hazy.

Dr. Petiot moved toward her, testing to see if touch
made her blink; it did. "Good," he thought, "it's better to
while she can still react." He reached for the buttons of he
nice clothes," he murmured to himself. "I don't want to d

The doctor continued stripping his victim. Her husb
an extra-heavy dose of medication; he could be left for lat
tim, Petiot thought of raping her—but there wasn't enoug
her into the triangular room and strapped her into positi
iron rings fixed into the wall. He could now watch throug
she awakened and realized her predicament. They usually
but it didn't matter, the room was soundproof.

He grew excited as he watched her awaken, her terror
roundings—and her vulnerability—sank in. Struggling v
called to her husband. "So much the better," he thought.
she wants." Moving to the husband's prostrate body, Peti
being careful to preserve the handmade suit. After binding
Petiot opened the door and dragged him into the cramped

smiled as he watched the woman's fear grow to panic, her nude, semi-
us husband at her feet. The doctor stood over him, holding a thin wire
n his hands. Crossing his hands, he looped it over her husband's neck
lled tightly. The man awakened enough to struggle as his eyes bulged
 face reddened. All resistance faded as Petiot ended his life.

azed with terror at the realization that her life and dreams were over,
tim's mind snapped as the doctor again caressed her body. "Too bad,
 of no further use to me," he said as he strangled her.

ter dragging the corpses to the kitchen in the basement, he hummed to
f as he methodically cut the bodies into small pieces and washed the
down the pipe to the sewer system below. He carried the remaining
to the furnace, where he fed them to the flames.

My wife will like the brooch that woman was wearing," he thought.

Vorld War II raged, German-occupied Paris became a dangerous place
vith collaborators, double agents, and Resistance fighters. Strange events
orrible atrocities were commonplace. Yet this tale may be the strangest,
iost ghastly, of them all.

n 1941, Dr. Marcel Petiot purchased a dilapidated three-story, nine-
i-century building that had been uninhabited since Princess Maria
redo de Mansfield had moved out in 1930. The once-elegant 15-room
ocated at 21 rue Le Sueur in a well-to-do section of Paris, also boasted
s and a courtyard. The doctor purchased the house in his son Gérard's
 for 495,000 French francs ($144,092 in 2002). (That same year, the
s transferred legal title for all of their 51 real estate properties to Gérard,
bly to avoid their seizure in the event of criminal prosecution.) The
 was a bargain; prices had dropped markedly since the German occupa-
f Paris. Strangely, although work was occasionally done on the house, all
ows facing the street remained shuttered.

On March 4, 1944, thick, greasy smoke spewed from the villa's chimney.
mount increased over the next few days. By Saturday, March 11, Jacques
ais was fed up with the nauseating stench that permeated his fifth-floor
ment across the street. But, when he went over to complain, he found a
on the door reading, "Away for one month. Forward mail to 18 rue des
bards in Auxerre." Monsieur Marçais called the police.

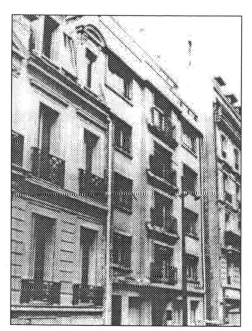

Dr. Petiot's house at 21 rue Le Sueur.

Soon, two bicycle policemen, Joseph Teyssier and Emile Fillion, arrived. There was no response when they knocked on the doors and windows, but a neighbor gave them Dr. Petiot's telephone number at his home, two miles away. When they called, his first words were, "Have you entered the building?" When told that they had not, but that there was a fire in the building, Petiot responded, "Don't do anything. I will be there in 15 minutes with the keys."

Thirty minutes later, Dr. Petiot had not appeared, so the policemen called the fire department. Fire Chief Avilla Boudringhin and several firemen entered a second-floor window. A pale and shaken Boudringhin soon exited the building. He later testified:

> After I had broken a window-pane, I entered the house and, guided by the smell, went down to the basement. Near the boiler, I saw human remains. The boiler was drawing rather noisily. It was burning human flesh. I saw a hand, at the end of a skeleton arm. It looked like a woman's hand. I made haste upstairs. I opened the street door for the police and said to them: "You'd better come and look, there's a job here for you."

The policemen then entered the basement, where they found two coal-burning stoves, one cold and the other roaring hot with a woman's hand dangling from its open door. Nearby, the bottom of a short staircase was littered with a head, skulls, arms, two nearly complete skeletons, shattered rib cages, feet, hands, jawbones, and large chunks of unrecognizable flesh. Teyssier quickly phoned his superiors.

Just then, a man arrived on a green bicycle. (Due to gasoline rationing in Paris, bicycles were a common form of transportation.) Hatless and wearing a gray overcoat, the rider was in his early forties and had dark, piercing eyes. Identifying himself as Dr. Petiot's brother, he accompanied the policemen to the basement. Viewing the human carnage without any discernible reaction, he commented, "This is serious. My head may be at stake."

As he left the building, he turned to Teyssier and Fillion and asked, "Are you Frenchmen?" Initially insulted by such a question, their attitude changed as the man explained:

> The bodies you have seen are those of Germans and traitors to our country. I assume you have already notified your superiors and that the Germans will soon learn of your discovery. I am the head of a Resistance group, and I have 300 files at my home which must be destroyed before the enemy finds them.

Officer Teyssier tipped his cap to the patriot and advised him to flee. Having been caught seemingly red-handed, Dr. Petiot climbed on his bicycle and leisurely rode away. Within a few days, the two policemen left France (and returned only after the Liberation), afraid of what both their superiors and the Germans would do to them because they had allowed the prime suspect in a serial murder case to escape.

Police superiors soon arrived and recalled the firemen to extinguish the fire in the stove so they could safely examine the building. Entering the house for a more thorough search, they found what had once been a large elegant home in nearly complete disrepair, with thick dust and cobwebs clinging to the piles of furniture, artwork, and junk that littered the premises. The main floor contained a horde of valuable antiques, museum-quality paintings, and sculpture. The two upper floors were strewn with a jumble of worthless goods.

The only clean and orderly spots were the doctor's office and the basement kitchen. The office was situated in a cramped L-shaped passageway, crammed between a staircase, a storeroom, and the stable. It contained a cabinet of medical supplies, a desk, a small round table, and two armchairs.

The large kitchen was designed much like a morgue. It had two sinks separated by a wooden table—one deep like a laundry tub and the other a longer, shallow sink into which a body might fit. The floor had a large drain that, unusually, was connected directly to the main sewer, which emptied into the Seine. A body could easily be eviscerated and dissected, and the blood, organs, and small bones quickly and efficiently washed directly into the sewer. This would explain the absence of viscera and blood in the furnace room.

In the garage and outside in the stable, they found pits half-filled with quicklime and human remains. John V. Grombach described the scene at the stable in his book, *The Great Liquidator*:

> A fetid odor rose from the depths, but the light of flashlights held by police did not reveal what lay there. A ladder led down to the depths,

however, and Commissaire Massu undertook to investigate. Down he went. Below him, a festering, bubbling mass almost caused him to strangle.

He set a tentative foot on the heap at the bottom. It was quicklime, steaming foully as it devoured a measureless heap of human remains. This, then, was a real charnel house. There were many more bodies here than in the furnace room—and God only knew how many altogether. Already most of the flesh and bones was [sic] past recognition.

But the horrors continued. A policeman investigating a canvas sack left on a staircase to the basement found the left side of a human torso, missing only the head, foot, and internal organs. A stained hatchet and a shovel lay nearby.

Early Years

Marcel André Félix Petiot was born on January 17, 1897, to 30-year-old Félix Iréné Mustiole Petiot and his 22-year-old wife, Marthe Marie Constance Joséphine Bourdon, both postal/telegraph workers. Marcel later believed that he was conceived prior to their marriage. His birthplace, Auxerre, was a rural town of 30,000 people, about 100 miles south of Paris. At an early age, Petiot was sent to live with his unmarried aunt, Mme. Gaston, in the same town. He grew up comfortably in a small brick house, and rarely had any contact with his parents.

Petiot demonstrated his cruelty early. He often vivisected dogs and cats; but no animal was spared. His nursemaid, for example, once found him dipping his beloved cat's paws in a vat of boiling water. Believing him remorseful, she allowed him take his pet to bed with him. The next morning, the suffocated cat lay in Marcel's bed; he was covered with scratches. Neighbors said that he routinely stole young birds from their nests, poked out their eyes with needles, and watched enchantedly as they flung themselves against the bars of a cage.

Petiot's intelligence was also evident at an early age, as were his odd interests. He devoured books on death and sex, including the 12-volume history of Casanova and books on the famous dualist/opera singer/bisexual Mlle. Maupin and the cross-dressing spy Chevalier d'Éon. Several books on Jack the Ripper were later found in Petiot's home in Villeneuve. Petiot made indecent proposals to male classmates and once fired a pistol at the ceiling in class. He was even found throwing knives, circus-style, around a schoolboy standing against a door. Luckily for both of them, he was amazingly accurate. Between the ages of 10 and 12, he saw a physician because of his sleepwalking, seizures, and bedwetting.

His mother died when he was 15 years old, and Petiot's behavior worsened. He was repeatedly expelled from schools for unruly behavior. In February 1914, he was caught stealing mail. Examined by a court-appointed psychiatrist, he was found to be "an abnormal youth suffering from personal and hereditary problems, which limit to a large degree his responsibility for his acts." Accordingly, the court found that "the accused appears to be mentally ill," and the charges were dropped. Petiot continued to be expelled from schools until, finally, he received his degree from a special school in Paris on July 10, 1915.

Six months later, with World War I raging, Petiot volunteered for the French Army. He wanted to serve in the medical corps since he planned to be a doctor, but, instead, was assigned to the Eighty-ninth Infantry Regiment and sent to the front in November 1916. On May 20, 1917, during bitter fighting, a hand grenade left a 7 cm.-long (almost 3″) gash on the top of his left foot and he was exposed to poison gas.

Ironically, he was sent to a local insane asylum that was being used as an acute care hospital. His foot healed well, but he began to demonstrate mental symptoms which would keep him confined to rest homes and clinics for almost a year. After a short incarceration for stealing blankets, he was sent to the psychiatric hospital at Fleury-les Aubrais. A physician there diagnosed him with "mental disequilibrium, neurasthenia, mental depression, melancholia, obsessions and phobias" and concluded that Petiot could not be held responsible for his actions.

Nevertheless, Petiot was returned to the front in June 1918. He soon had a nervous breakdown and shot himself in the foot; for the next year, he was in and out of psychiatric hospitals. In March 1919, a psychiatrist at the Rennes military hospital recommended that Petiot be discharged from the army due to neurasthenia, amnesia, mental unbalance, sleepwalking, severe depression, paranoia, and suicidal tendencies.

The French *Commission de Réforme* that governed pensions and discharges agreed and released Petiot from the army on July 4, 1919, with a 40 percent disability. This was increased to 100 percent disability a year later when the *Commission* psychiatrist confirmed the previous findings and determined that Petiot was unable to perform any physical or intellectual work. He suggested that he might best be placed in a psychiatric hospital for continuous observation. The following year, Petiot's grandmother testified before another board, saying, "My grandson was a very strange child. From an early age he was extremely intelligent but told exaggerated stories about himself and his importance."

Petiot, meanwhile, had completed an accelerated medical school didactic program designed for veterans in only eight months. He received his degree from the *Faculté de Médecine de Paris* on December 15, 1921, and spent the next two years in clinical training, assigned to the very hospitals in which he had earlier been confined with a diagnosis of "dementia praecox" (schizophrenia). He had, as his lifelong friend René-Gustave Nézondet believed, achieved his goal: a position with power over life and death.

Petiot continued to receive annual psychiatric examinations, under protest, through 1923. Although he was having seizures about twice a month, his disability payments were decreased by half. Petiot continued to draw his Army disability until his execution in 1946.

Life as a Country Doctor

The new doctor moved to the historic village of Villeneuve-sur-Yonne, only 25 miles from his birthplace, to set up practice. Villeneuve was an old fortress town and contained a royal residence built in 1163, although the original village had been established before the Romans arrived. Surrounded by a high wall and a moat, and complete with a drawbridge and watchtowers, Villeneuve had become the capital of Yonne.

Two elderly physicians served the 4,200 townspeople. Petiot immediately upstaged them by distributing leaflets proclaiming:

> Dr. Petiot is young, and only a young doctor can keep up to date on the latest methods born of a progress which marches with giant strides. Petiot treats, but does not exploit his patients.

An astute diagnostician, he seemed to be as good as his word. He treated people well, listened sympathetically, kept office hours on Sundays, and charged the indigent a minimal fee. What his patients didn't know was that he had enrolled them in "Medical Assistance" (public aid), and thus was paid at least once for each patient—and twice for many.

Many of Petiot's prescriptions were for potent narcotics, what Villeneuve pharmacist and sometimes mayor Paul Mayaud referred to as "horse cures." When the strong doses were questioned, Petiot's true nature emerged. Responding to a pharmacist's query about a child's prescription that was sufficient to kill an adult, Petiot replied, "What difference does it make to you anyway? Isn't it better to do away with this kid who's not doing anything in the world but pestering its mother?"

Petiot was an austere and private person, and lived modestly, even shabbily. He abstained from smoking and drinking, and avoided the cafés that were at the center of the town's social life. His primary distraction was his light-yellow sports car, which he would drive at night without headlights. This practice caused dozens of accidents and, eventually, the car lost its bumpers, mudguards, and paint. He read voraciously, consuming up to 300 pages an hour of police stories and pulp fiction, and often quoted long passages from memory. The doctor had few friends; those who knew him described him as scornful of other people, institutions, sickness, danger, life, and the law. The ancients described this viewpoint as "solipsism," a belief that everything outside oneself is illusory and exists only to fulfill one's needs—not a particularly good attitude for a physician.

People noted another oddity: Dr. Petiot was a kleptomaniac who constantly stole small things of no importance and for which he had no use. He also defrauded his landlords out of an antique stove worth F25,000, replacing it with an imitation. When they threatened him with a lawsuit, Petiot replied that he was a certified lunatic and couldn't be held responsible for his actions.

It is unlikely that he could have successfully used this defense in court, however. But this was not to be tested: Police did not adequately investigate the disappearance of his 26-year-old, apparently pregnant, housekeeper-mistress, Louisette Delaveau, in mid-May 1926. At the time, police received a report that Petiot was seen loading a large trunk into his car, but they did not investigate. Just such a trunk, with the decapitated and unidentifiable corpse of a young woman, was subsequently found on an abandoned farm outside town.

Petiot's Political Career

Petiot once told an acquaintance, "To succeed in life, one must have a fortune or a powerful position. One must want to dominate those who might cause one problems, and impose one's will on them."

With his medical practice thriving, he was now ready to gain more power, so he entered the mayoral race as a Socialist (a major political party in France) candidate. He was an excellent speaker who could enthrall crowds, and had a natural edge in the election, since many of the townspeople were his satisfied patients. However, he could not avoid skullduggery. Near the end of the campaign, he arranged to be the first speaker at a large gathering. After he finished, at exactly 9:45 P.M., an accomplice short-circuited the town's electricity, plunging the area into darkness and silencing the microphone his opponent was about to use. On July 25, 1926, Petiot became Villeneuve-sur-Yonne's mayor in a landslide victory.

His opponent, Monsieur Gandy, complained that Petiot had boasted of feigning mental illness to escape the army with a pension. The *Commission de Réforme* reviewed its findings and confirmed that they had certified the new mayor as, essentially, a part-time lunatic:

> The very fact mentioned by Monsieur Gandy—the alleged admission of a fraud perpetrated to obtain a pension—is but another manifestation of the subject's mentally unbalanced state . . .
>
> This form of mental disorder can very easily escape detection by lay persons who are inclined, as Monsieur Gandy, to attribute the same significance to the words and actions of someone mentally ill as they would to those of a perfectly normal individual.
>
> In addition, to fully appreciate this sort of infirmity, one must take into consideration the fact that in the course of its evolution, the affliction can show rather long periods of remission which might lead lay persons to believe it has actually been cured.

Although theft, mismanagement, autocracy, and many other irregularities characterized Mayor Petiot's tenure, the townspeople and, in particular, the town council continued to support him. Some years later, Dr. Eugène Duran would testify about Petiot:

> [He] was a politician to the depths of his soul, knowing how to flatter the people and make them love him. Nonetheless, his altruism was but an appearance, since his overriding passions were money and personal power. He was very intelligent, but had occasional mental lapses which made him seem truly abnormal . . . He was never honest as a mayor, as a doctor, or as an individual.

For a while, Petiot's private life seemed to settle down. On June 4, 1927, he married Georgette Valentine Lablais, the "lovely and petite" 23-year old daughter of a wealthy local landowner and Parisian restaurateur. The following April, their only child, Gérard Georges Claude Félix Petiot, was born. But trouble was not gone for long.

On January 29, 1930, a local court sentenced him to three months in prison and imposed a F200 fine for attempted fraud. Although he received a suspended sentence due to his mental condition, Petiot temporarily lost his mayoral post because of the conviction.

Petiot's legal troubles continued. On March 11, 1930, Henriette Debauve, the wife of the local dairy cooperative's director, was found murdered in her burning home. The house had been robbed while her husband was away collecting the cooperative's monthly earnings. Police found muddy footprints leading toward the village. A few weeks later, a Monsieur Fiscot told neighbors that he was going to tell the police that he had seen Mayor Petiot near the Debauve home at the time of the murder. Before he could notify them, however, Petiot persuaded the man, who suffered from severe arthritis, to come to his office for a miraculous new medicine from Paris. Fiscot died three hours after receiving the injection. Petiot signed the death certificate, stating that the death was due to an aneurysm.

Mme. Debauve's murder remained unsolved. Police investigating the rue Le Sueur deaths did not find the case file until after Petiot's 1946 trial and, as *Commissaire* Massu commented, "By then no one particularly cared whether he had murdered one person more or less."

In mid-July 1931, a routine audit of the town's records found sufficient irregularities to again remove Petiot from his mayoral position. As he had before, Petiot blamed his "political enemies." Demonstrating their loyalty, the town council members all resigned. Petiot ran for mayor again later in the year, but was defeated. By then, however, he had been elected as a "General Councilor" for the entire Yonne region, a position comparable to that of a U.S. Congressman. A modern student of the Petiot case, Pierre Maniere, wrote that while in that position, Petiot was

> dynamic, conscientious, attentive to all departmental problems and particularly to those concerning his electors. [He presented] a sympathetic and reassuring image—one that he maintained throughout his participation in the departmental assembly and that hardly led one to suspect any hidden Machiavellianism in his character.

Unable to stay out of trouble, Petiot was convicted on July 19, 1933, of altering an electric meter to obtain free power. Even though the 15-day jail sentence and F100 fine were suspended, this effectively ended his political career. He was officially removed as General Councilor on October 17, 1933, although he continued to list this position on his résumé.

Medical Practice in Paris

His political career ruined, Petiot moved to Paris with his family to resume his medical career. He bought an apartment in a busy commercial district on rue Caumartin, where he spent several months starting a practice.

As in Villeneuve-sur-Yonne, Petiot printed leaflets with exaggerated credentials and claims and placed them in every mailbox in the area. He asserted that he could: provide painless childbirth, drug cures, and pain relief for a variety of disorders; remove tattoos, scars, and tumors; and cure fungi, goiters, anemia, obesity, diabetes, arthritis, tuberculosis, ulcers, syphilis, arteriosclerosis, heart and liver disease, and, even, fatigue. These claims were so outlandish that, during his murder trial, the court president commented, "This is the prospectus of a quack!" To which Petiot replied, "Thanks for the advertising." Nonetheless, Petiot again acquired a large and devoted cadre of patients. When French police later interviewed nearly 2,000 of them, they had only high praise for the doctor's selfless devotion.

During the next several years, he was the subject of multiple investigations for violating the narcotics laws, for possibly performing illegal abortions, and for possibly stealing F74,000 from a patient's desk while in the home to pronounce him dead. There was also the unusual death of a 30-year-old woman who had been given anesthesia in his office. Raymonde Hanss had come to have an abscess drained, but, when she never awakened from the anesthetic, Petiot drove her to her home, where she died a few hours later. Although the coroner found an enormous amount of morphine in her body, the case was dismissed.

On April 4, 1936, Petiot became embroiled in serious legal difficulties over a relatively minor incident. After being caught absentmindedly walking out of a bookstore with a book under his arm, Petiot threatened the store detective, tried to strangle him, and then fled. The detective filed a complaint with police and, since Petiot had given the detective his correct name, they were able to track him down.

Petiot eventually turned himself in at the police station, and offered a rambling letter stating that he had been wandering despondently through the bookstore while working out the details of a machine to cure chronic constipation, as well as plans for a perpetual-motion machine "based on a very simple principle and which will run until the end of time." The police found his behavior, not to mention the letter, peculiar and even dangerous, so they ordered a psychiatric examination. The psychiatrist, Dr. Ceillier, found the agitated, sobbing Petiot to be not only depressed but also "dangerous to himself and others." This was sufficient to involuntarily commit him to a psychiatric hospital. Petiot would later say of this episode, "You never know how mad you are. It's all a matter of comparison."

Georgette Petiot arranged for her husband to be placed in a private facility rather than the state mental hospital. Petiot believed that he could dupe the easygoing director, Dr. Achille Delmas, and he was correct. As soon as the legal charges were dropped, he convinced Delmas, who had initially diagnosed Petiot as manic-depressive, that he was sane. Delmas petitioned the court to allow Petiot's release. The court-appointed psychiatrist found Petiot to be "chronically unbalanced" but suitable for release. Nevertheless, Petiot remained incarcerated for reasons that are unclear. After he sent letters complaining about unjust and inhumane treatment to the judge, the prosecutor, and even the president of France, the court appointed three well-known psychiatrists to examine him and determine whether he should be released.

All three found that Petiot's version of the events did not correlate with the objective facts, thus "leading to strong doubts as to his good faith at any point during this affair." For example, despite his multiple run-ins with the law, Petiot claimed he had never before had any legal difficulties. When questioned about Raymonde Hanss's death, he replied by disparaging both her and her mother. The psychiatrists believed that Petiot had lied to them and feigned mental illness for his own benefit:

> But in our present report . . . the aim . . . was to present the true nature of Petiot, who is an individual without scruples and devoid of all moral sensibility . . . This picture of an amoral and unbalanced person . . . deemed that Petiot was no more or less sick, no different than he had been throughout his life, and, we might add, from what he shall be for the rest of it.

Despite their conclusions, the psychiatrists found that Petiot did not meet the criteria for involuntary commitment. However, they stated that if he committed additional criminal acts, he should not be allowed to use the insanity defense. (He never did.) Seven months later, on February 20, 1937, Petiot was released from the psychiatric hospital.

For the next several years, the doctor was not accused of any wrongdoing except for cheating on his income tax. In 1938, for example, he had an income approaching F500,000 (more than $100,000 in 2002), of which he declared only F29,700. He deducted office expenses from that amount, and paid taxes on only F13,100 (about $2,600 in 2002). Despite the passionate, and often ridiculously perjurious, defense he presented, Petiot was finally convicted of fraud and had to pay the F25,000 fine.

A Gruesome Discovery

After police discovered the ghastly scene at the rue Le Sueur house, they called *Commissaire* George Massu. Thirty-three-year-old Massu had only recently been promoted to chief of the *Brigade Criminel* (homicide squad) of the *Police Judiciaire*, the detective unit for Paris that paralleled the *Sûreté Nationale* in the rest of France. Although young, the *Commissaire* had already made 3,257 arrests during his career. At about 9:30 P.M., he was awakened to participate in what he later called "the greatest criminal affair of the century."

Other than the peculiar location and extraordinary neatness of the consulting room in the midst of a chaotically filthy residence, nothing more seemed out of place—with the exception of the body parts, of course—until police made a startling discovery: A narrow corridor joined the office to a triangular room, just six feet at its base with two eight-foot sides. The room appeared to have two entrances: the one from the passageway and, opposite to it, a double door with an adjacent electric doorbell. The wooden door appeared to exit onto the street, but, after police forced it open, they found only a solid wall behind it with the wires from the doorbell dangling uselessly behind the jamb. The door from the corridor had no inside handle. Except for a naked light bulb hanging from the ceiling, the empty room had only one functional apparatus: eight heavy iron rings firmly attached to one wall.

Searching for clues, a policeman ripped off some wallpaper and discovered an eyepiece similar to those used to identify visitors in a hotel or apartment. The other end of the viewer was situated about six feet above the floor in the adjacent stable, and it was perfectly positioned to observe the face of someone restrained within the iron rings. Massu came to believe that Petiot had lured unsuspecting victims, possibly patients sedated with drugs or gas, into the nearly soundproof chamber. Then he probably lashed them between the iron rings and watched as they struggled to get free.

Police later talked with the construction workers and two masons who had built the triangular room and a wall around the courtyard in October 1941. A friendly Petiot had told them that the room would be used after the war for electrotherapy and that he planned to monitor the patients through the spy hole. The masons had charged Petiot F14,458 ($4,209 in 2002) to build his torture chamber.

When police interviewed Victor Avenelle, a professor of Romance languages who lived at 23 rue Le Sueur, he said that he frequently heard muffled, terrifying cries for help coming from 21 rue Le Sueur, always at about

11:30 P.M. Other neighbors had also heard such cries, always between 10 P.M. and midnight. They had all decided that because of the Occupation and the possibility that the Gestapo was involved (the French Gestapo headquarters was located only a few blocks away), they should ignore it. As was frequently said, "The best policy in occupied Paris was to hear nothing, see nothing, and mind one's own business."

Massu and his men diligently searched the consulting room for needles, drugs, and gas that could have been used to sedate the victims; none were found. At 1:30 A.M., as the police were preparing to leave, Massu received a telegram from headquarters: "Order from German authorities. Arrest Petiot. Dangerous lunatic."

The message was clear; however, the police in occupied Paris operated under rules meant to aid, whenever possible, the *Maquis* (the French Resistance, made up of men and women who secretly battled the Germans and French collaborators in their homeland during World War II). Whenever German authorities showed an interest in a case, Parisian police would display almost farcical behavior, including delays, omissions, and mistakes. Rather than spurring Massu to action, the Germans' order encouraged him to declare that he was too tired to pursue the case just then, and to instruct the two inspectors with him to wait until morning to investigate further.

The next morning, the police continued their delaying tactics by investigating minor, irrelevant details of the case. Finally, late in the morning, they went to the doctor's rue Caumartin apartment, where the concierge's 12-year-old daughter, Alice Denis, said that she had not seen Dr. and Mme. Petiot since 9:30 the prior evening. They knocked on the apartment door and found it unlocked and empty; the bed looked as if it had not been slept in.

In reality, the Petiots had left just 30 minutes before the police arrived; Mme. Petiot had persuaded Alice to lie about their movements. The Germans told Massu that they were astonished that Petiot was not yet in custody. He replied that he could not understand their reaction, since he had obtained files indicating that the Germans had incarcerated Petiot for eight months but had recently released him. Massu's indifference was soon replaced with real police work, however, when he realized that Petiot's crimes had not been committed in the name of France, but were, instead, of a very personal nature. Unfortunately, by that time the police had lost the trail—Petiot had vanished.

On Monday, March 13, banner headlines in every French newspaper screamed the sensational findings at the rue Le Sueur house. Reporters blindly estimated that as many as 60 women had been killed and butchered in the home. They claimed that Petiot was a drug addict, an abortionist, a sadist, and a lunatic, and dubbed him the "new Landru." (Henri Désiré Landru, known as "Bluebeard," had been guillotined in 1922 for seducing and murdering at least ten women for personal gain and killing one boy, and then burning their corpses in his kitchen stove. At the time, he was happily married and had a young mistress.) Reporters concocted bizarre schemes as to how Petiot enticed and then killed his victims. Some even claimed that the women had been made to stand in the quicklime pit, slowly dissolving while alive. The Petiot case quickly became the primary topic of Parisian conversation.

Police continued to search the rue Le Sueur house, finding a jumble of personal items that included 22 used toothbrushes, 7 pairs of eyeglasses, 15 women's combs, 9 fingernail files, and 5 gas masks. Only a few items, however, had markings that could be used by police to identify their owners. These included a black satin evening gown embroidered with golden swallows that retained its manufacturer's label, a man's white shirt with the initials "K. K." inexpertly removed, and a distinctive hat made by a Parisian designer.

Most of the human remains were taken to the *Institut Médico-Légal,* the world's first scientific forensic laboratory. Police hired four gravediggers from Passy Cemetery for the gruesome task of sifting the quicklime piles for additional body parts. All remains were examined by the *Institut*'s forensic team led by Dr. Albert Paul, a noted expert "whose macabre humor and love of morbid detail made him as popular at social affairs as in court." Assisted by two physical anthropologists, the team spent several months trying to piece together the remains to determine the number, gender, age, and, if possible, the identity of the victims. So much material was missing, however, that in their 150-page report they could only guess what had occurred.

The team determined that there had been at least ten victims—five men and five women. This number, according to Dr. Paul, was "vastly inferior to the real one." He suggested that there could be as many as 30 victims. He based this on the human remains that they were unable to allocate: 33 pounds of badly charred bones, 24 pounds of uncharred fragments, 3 garbage cans full of body pieces too small to identify, and 11 pounds of hair, including 10 entire human scalps.

Some of the bones were so crudely broken that Dr. Paul surmised that they had been wedged between a door and its jamb and smashed, either to hide evidence of old fractures or, more likely, to make it easier to put them in the stove. It was clear that someone familiar with anatomy had dissected the bodies. When Petiot's lawyer, *Maître* Floriot, commented that Petiot never took a dissection course in medical school, Dr. Paul replied, "That's a shame, because he dissects very well."

Of the ten victims the team could isolate, the youngest was a 25-year-old woman and the oldest, a 50-year-old man. Attempts to identify most of the victims by means of old fractures and dental work proved fruitless. X-rays did not demonstrate any bullets or other identifiable foreign bodies. Because of the bodies' advanced state of decomposition, toxicologists could test only for heavy-metal poisons such as lead, mercury, and arsenic. Unfortunately, they could not test for the more common organic chemicals that could be used as poisons, such as those found in Petiot's home.

Petiot later testified that "of the 63 persons I liquidated, 30 were Boches [German soldiers] in uniform. Ten of the dog tags of these 30 Germans are in the hands of my lawyer." But no German uniforms were found at the rue Le Sueur house, and *Maître* Floriot never produced any dog tags.

Eight-six cadavers and many dissected body parts—51 men and 35 women, including 9 severed heads—were found in the Seine between 1941 and May 1943, when the Gestapo arrested Petiot. None of these bodies could be identified, since their fingerprints, faces, and scalps had been expertly removed. Dr. Paul concluded that most bore the mark of the same expert hand as the rue Le Sueur bodies; unique marks on all the victims' thighs also pointed to the murderer being the same. Over the next several years, additional bodies and body parts bearing similar markings were unearthed in trunks, fields, and abandoned houses.

The First Victims are Identified

Police easily identified two of the victims: Jean-Marc Van Bever and Marthe Khaït, who had disappeared just before they were to testify against Dr. Petiot on two separate narcotics charges.

In 1942, the *Police Judiciaire* vice squad impounded all Parisian pharmacies' account books in an attempt to identify narcotics abusers and the doctors who supplied them with drugs. With France's borders tightly sealed, physicians and pharmacies provided nearly the only access to these controlled substances. Based on this information, police arrested Jean-Marc Van Bever and his mistress, a licensed prostitute named Jeannette Gaul, on February 19, 1942. Van Bever was the educated but dissolute son and nephew of well-known French artists. Having squandered his inheritance, he had his first full-time job, at the age of 41, delivering coal for F60 to F120 a day. He had saved about F3,000, which he always carried with him.

Although Jeannette Gaul had given up prostitution when she moved in with Van Bever, she was still a heroin addict. She had arranged for five doctors to each prescribe enough narcotics to gradually wean her off the drug. This was a legal method of treatment at that time, although only 25 Parisian physicians used it. One was Dr. Petiot, who, in 1942, ran a general practice from his apartment at 66 rue Caumartin. Given the previous investigations into his prescribing practices, Petiot was considered highly suspect when Gaul, one of his addict-patients, was found to be receiving an abundance of drugs.

In this instance, Petiot was probably innocent. In his statement, he said that he only charged Gaul and Van Bever F50, a small sum consistent with a routine office visit, and certainly not what anyone would charge for illicit drugs. (In fact, throughout his career, Petiot remained relatively law-abiding when practicing medicine.) Van Bever and Gaul continuously changed their stories, seemingly in an attempt to implicate the doctor. They accused Petiot of dispensing the prescription without first examining Van Bever—a serious charge that was bolstered when, initially, the doctor could not find his examination record.

Bewildered, the judge indicted all three and set the trial date for May 26, 1942, although he immediately released Petiot. Ten months later, a stranger visited Van Bever, who had been released from prison on bail, with a message from his still-jailed girlfriend. Van Bever disappeared, leaving behind everything he owned. Two letters signed by him, which police later found to be forgeries, subsequently arrived at his lawyer's office. Police questioned Petiot, who denied any knowledge of Van Bever's whereabouts. Ten days later, the doctor suddenly "found" the missing report of Van Bever's physical exam. At Petiot's murder trial, the prosecutor speculated that the extremely detailed report was the result of an autopsy, rather than a physical exam.

Jeannette Gaul was tried on the drug charges and received a six-month jail term, after which she resumed her life of prostitution and drug use; she died of tetanus three months later. At the same trial, Van Bever received, in absentia, a one-year sentence, while Petiot received a suspended one-year sentence and a F10,000 fine, which was subsequently reduced.

A strikingly similar case helped identify another of Petiot's victims. On March 5, 1942, police arrested a young woman, Raymonde Baudet, for altering a tranquilizer prescription from Petiot to read "14 ampules of heroin." For her "cure," Baudet had received four prescriptions from him under her mother's name, Marthe Khaït. She also was getting heroin under this ruse from a number of physicians. Probably concerned that the police would implicate him as a drug pusher, Petiot convinced the mother, over her policeman-son's objections, to receive a dozen "dry injections" (without medications) in her thigh to show that she also was a drug user and that the prescribed drugs had been for her.

Several days later, Marthe Khaït changed her mind and visited her own doctor to explain what was going on. Dr. Pierre Trocmé was aghast that a French physician would act in that manner, and he urged her to go to the police. Trocmé later refused to testify against Petiot on the grounds of "professional privilege." On March 25, only three days after Van Bever disappeared, Mme. Khaït went to see her daughter's lawyer, *Maître* Pierre Véron, who had been recommended by Dr. Petiot (and who would prove to be the most effective of the prosecuting lawyers in Petiot's murder case). She took nothing with her, obviously expecting to be gone only a short while, because she left a pot of water heating on the stove to use for the laundry. She never came home.

The next morning, her husband David found two letters under the door. They appeared to be from Mme. Khaït, and stated that she was going to unoccupied (Vichy) France until her daughter's trial was over. The letters also stated that, unknown to her family, she had been a drug user for several years. After discussing the situation with Petiot, who said he had aided her, her husband came to believe the story. Sadly, he never saw Petiot come to trial, since he was subsequently deported to a Jewish concentration camp, where he died. On May 7, Mme. Khaït's son and his father (Khaït's first husband) filed a missing person's report with the police.

Police Inspector Roger Gignoux, who had also been assigned to the Van Bever case, found the two cases to have remarkable similarities—including the involvement of Dr. Petiot, narcotics, and the sudden disappearance of witnesses. Ultimately, he concluded that one person (probably Petiot) had written the letters that both victims had supposedly sent after they disappeared.

Raymonde Baudet, also known as Mlle. Khaït, was found guilty on the drug charges and sentenced to the four months she had already been in prison. Petiot received another one-year suspended sentence and a F10,000 fine. His lawyer subsequently got the fines for both drug convictions reduced to a total of F2,400 (about $700 in 2002).

Although the investigating magistrate in both cases, *Juge d'Instruction* Achille Olmi, did not take the cases seriously, Raymonde Baudet's attorney,

Pierre Véron, did his own investigation and pressed Olmi to indict Petiot on kidnapping or murder charges. Olmi, considered "one of the less efficient and scintillating magistrates in Paris," did not consent to conducting a search of Petiot's waiting room and office until a year later. At that time, he allowed only a superficial search and notified Petiot of the search team's pending arrival several days in advance. Even then, when the doctor protested, Olmi's assistant reassured him: "Please, Dr. Petiot. We are not accusing you of anything. This is all mere formality. We really don't suspect you of burning Van Bever and Marthe Khaït in the furnace of your central heating."

Véron kept up the pressure for an indictment, but Olmi ignored him. A year later, and two days after the discovery at rue Le Sueur, the lawyer confronted Olmi with evidence of the lives lost due to his blundering. Olmi could only say, "I was going to arrest Petiot tomorrow—I really was! But they took the dossier away from me. I don't understand why."

Searching for Dr. Petiot

The search for Dr. Petiot began in earnest on Monday, March 13, 1944, when Chief Inspector Marius Batut and a subordinate obtained, with great difficulty, the use of a car and sufficient gasoline to travel to Yonne, the doctor's native province. Based on the address that had been tacked to the rue Le Sueur house's front door, they headed for Auxerre, where Petiot's brother, 37-year-old Maurice, lived and owned a radio store. Maurice was a decade younger than his brother. While a chronic failure at business before the war, he had recently paid large sums for furniture, art, jewelry, and real estate, although it was unclear where the money had come from. They found Maurice at his store, which a horde of reporters had invaded earlier in the day. Obviously upset, Maurice claimed that he had not seen or heard from Marcel since late February.

Nevertheless, police were watching the Auxerre train station and, the next morning, they recognized Marcel's wife, Georgette, on the platform. They arrested Georgette and her brother-in-law Maurice. Accompanied by *Commissaire* Massu, they all returned to Paris. Photographers mobbed Georgette Petiot as she arrived at *Police Judiciaire* headquarters. When questioned by police, she claimed to know nothing that could help them:

> I did not know the house on the rue Le Sueur very well. I only went there once, and I didn't like it; it was too large. I don't even remember the previous owner's name. I know that he [her husband, Dr. Petiot] had some

work done there, but I don't know what kind. My husband has always been a very gentle person, but he never told me anything about his business affairs, something that I complained about frequently.

Georgette alleged that on the day the police discovered the rue Le Sueur bodies, inspectors had called their home at 7:30, as she and her husband were eating dinner. The doctor said only, "All right, I'm on my way," and then quickly left. She claimed that her husband had not returned that night. The next morning, fearing that the Germans had arrested him, Georgette tried to take a train to Auxerre where her son went to school, but there were none running. Only that evening while reading the newspaper, she asserted, did she discover the horrors her husband had been accused of committing. She said that she spent the night sitting on the stairs at 52 rue de Reuilly, a building that her husband owned.

Maurice was sent directly to Paris's Santé Prison, charged with conspiracy to commit murder. He claimed he did not to know his brother's whereabouts. When questioned, Maurice admitted that he had been to the rue Le Sueur house several times to supervise some construction while the Germans had his brother incarcerated. He had also paid some utility bills for the property. He said he toured the entire building in January 1944 to check for water leaks with an architect, who confirmed the story. Both claimed they did not see or smell anything suspicious—even though the stench was pervasive when the police arrived on March 11. They also claimed that heavy marble slabs had covered the manure pit later found to contain quicklime and body parts.

Maurice denied delivering quicklime in February 1943, and challenged the police to "prove it!" They did just that. Jean Eustache, an Auxerre trucker, described taking Maurice to the quarry at Oise-sur-Armançon on February 18, 1943, to collect 660 pounds of quicklime, which they then delivered to the rue Le Sueur house. Maurice reluctantly admitted that this was true, saying that he did it at his brother's request. He needed lime to exterminate cockroaches—or was it to whitewash the façade? He couldn't quite be sure.

On Friday, March 17, police escorted Maurice and Georgette Petiot to the rue Caumartin apartment for a brief search. They had to force their way past a crowd of gawkers and reporters, all shouting questions at Georgette, who turned and screamed, "You are assassins! You're making fun of my misery! You know that I only went to the Yonne [Auxerre] to see my son!"

Although police found no drugs at the rue Le Sueur house, Petiot's apartment-office contained a supply of scopolamine, chloroform, strychnine, digitalis and ouabain (a similar medication), and 504 ampules of morphine—

at least 50 times the normal physician's stock of drugs. They also found the not-unexpected personal supplies of black-market coffee, sugar, and chocolate. All the money and jewelry, however, had been taken by the doctor when he fled. Georgette learned several days later that she was officially under arrest for "accepting stolen goods"—a five-carat diamond from her husband.

The Investigation

About this time, French police obtained the file describing Petiot's arrest by the Gestapo. In early 1943, an informer had told the Germans that a mysterious "Dr. Eugène" was running an organization to help Jews and downed Allied pilots escape from occupied France. Operating out of a barbershop, the group supplied their "customers" with false passports and a safe passage to Spain or South America. Following this lead, the Gestapo arrested Dr. Petiot and his close friend, René-Gustave Nézondet. They also arrested Edmond Pintard, alias Françinet, a 56-year-old burned-out actor described as "a comically lean Ichabod Crane type," as well as Pintard's friend, Raoul Fourrier, a 61-year-old barber. All but Nézondet, who was released two weeks later, had been held in Fresnes Prison from June 1943 until January 1944.

Soon, a new character entered the picture: Roland Albert Porchon, an overweight, middle-aged man who ran a trucking company and a used-furniture store. He told police that he had sent René Marie and his wife Marcelle to Dr. Petiot so they could escape occupied France. Petiot set the price at F45,000 each, which Porchon offered to help them raise by buying all their possessions for F220,000. The Maries, bothered by the doctor's reputation, declined his offer. As soon as Petiot's crimes became public, Porchon first asked the Maries to keep silent about his role and then went to a policeman friend saying that he was involved in a Resistance-led escape organization. When that story proved false, Porchon was taken into custody.

Taken before the *Juge d'Instruction* on March 17, 1944, Porchon claimed that Nézondet had told him, "Petiot is the king of criminals. I never would have thought him capable of such a thing." Nézondet had also spoken of seeing "sixteen corpses stretched out" at the rue Le Sueur house, "completely blackened; they were certainly killed by poison or injection ... I suppose he asked them for money to pass them into the free zone and instead of helping them escape, he killed them." Supposedly, Nézondet told Porchon to remain silent; he would go to the police after the war.

Actually, as early as August 2, 1943, while Petiot was in the Gestapo prison, Porchon had talked to *Commissaire* Doulet:

> A Parisian doctor who, under the pretext of passing young people out of the country, asked them for sums of money between F50,000 and F75,000 and then did away with them after payment. This doctor supposedly got rid of the bodies by burying them in the courtyard of his building.

Porchon claimed that he had heard this from the Gestapo, "who did not want to interfere since it was a purely French matter." At *Commissaire* Doulet's urging, Porchon retold his story to an officer at the *Police Judiciaire*, who did not investigate further.

Both Porchon and Nézondet later testified that Paris police told them that "the Germans have let him [Petiot] knock off 30 or 40 travelers and there is nothing we can do about it." In fact, after the Germans released Petiot in January 1944, Nézondet claimed that the *Police Judiciaire* told him, "The Petiot affair is over; besides, we can't follow him." One inspector muttered, "I wouldn't be surprised if there were 30 or 40 victims in this case," suggesting to Nézondet that the police knew about the rue Le Sueur corpses at that time.

It remains unclear whether, as lawyers claimed in court, Petiot actually worked for the Germans or, as some writers now claim, he worked for the Communists. Petiot's relationship with the Communists is uncertain, although he did join the French Communist Party as a student and knew both Maurice Thorez (leader of the original French Communist organization in Paris) and Nguyen Tat Thanh (Ho Chi Minh). When he was captured, he was carrying a multitude of identification papers, including a Communist Party membership card.

Initially, Nézondet denied everything when questioned in March 1944. However, his mistress's friend, Mme. Marie Turpault, said that in December 1943, she had asked Nézondet about Dr. Petiot, and he replied, "He's in prison right now, and he should stay there." According to Mme. Turpault, Nézondet claimed that Maurice Petiot had asked him to help dispose of a book with names of supposed victims, remove the bodies Maurice had found in a pit at the doctor's rue Le Seuer house, and build a wall to hide the corpses. Nézondet told her that he refused.

When confronted with Mme. Turpault's story, Nézondet maintained that she was also confabulating, although her story matched much of Porchon's testimony. Finally, on March 22, Nézondet admitted that Porchon and Turpault had been truthful. While Petiot was still in prison at Fresnes, Nézondet said he met Maurice Petiot in November or early December 1943.

Maurice told him, "I have just come from my brother's house. There's enough there to have us all shot." Nézondet asked if he had found weapons or a secret radio, and Maurice replied:

> I wish that's all it was. The journeys to South America begin and end at the rue Le Sueur. There are bodies piled in a pit, with their hair and eyebrows shaved off. I found a book where he [Marcel] wrote down the names of his victims; there must have been 50 or 60 of them.

Maurice told him that the doctor killed his victims with a poison-filled syringe that he could operate remotely. He had also found piles of civilian clothing and German uniforms, which he had crated up and removed in a five-ton truck. During a dinner at his apartment a few weeks later, Nézondet said he told Georgette Petiot about the horrors at rue Le Sueur that Maurice had recounted to him.

When questioned by police, Maurice and Georgette claimed they knew nothing about Nézondet's activities. To keep him safe and available, the police charged Nézondet with "non-denunciation of a crime" and locked him in Santé Prison for the next 14 months. During the subsequent trial, the Petiot family called Nézondet a buffoon and a lunatic.

The "Escape" Network

The police also confronted two of the doctor's accomplices identified in Gestapo files: Edmond Pintard and Raoul Fourrier. Both reluctantly revealed that they had unwittingly helped send a dozen people to a horrific death at Petiot's hands. Fourrier had been the doctor's barber and his patient. The doctor had told Fourrier that he had an organization that could get people safely to South America. When asked the price, Petiot replied, "Twenty-five thousand francs per person, false papers supplied, all costs included. If you know people who need to escape." Thinking that he could make some easy money, Fourrier mentioned the network to his friend Pintard, who began to actively recruit customers.

Massu now had to consider whether the murders he was investigating were committed under the guise of providing an escape from France. This idea seemed to be confirmed when the business partner of Joachim Guschinov, a Polish Jew, revealed the story of Guschinov's "escape" from France. He told Massu that Petiot, Guschinov's doctor and neighbor, had offered to use a fake Argentinian passport to get the man to South America for F25,000 ($5,075 in 2002).

Guschinov had accepted Petiot's offer. After removing all identifying marks from his clothing, he had sewn $1,000 in U.S. currency into the shoulder pads of his suit. In his baggage, he had secreted silver, gold, diamonds worth F500,000 to F700,000, another F500,000 in cash, and five sable coats. The night he left, he had dined with his wife, who then accompanied him to a corner near the place where he was to meet Petiot. Saying that he had to continue alone, they had kissed and parted. Mme. Renée Guschinov later testified:

> Petiot advised my husband to flee. On January 2, 1942, my husband left home. He told me Petiot was going to get him to Argentina, and that he had to have some injections because of health regulations ... My husband said he was worried about these injections.

When she asked Petiot for news of her husband two months later, the doctor showed her an undated note in Guschinov's handwriting saying that he had safely reached Buenos Aires. Mme. Guschinov added:

> [Petiot] told me all sorts of stories about the passage, and said my husband's business was going well in Buenos Aires and that I should join him there. Petiot said he couldn't show me the letters, because they were too compromising and he had destroyed them. I cabled to some friends of ours there, and they said they hadn't seen my husband.

Justifiably suspicious, she declined Petiot's assistance to join her husband. Although her husband's letters ceased coming, being a Jew, she was afraid to voice her suspicions to the police. She reluctantly came forward only after the Petiot affair was publicized.

Escaping from occupied France was not easy. The initial goal was to get to Spain, and from there go to England, Africa, or South America. But skilled mountain guides were needed to cross the Pyrenees Mountains through Andorra. Going by boat was even more difficult, since one had to avoid detection by the numerous patrol boats. Only about one-third of those who attempted to escape to Spain arrived safely. Many were caught by the Germans or killed by dishonest guides. By the fall of 1942, only those using one of the established escape networks could hope to get out. At that time, the charge was about F50,000, but the price rose as the war progressed.

Underworld Victims

The first customer Pintard and Fourrier recruited was Joseph Réocreux, alias Iron Arm Jo or Jo le Boxeur, an underworld figure who, after executing several robberies dressed as a Gestapo officer, felt it was time to leave France. The two quoted a price of F50,000—double what Petiot charged. Petiot found out and threatened to dump his procurers if they didn't stop such thievery. They apologized and took Jo to meet "Dr. Eugène" (in reality, Petiot). (Despite their protestations, the two later boosted their price for other potential "escapees.")

Jo told compatriots that the doctor's eyes had made him extremely uneasy, and he persuaded a friend, François le Corse, to escape first and take Jo's mistress. They and their luggage disappeared with Petiot. Several weeks later, Petiot showed Jo a letter that was supposedly from François in Argentina. Convinced that the route was safe, Jo prepared to leave France. He put gold plaques into the heels of his shoes, sewed F1.4 million into the shoulder pads of his suit, and loaded the two prostitutes who would accompany him with jewels. They met Petiot and departed. Several days later, Petiot was seen wearing Jo's gold wristwatch—an item no one believed that he would voluntarily surrender. A telegram "from Jo in Argentina" arrived several weeks later and Pintard passed this around to help drum up new business.

Adrien "le Basque" Estébétéguy was the group's next victim. He was one of Jo's underworld friends and had served eight prison terms. He also had seven outstanding warrants that had not been served because he was under Nazi protection. In early 1943, he had fallen out with both his German protectors and the French police, and decided his best move was to leave France. He was joined by his friend, Joseph Didioni Sidissé Piereschi (alias Dionisi or Zé). Zé was a convicted murderer who had served three years in a penal colony. He later deserted from the French Army (twice) and engaged in arms trafficking, train robbery, and running a brothel for German soldiers. Having escaped from prison after a robbery that netted him nearly F1 million, he also thought it best to leave France.

Accompanying the men were their mistresses, 35-year-old nightclub singer and model Gine Volna, alias Gisèle Rossny, and a 24-year-old prostitute, Joséphine-Aimée Grippay, alias Paulette la Chinoise. Grippay packed her favorite evening gown—a distinctive black satin dress with golden swallows embroidered on the bosom—for her trip to South America.

Petiot told Fourrier that the signal that the group had gotten safely out of France would be a sun surrounded by flames drawn on a F100 bill, which would be ripped in half and sent to Petiot. Soon after their "departure," Petiot proudly showed the half bill to his comrades. Police later found the other half at the doctor's house on rue Caumartin.

The Gestapo Files

Pintard was not very subtle with his recruiting efforts, and the Gestapo soon learned about the "escape" organization. They described it in a report dated April 8, 1943:

an organization which arranges clandestine crossings of the Spanish border by means of falsified Argentinian passports ... A group leaves for Spain every three weeks. The interested party must pay F50,000 ... subjects are taken to the train station and turned over to two other members of the organization, who give them their false passports in exchange of the F50,000. All liquid cash—particularly foreign currency—and jewels must be surrendered, and are returned only at the Spanish border. Each traveler is free to take with him as much money as he chooses.

Robert Jodkum (an alias) from the Paris Gestapo's Jewish Affairs Section simultaneously reported:

According to my informants, the doctor in question does not deal solely with Jews, but with anyone who comes to him, and it is said that he has abetted the escape of certain suspicious persons, notably terrorists, and even army deserters ... It would be interesting to be able to organize a surveillance.

Jodkum decided to infiltrate the network using Yvan Dreyfus, the Jewish head of a large electronics firm. Dreyfus had returned from his studies in the United States to serve in the French Army, saying, "I am a Frenchman ... Now that France is in trouble, I cannot desert her." He supplied the Resistance with transmitters, and was trying to flee to Britain to join de Gaulle's Free French forces when he was captured. He had been scheduled to be deported to the death camps, but was released after his wife, Paulette, paid about F5 million (about $1 million in 2002) ransom and he agreed to betray any organization smuggling Jews out of France.

Jodkum put Dreyfus in touch with the Petiot organization, but, apparently to protect the Resistance, Dreyfus never allowed the Gestapo to meet with "Dr. Eugène." When Petiot met Dreyfus with his bags and money on May 19, 1943, the two eluded Gestapo pursuers. Dreyfus vanished. (During his trial, Petiot tried to imply that Dreyfus was a collaborator, prompting a telegram from Pierre Mendès-France, one of De Gaulle's ministers, which was read in court: "I learn with stupefaction [that] Petiot dares sully [the] memory [of] Yvan Dreyfus." Taken aback, Petiot, for the only time in the trial, remained silent during Paulette Dreyfus's testimony.)

The Gestapo section charged with security for the occupied territories also tried to infiltrate the network. Charles Beretta, a French collaborator, met with Petiot. He questioned Beretta, checked his identity papers, and then requested F100,000 for transportation and travel documents. They finally agreed on F60,000. Petiot told Beretta to pack two suitcases and bring a blanket. Fourrier and Pintard collected the money (the Gestapo had recorded the serial numbers) from Beretta the next day. On Friday, May 21, 1943, when Beretta showed up for his "escape," the Gestapo burst in and arrested Fourrier and Pintard. Learning Dr. Petiot's identity and whereabouts, they arrested him at his rue Caumartin apartment.

Petiot was questioned and beaten that night and the next day. Confessing that he was part of an escape organization, he claimed he did not know any other network members, saying only that he sent escapees to a person known as "Robert Martinetti," but had no way of contacting him. Petiot repeated this story, even after the Germans tortured him for days at a time. He was beaten so badly that he spit up blood for a week and had dizzy spells for six months. They also attempted psychological torture, showing him one dead man and another whose face had been pulverized and claiming that they were members of Petiot's escape network.

Nézondet, arrested with Petiot at his apartment, was soon released. Just before his release, Petiot told him, "Tell my wife to go where she knows to go and dig up what is hidden there." Georgette claimed not to understand the message, but she relayed it to Maurice, who quickly went to the rue Le Sueur house.

Fourrier, Pintard, and Petiot were held in various French jails for eight months. Two days after they released Fourrier and Pintard, the Gestapo inexplicably freed Petiot on January 13, 1944. Maurice had paid them F100,000; even so, the Germans would normally have shot someone like Petiot, if not for being an admitted Resistance member, then for the insolence he constantly showed. Petiot told his jailers he didn't care about life, since he had "terminal cancer." (Actually, it was his brother who had cancer.) Maurice later told a judge:

> There were only two things they could do with him [Dr. Petiot]: convict him and deport him to the salt mines, from which he would never return, or execute him; or else free him—they could no longer just hold him in prison . . . [A policeman] told me: "Your brother is sick, you will take care of him; I cannot bring myself to liquidate a man such as he."

It is possible that they released Petiot so that they could track his movements, but they were obviously unsuccessful. The rue Le Sueur bodies were discovered only two months later.

Dead Men's Luggage

Although Dr. Petiot could be linked to 13 deaths, the piles of human parts and discarded personal items at the rue Le Sueur house suggested that there were many more victims. But there were only a few items that could be used to identify them. Joséphine Grippay's black silk embroidered dress and a picture of Jo "le Boxeur" Réocreux were two.

A woman who lived directly across from 21 rue Le Sueur remembered seeing at least 47 suitcases and trunks removed from the house the previous summer, in a van marked "Transports-Avenue Daumesnil." The police tracked down the company and discovered that on May 26, 1943 (five days after the Germans arrested his brother), Maurice Petiot had sent 45 suitcases to Auxerre. Maurice confessed only to removing the suitcases, which were stored at his friend's house in Courson-les-Carrières. Police searched the Courson house and found 49 pieces of luggage; 37 were from the delivery in May. The police eventually discovered 83 suitcases filled with nearly three tons of travel items, all presumably from Dr. Petiot's victims. Some victims, such as Van Bever and Mme. Khaït, left home without any baggage.

The clothing bore two dozen different laundry marks and 48 sets of initials; most could not be matched with the few known victims. It didn't help that conducting investigations was extremely difficult in occupied France. Nevertheless, some of the suits and shirts could be matched with Estébétéguy, Réocreux, Piereschi, le Basque, and their companions.

Police were inundated with anonymous letters containing "clues" about the case, but one identified more possible victims. Several of the shirts had been made in Amsterdam and were marked "Wolff" or "Made for Monsieur Wolff." The letter's author knew of a Jewish family that had arrived in Paris from Holland in August 1942, encountered the Gestapo, and wished to flee France. They met a physician who claimed that he could get them to South America, but first they would have to convert their assets into gold and precious gems. "Madame W.," "Maurice W.," and his wife "L.W." met the doctor in December 1942, and were never heard from again. The writer also thought that "the family B.," an elderly couple, and two couples in their twenties had all disappeared after meeting the doctor the following January.

After a public appeal, the letter's author, Ilse Gang, came forward and testified. The "W's" turned out to be a wealthy Jewish family from Königsberg, Germany. Herr Wolff had run the Incona Lumber Company which had branches throughout Europe. Soon after Hitler came to power, the family moved—his son Maurice and his wife went to France; Herr Wolff, his wife, and his other son went to Amsterdam. The youngest son escaped to the United States and the rest ended up in Paris. Through their old friend, Ilse Gang, they made contact with the mysterious "Eryane" Kahan.

Kahan, reputedly a former prostitute and probably a Gestapo informant, learned that the Wolffs wished to flee France. In December 1942, she put the Wolffs in touch with her physician, Dr. Louis-Théophile Saint-Pierre, whom the police wanted for fraud and performing illegal abortions. He, in turn, steered them to Pintard, who introduced them to "Dr. Eugène."

Petiot met them in a friend's apartment, had tea, and spoke of music and art, appearing to be, as their lawyer later said, "a man of vast culture and fine sentiments, whose magnanimity and character fully explained his devotion to the noble cause of clandestine passages." Petiot told them that he could smuggle them out of France and that they could take as much money as they wished but only two suitcases apiece. He also warned them not to carry any identification papers or other means of identification, a warning they ignored since most of their belongings were embroidered with their initials. Kahan later said that the Wolffs "were in deathly fear of the Germans. They were so happy about the possibility of escaping that they considered Petiot their benefactor—almost a god."

Near the end of December 1942, the Wolffs spent what was to be their last day in Paris with Ilse Gang, telling her about their pending adventure. They had sewn jewels into Maurice's jacket, and were eager to begin a new life. No one heard from them again. Two months later, Kahan stopped by Ilse Gang's apartment to ask if she wished to take the same journey as the Wolffs; wisely, she declined the offer.

Others were not as lucky. Some of the Wolffs' friends, the Bastons (a pseudonym for Basch), also wanted to flee France, along with four relatives. Eventually, they met Robert Malfet, a former chauffeur who specialized in escapes from France. He left them with Kahan in early January 1942; she then steered them to Petiot. They were never heard from again. Kahan later told Malfet that he would benefit by directing others to her and "the doctor" for trips to South America. After his arrest, police found F315,000 ($14,555 in 2002), expensive jewelry, and 55 newspaper articles about the Petiot affair in Malfet's apartment. At trial, Petiot admitted: "Yes, I killed the Basches and the Wolffs. I didn't know they were Jews, but I knew they were German spies sent by Eryane Kahan."

In April 1943, Malfet produced another family interested in escaping, Michel and Marie Cadoret de l'Epinguen and their young son. Directed to Kahan, they soon met "Dr. Eugène" and gave him a F50,000 down payment. As Michel later explained:

> The doctor gave us details about the method of passage, pointing out that we would leave when space was available and that he was helping us only as a special favor . . . He specified that we would have to receive injections . . . Finally, he advised us to take the maximum amount of money but not more than 50 kilograms of luggage.

Mme. l'Epinguen, herself a physician, found Petiot to be uncouth and slovenly. She later testified:

> Petiot told us that . . . we would be furnished with false identity papers. There was something very suspicious about the whole arrangement. Petiot told us we would need vaccinations to get into Argentina. He said, "These injections will render you invisible to the eyes of the world."

This, combined with a vague mistrust of Eryane Kahan, led them to cancel their deal with the doctor. Surprisingly, Petiot returned their money. They found another means of escaping France, and the l'Epinguens were shocked to learn, on their return in 1945, that "Dr. Eugène" was actually the Dr. Petiot on trial for murder. (The foreign press gave little coverage to the event.)

After Dr. l'Epinguen described Petiot's plan for injections at the trial, Petiot sarcastically replied:

> I see it all now. The mad doctor with his syringe. It was a dark and rainy night. The wind howled under the eaves and rattled the windowpanes of the oak-paneled library.

At that point, the judge stopped him from continuing. Foolishly, Petiot then asked her, "Weren't you asked for F90,000 at first?" When Dr. l'Epinguen said that she couldn't recall, he countered, "Think. It's very important. That's what saved your life." The audience in the courtroom gasped at this guilty admission.

Between June 1944 and August 1945, police identified five more of Petiot's victims. One, Nelly-Denise Bartholomeus, was a newlywed who had apparently gone to Paris for an abortion (at that time, a capital offense in France). On June 5, 1942, a midwife sent her to Dr. Petiot for treatment. She disappeared.

Another victim was Dr. Paul-Léon Braunberger, a 62-year-old Jewish physician who had been advised by the Germans in June 1942 that he would soon have to close his practice. Following a mysterious phone call, he disappeared, taking only his medical bag. His family and acquaintances received letters with preposterous requests, which the police determined had been written under duress. Braunberger's only known connection to Petiot was a party they had both attended some years before, and the first letter went to the party's host—a man whom Dr. Braunberger detested. Among the luggage found at Courson-les-Carrières were a custom-made shirt and a hat with the initials "P. B." Mme. Braunberger identified these as the clothes her husband was wearing when he disappeared.

In August 1945, the French minister of justice received a letter from the American Joint Distribution Committee in New York inquiring about the whereabouts of three members of a family that had lived in Paris. Kurt Kneller had immigrated to France from his native Germany in 1933. After marrying Margeret "Greta" Lent and having a son, René, he applied for French citizenship in 1937 and joined the French foreign legion until disarmament in 1939. Being a Jew, he was fearful for his family's well-being and planned to leave France. He told a friend that his doctor was going to help them. In mid-July 1942, Petiot came to take them on their journey. Afterward, the only news ever received from them was a letter with unusual handwriting and strange grammar saying that they had arrived safely.

The day he left, Kurt Kneller was wearing a shirt embroidered with "K. K." and his son was wearing pajamas that were later found at the rue Le Sueur house. Three weeks after the Knellers disappeared, the head, legs, feet, and other body parts of a boy the same age as René were found floating on the Seine. Nearby were the head, femurs, pelvis, and arms of a middle-aged woman. Three days later, a man's head was found nearby. All had been dead for about three weeks, but the remains were too decomposed to be identified.

It should be noted here that throughout the war, investigations into disappearances and searches for criminals were complicated by France's division into German-occupied France and Vichy France. The Vichy government nominally controlled the southeastern two-fifths of the country that was not occupied by the Germans until November 11, 1942. (Despite the signing of the Franco-German Armistice on June 22, 1940. The demarcation line, however, remained in effect until February 1943.) Special permission was required to cross the line, although it was relatively easy to use forged papers or to sneak across at poorly guarded locations. The Vichy government continued to collaborate with the Germans, supported by French citizens, until it was clear that Germany was losing the war.

The Arrest

Although police initially could not find Dr. Petiot, they jailed nine conspirators in spring 1944, including Maurice and Georgette Petiot, Fourrier, Pintard, and Nézondet, on charges ranging from murder and conspiracy to receiving stolen goods. All charges were ultimately dropped. When signing Maurice and Georgette's release, the prosecutor consoled himself with the idea that "even if Justice can do nothing against them, the name that they bear and whose sad reputation affects them personally, may serve as a constant source of shame unless Petiot's amoral numbness has conquered them as well." Maurice may actually have been released because he had terminal cancer; he died shortly after his brother's trial.

Dr. Marcel Petiot had disappeared on his bicycle the night that police discovered the macabre scene at the rue Le Sueur house. Although his picture had been on the front page of most French newspapers, he could not be found. The police were deluged with clues. Petiot supposedly had been spotted at the Spanish and Belgian borders, boarding a ship to South America, and in every part of France. One tip actually led them to a Marcel Petiot—but it was a different man. Then, in mid-1944, the war and its aftermath intervened to suspend the search.

On June 6, 1944, the Allies landed at Normandy and chaos resulted. August 19, the Paris police went on a strike which ended with German tanks attacking their headquarters. The Resistance began to fight in the streets and, by August 25, Paris had surrendered to the Free French Army. What followed was a confusing bloodbath. Up to 40,000 collaborators were summarily tried and executed, and hundreds of thousands more were relieved of their positions, jailed, or simply disgraced by accusation. France tried to rebuild in the face of 500,000 dead, 3 million people returning from prison and labor camps, and 1.5 million homes destroyed. It was a chaos that benefited Dr. Petiot.

The search for Petiot had ground to a halt and *Commissaire* Massu decided to try to flush out the paranoid killer. He gave the press the "confession" of "Charles Rolland," an invented acquaintance who identified Petiot as a cocaine pusher, sexual voyeur, and collaborationist. It was published on September 19, 1944, under the headline "Petiot, Soldier of the Third Reich." Dr. Petiot took the bait. He responded with a letter protesting his innocence, and which included enough details to indicate that he was still in Paris and serving as an officer with the French Forces of the Interior (FFI). As police painstakingly began to compare the handwriting in the letter with that of potential suspects, they also distributed Petiot's description to several key FFI officers, including Captain Henri Valéry, chief of counterespionage and interrogations at Reuilly (Paris) Army Base.

As it turned out, Captain Valéry was actually Petiot. How did the doctor evade police and join the FFI? After initially staying with friends, Petiot cajoled an acquaintance and patient, house painter Georges Redouté, to let him stay in his apartment. (Redouté spent months in prison before authorities recognized that he was an innocent pawn of the doctor.) Petiot regaled Redouté with stories of his fictional Resistance exploits and persuaded him that the rue Le Sueur bodies were a result of his patriotic deeds. During the months that Petiot stayed with Redouté, he slept on the floor, went out only at night, and read newspapers during the day. The apartment's concierge recalled:

> Henri Valéry rarely went out in the daytime. He only went out for food and books. Once there was a bad leak in the house and the fire department and plumber tried to get into the apartment where Valéry was staying. I had a very hard time convincing him that the men were not after him. He was very *engageant*, very nice in manner, and a convincing talker.

A few days after the liberation of Paris, Petiot finally emerged and decided to join the FFI, both as cover while in Paris and so that he could easily move out of France to safety. To accomplish that, he needed another identity, preferably that of a doctor so that he would continue to have the prestige he desired. Petiot discovered that the Gestapo had arrested Dr. François Wetterwald for his Resistance activities on January 15, 1944, and then sent him to a concentration camp. Going to the Wetterwald home in the guise of an International Red Cross official, Petiot persuaded his mother to show him Wetterwald's identity papers, some of which he stole. He then enlisted in the FFI as "Dr. Wetterwald," but asked, supposedly for security reasons, that he be allowed to use the name "Henri Valéry," which was the name of the physician who had formerly occupied Petiot's rue Caumartin apartment.

Petiot/Valéry functioned superbly in his new military position, and he was soon promoted to captain. Co-workers saw him as a tireless and dedicated officer bent on rooting out collaborators and traitors. He boasted of his Resistance activities, saying that he had killed 63 "collaborators," including a "boxer." Few knew that Petiot was using his subordinates in the agency to seize property from rich citizens after jailing them on trumped-up charges.

About six weeks after "Rolland's" fictitious confession was published, Petiot was delivered into police custody under mysterious circumstances. On October 31, 1944, three military officers, including a Captain Simonin,

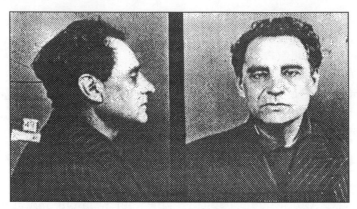

Police Judiciaire mugshots of Dr. Marcel Petiot. (Archives de la Ville de Paris)

violently subdued and captured Petiot at Paris's Saint-Mandé-Tourelles metro station. After interrogating Petiot at length, Captain Simonin turned him over to military security, which delivered him to *Police Judiciaire* headquarters. What Captain Simonin learned from Petiot would never be discovered, because he disappeared. In reality, the "Captain" was a notorious collaborator named Soutif who had been instrumental in hundreds of deportations and in the death of dozens of Resistance members.

Police did discover that Petiot had tried to cover up a murder and large-scale robbery by three of his subordinates in the FFI. One of these, Corporal Jean Salvage, had previously worked for the mysterious Captain Simonin. When police tried to question Salvage, the military refused to cooperate, saying he had been sent on a secret mission. He was never found.

When apprehended, Dr. Petiot was carrying a loaded 6.35-mm automatic pistol, F31,700, and 50 documents, including identity papers in the names of Valéry, Wetterwald, Glibert, de Frutos, Bonnasseau, and Cacheux. He also carried military orders that authorized his effective disappearance to French Indochina. The item that would prove the most damaging, however, was a ration card that had been altered to insert the name "Valéry" after the first name "René." It also had a birthdate of May 8, 1935, and a birthplace of Issy-les Moulineaux—information that matched one of his victims, eight-year-old René Kneller.

The press, in the midst of post-war chaos and tragedy, was no longer interested in Petiot's story. As the editors of the formerly underground newspaper, *Combat,* wrote:

> We refuse to glorify an affair which is repugnant from so many points of view. Too many tragic or urgent problems demand out attention for us to permit ourselves to go into the scandalous details of sensational news items.

Police were left to toil in obscurity for the next 18 months—that is, until the trial began.

Petiot's Strange Tales

Housed on Santé Prison's death row (although he had not yet been convicted), Dr. Petiot, in a totally unexpected move, admitted to some of the killings. However, he justified them by saying that the victims were collaborators and, since he was a Resistance member, slaying them was his duty. At that time, no justification could have been more acceptable. The French were appalled and embarrassed by collaborators, while pride and honor were reserved for those who had worked with the Resistance (and whose numbers seemed to multiply with each passing day).

Skilled at arguing his position, despite obvious facts to the contrary, Petiot repeatedly told his preposterous tales with unruffled calm, all the while dangling a cigarette from his mouth. *Juge d'Instruction* Ferdinand Goletty, the investigating magistrate, heard a tale fuzzy on details and more akin to that of a comic book super hero.

The doctor claimed that he had begun his Resistance activities in 1940 by joining a group of anti-Franco (anti-fascist) Spaniards based in Paris. "I did some very good things with these people," Petiot claimed, "but I do not want to tell you about them since my case is a simple one and I have no desire to complicate matters." He claimed that he had developed a silent short-range weapon, which was ideal for sniper operations, and that he had used it on two Germans (actually, both appeared to have died from natural causes). According to Petiot, the plans had been turned over to the American Consul in Paris in 1941 (in reality, the consulate had already relocated to Vichy France.) But he refused to give Judge Goletty a detailed description of the weapon.

Petiot also described how he had learned self-defense and the use of various weapons, such as guns, grenades, and plastic explosives, although he was unable to remember the name of the Resistance operative who had trained him. He said that through his medical practice he had gathered information on German troop movements and weapons development, including a boomerang device that not even the Germans had heard of.

Petiot claimed that he was in charge of a cell to root out informers, or *mouchard* (from *mouche*, French for "fly"), who had infiltrated the Resistance. His group, named "Fly-Tox" after a common brand of fly-killer, sought out and killed collaborators wherever they found them. "Fly-Tox" operatives would follow any non-uniformed people who left the Gestapo office. Claiming to be plainclothes German police, they then "arrested" and interrogated them; they clubbed to death those who worked for the Germans. Petiot said the bodies were buried west of Paris, but the only two corpses found at the location he specified had been killed by known vigilantes who had confessed. While he admitted killing François le Corse, Adrien le Basque, Jo le Boxeur, and their friends, he justified this by saying that they had all been collaborators.

In what one author described as "this delirious proliferation of noble acts," Petiot also imagined himself to be a saboteur who destroyed German boxcars with explosive devices that he had invented. *Maître* Pierre Véron, a well-known Resistance fighter who blew up bridges throughout France during the war and who represented Yvan Dreyfus's family, had the following exchange with Petiot at the trial:

Véron: What are plastic explosives?

Petiot: (No answer.)

Véron: How do you transport plastic explosives?

Petiot: Wait a minute, it's coming back to me. Several comrades filled a suitcase with plastic explosives and detonated them with a bomb with a timer, and then came to hide at my house.

Véron: What is this "bomb with a timer"?

Petiot: A German grenade ... you know ... the ones with the handle. We heard the explosion 30 minutes later ...

Véron: German fragmentation grenades have a seven-second fuse!

Petiot: (Mumbled something incoherent and glowered at Véron.)

Petiot's lawyer, Floriot, jumped up and demanded to know whether this was "a trial or an entrance exam for the Polytechnic Institute?" Véron replied, "This is an examination on the Resistance, and it didn't take long to show that your client is an impostor."

Several days later, Véron and Petiot would reprise this conversation while Captain Henri Boris, General Charles de Gaulle's wartime director of aerial operations, was on the stand.

Véron: Petiot, how did you obtain your plastic explosives?

Petiot: We got sheets of it from ...

Véron: Plastic explosives don't come in sheets.

Petiot: I knew about detonators when you were still breastfeeding. You've never even seen plastic explosives.

Véron: No, I've only driven around with 150 kilos of them in the trunk of my car ... How did you detonate your plastic explosives?

Petiot: I put them between two German grenades and set them off.

Boris: You couldn't detonate plastic explosives like that.

Petiot: They didn't go off.

These exchanges are typical of those that investigators and lawyers had with Petiot. No matter how many obvious untruths and contradictions there were, Petiot fabricated more stories about his exploits. In addition, Petiot refused to name anyone who had worked with him in the Resistance except those who could not verify his statements. Those he did name probably never existed or else they were dead, as were Pierre Brossolette, Lucien Romier, and Jean-Marie Charbonneaux, known as "Cumuleau." (Petiot probably heard about these dead heroes when he shared a cell at Fresnes Prison with a real Resistance fighter.) At the trial, Judge Leser told Petiot, "It would certainly help your case if you gave us the names [of your Resistance comrades]," to which Petiot replied, "All right. I'll give them to you ... As soon as I'm acquitted." The judge sardonically replied, "I rather doubt that you will be."

As for the bodies found at the rue Le Sueur house, Petiot claimed that those individuals were killed by the Germans; he asked his brother for quick-lime only so he would not be blamed for the deaths. After arriving at the house on the evening when police discovered the bodies, Petiot "saw that the police and fireman, with typical impertinence, had broken open the doors." He fled to rejoin the Resistance where, he proclaimed, he was given a new code name, "Special 21."

During the pre-trial inquiry, Judge Goletty asked why Petiot had not turned himself in after the liberation of Paris. Petiot answered:

I felt that the accusations against me were so manifestly false, I was so convinced that my innocence would be obvious to anyone who gave the least bit of thought to the matter, that I did not imagine I ran any risk of imprisonment. Nonetheless, I did not go to the police because the police had not yet been purged of collaborators, and because I was more useful to France continuing the fight than discussing my personal affairs.

Lieutenants Albert Brouard and Jacques Ibarne from the *Direction Générale des Etudes et Recherches* (military security) were given the unenviable task of investigating Petiot's alleged Resistance activities. Ibarne was especially qualified to do this, as he had served in the Resistance under the pseudonym Jacques Yonnet. They actually had more data available for their inquiry than might be supposed. A post-war record had already been compiled of the names, address, and photographs of all official Resistance members. Petiot and his group were not listed. Petiot explained this absence by charging:

> Those who compile these dossiers [of Resistance groups] are either lunatics or criminals. Surely they know that some DGER [military security] officers are former Gestapo members. On the first day of the next war, the first people the spies will execute are the people on the lists, thanks to those lists.

Ibarne and Brouard also found that Petiot's description of his "pal" Cumuleau was completely wrong. In fact, Jean-Marie Charbonneaux had begun using that pseudonym after Petiot was already in a German prison, and he was dead before Petiot was released. Their investigation did find one Spanish anti-fascist cell in the area of Paris that Petiot specified, and the members did know him—but only as the doctor who had delivered a member's baby. No one in any Resistance group had ever heard of "Fly-Tox," and the code names and procedures Petiot cited were incorrect.

On May 3, 1945, Ibarne and Brouard submitted their official report concluding that Petiot's tales should be rejected:

> Petiot's statements, his hesitations, his contradictions, his glaring ignorance of the structure of the Resistance and even of the nature and operation of those sectors for which he pretends to have worked, the numerous improbabilities in his declarations, his systematic habit of mentioning only Resistance comrades who are either dead (Cumuleau, Brossolette) or who cannot be found (the members of Fly-Tox) lead one to believe that Petiot was not at any time in serious contact with any Resistance organization whatsoever. He has simply exploited information he possesses ... We formally reject the hypothesis that the accused played even the remotest part in the Resistance.

It should be noted here that in France, the formal inquiry, or investigation, is conducted *after* the suspect has been arrested. This inquiry is led by a *Juge d'Instruction*, who determines if the case warrants prosecution.

Over the next year, *Juge d'Instruction* Goletty questioned Petiot every few days in his chambers. Petiot kept repeating the same stories until, on October

30, 1945, he said, "I refuse to answer any more questions because I wish to explain myself in public, in court, as quickly as possible." Petiot remained firm, so Judge Goletty submitted his dossier, which weighed 66 pounds, to a three-judge panel. They decided that there was sufficient evidence to go to trial on charges that Petiot had murdered 27 people for personal gain estimated at F200 million (about $50 million in 2002). The case was then turned over to the office of the *Procureur Général* for trial.

Unwilling to become involved in any case that dealt with the Resistance, the *Procureur Général* passed the case to his assistant, who, in turn, passed it "downhill." Finally, the case landed on the desk of the newest— and, at 30 years of age, the youngest and most inexperienced—lawyer in the office, *Avocat Général* Elissalde. Elissalde had already familiarized himself with the case, and he shepherded it through the Assize Court, which set a trial date. At that point, *Avocat Général* Pierre Dupin, a mediocre courtroom attorney, was assigned to prosecute the case. He had only six weeks to familiarize himself with the voluminous case materials and prepare for trial.

Dupin was no match for the defense team, led by France's greatest living criminal attorney, René Floriot, who had defended many high-profile clients. He had an excellent courtroom record, and often won acquittals or lighter sentences for his clients. It was said that his life was the law: he abstained from marriage, tobacco, and, other than a glass of champagne before his closing statements during trials, alcohol. Georgette and Maurice Petiot had hired him in March 1944, and he was present during each of the doctor's interrogations. As he was intimately acquainted with the case, he was prepared and anxious to go to trial. So was Dr. Petiot; he told his guards that it would be a wonderful and amusing trial—he would make everyone laugh.

The Trial

On March 18, 1946, the trial of Dr. Petiot began at the *Palais de Justice*. It would last 16 days, use 12 legal teams and 90 witnesses, and produce 3 tons of evidence and 660 pounds of documents. Hundreds of trunks, hatboxes, and suitcases containing evidence were crammed from the floor to the ceiling along one wood-paneled wall, making the courtroom look to observers like a railway luggage room.

The trial was presided over by Judge Marcel Leser, the president of a three-judge tribunal. These scarlet-robed judges, of whom only the president was allowed to actively participate during the trial, and seven jurors would deliberate on Petiot's fate. Under French law, only a two-thirds majority (six votes) was necessary to convict on any count, and there were 135 separate counts to Petiot's indictment. The doctor was charged with killing 27 people and, for each of these, he was charged with:

1. Fraudulent appropriation of clothing, valuables or other personal items.
2. Willful murder in Paris or elsewhere in France.
3. Committing murder with malice aforethought.
4. Committing murder with premeditation.
5. Committing murder to appropriate valuables.

The majority of the charges were capital offenses, so the prosecutor only had to prove one of the charges to send Petiot to the guillotine.

The prosecution and defense were not the only lawyers present. Under French law, lawyers representing each victim are allowed to aid the prosecutors and, if the defendant is found guilty, to request that the court assess civil damages. In this trial, these civil lawyers were often more effective than the state's attorney.

The courtroom was packed with the victims' families and their attorneys, visiting lawyers and magistrates, 100 journalists, more than 400 spectators, and enough police to control the crowd. Spectators needed special yellow passes to gain entrance, but forgery had become commonplace during the Occupation and hundreds of fake passes were sold on the street. The trial started at 1:20 P.M. and, by 1:50 P.M., the jury had been selected. Petiot entered the courtroom wearing a blue-gray suit, a purple bow tie, and a gray overcoat. His sallow complexion and hollow eyes contrasted with his wavy dark hair. The beard he had worn when passing as Captain Valéry was gone.

Petiot's hands became a focus of the journalists' attention. Throughout his life, he had an "intense and excitable air" and "constantly rubbed his hands together." Petiot's hands were large and dark, with out-curving thumbs, bony fingers, and rough skin. The press characterized them as powerful hands, "the hands of an assassin; the hands of a strangler," but certainly not those of a physician. As the clerk read the long indictment, Petiot looked bored and used his hands to draw caricatures of the prosecutors.

French criminal trials begin with a summary of the defendant's life, which, in Petiot's case, police had spent nearly 18 months compiling. As Judge Leser started to read, Petiot began what would become his courtroom trademark—supercilious outbursts challenging anything negative that was said about him. To the statement "As a child, you were noted for your fits of violent temper," Petiot angrily replied, "Oh, come now, if we start like this, we shan't get on very well." After several such outbursts, an exasperated Judge Leser said, "Next you're going to tell me the whole dossier is false." Petiot replied:

> No, I wouldn't say that. Only eight-tenths of it is false ... Why don't we stop this farce right now? This story was made up by all the bigots and idiots in the country ... I don't care to be treated like a criminal. And I beg the gentlemen of the jury, who will be the final arbiters of this fight, to carefully note all the lies in the dossier.

Throughout the trial, observers never believed that Petiot was either innocent or truthful, but the prosecutor was so incompetent that he could not catch Petiot in a lie. That task would be left to the judge and the other lawyers. Reporters began to score each day's events—the prosecution nearly always lost.

At the end of the second day, in an almost unheard-of breach of procedural propriety, Judge Leser and two jurors gave interviews to the *New York Herald Tribune*. Leser was quoted as saying that Petiot was a "terrifying monster, an appalling murderer." One juror got it exactly right, saying, "He is mad. But of course he is mad. He is intelligent, though. He has a terrible intelligence. He is guilty, and the guillotine is too swift for such a monster." The other juror added, "We are only hearing about the bodies that were found, but how many more he killed, and how many bodies he hid, we shall never know." Floriot, Petiot's lawyer, immediately demanded a mistrial. The appellate court, however, simply replaced the two jurors with alternates, reprimanded the reporter, and allowed Judge Leser to continue.

Petiot was again asked about his Resistance activities. He repeated his claims to head "Fly-Tox," and had a heated exchange with *Maître* Véron about his explosives experiences. Petiot's repeated claims to have worked for the Resistance and his obviously false stories soon irritated the real hero, *Maître* Véron, who exclaimed, "I won't tolerate having you dirty the name of the Resistance for your own ends!" The audience applauded.

Petiot then began the diatribes that would undermine his skilled lawyer's work. "Shut up, you defender of Jews," he shouted at Véron. "You're working for the traitor Dreyfus and you're a double agent yourself!" Aghast, Véron moved toward Petiot with raised fists, shouting, "Take that back or I'll knock your teeth in!" The judge soon restored order.

On the trial's third and fourth days, witnesses appeared on behalf of Petiot's many victims. The doctor alternated between acting bored with the proceedings and verbally challenging or abusing the witnesses. (In France, defendants are allowed to question witnesses in criminal trials.)

On the fifth day, the court took the unusual step of moving to the 21 rue Le Sueur house so the jurors could see the site of the murders, or at least the body dispositions. Three hundred *gendarmes* attempted, often unsuccessfully, to hold back the throngs of people hoping for a look at Dr. Petiot. As the hand-cuffed Petiot was led into the house, he said, "Peculiar homecoming reception, don't you think?"

The visit was a chaotic affair. Judge Leser kept screaming to keep the door open so that the official visit would "be public." He also reportedly ran around the house yelling, "No smoking in the courtroom!" and "Silence in the court!" No one had thought to restore the electricity, so the examination was conducted by candlelight, prompting Petiot's sarcastic comment, "Truly this is enlightened justice!" Later, when they examined the triangular room, that was thought to be Petiot's execution chamber, he exclaimed:

> I admit that I executed several people, so what difference does it make whether they were killed here or there? Why do you keep harping on such silly things? The rest of the world really is going to think we're a bunch of imbeciles in France!

The visit had a much greater effect on the jurors than anyone had expected; several said that they had nightmares for days afterward.

On the sixth day, the courtroom was crowded with so many reporters that some had to sit with Petiot in the prisoner's box. Spectators included Prince Rainier of Monaco and Mme. Gouin, the wife of the provisional president of France. Petiot, as usual, was out of control. At one point, Judge Leser asked him, "Petiot, can't you try to control yourself a bit?" Petiot replied, "We've known each other for six days now. Do you really think I can control myself?"

During a coroner's testimony, Petiot demonstrated both his intelligence and his knowledge of advanced forensics when he asked about estimating the time of death using insect larvae. Dr. Piédelièvre replied that the fire had destroyed the evidence. Petiot told Piédelièvre, "If you will permit me, I would like to drop by and discuss it a bit further after the trial is over." But, as the trial progressed, Petiot became more irritable, at one point telling the judge, "The further this trial goes, the more confusing it becomes." "Voilà," replied Judge Leser as laughter filled the courtroom.

Dr. Génil-Perrin, one of the psychiatrists who had determined that Petiot was sane enough to stand trial, testified next:

> I have examined Petiot and found him to be remarkably intelligent, and endowed with an extraordinary gift for repartee [at which point court-room observers burst into laughter, having been regaled with the doctor's

outbursts for a week] ... but a stunted moral development. He is entirely responsible for his acts.

Another psychiatrist, however, complained that he had trouble examining Petiot, since the doctor had wanted to ask all the questions. Petiot rolled his eyes and, again, the courtroom erupted with laughter.

On the thirteenth day of the trial, which was April Fool's Day, the defense called their witnesses. (Rumor had it that the American judges from the Nuremberg trials, which were being held at the same time, would attend as guests, but they never arrived.) Most of those who testified were character witnesses with moving tales of Petiot's devotion to his medical practice, but they could not substantiate any of Petiot's claims about his Resistance activities. Petiot's accomplices, hesitant to say anything incriminating, provided no new information. His brother Maurice, nearly dead from throat cancer, shuffled to the stand to offer a muted defense of his brother.

The only substantive defense witnesses were three of Petiot's fellow prisoners at Fresnes. Lieutenant Richard l'Héritier was a French paratrooper who, after being captured by the Germans, shared a cell with Petiot for five months. Both he and another cellmate testified that Petiot had repeatedly spoken of his "Fly-Tox" group and of the escape organization. Both said that Petiot, unmindful of his own safety, was constantly sarcastic to the German guards. Mme. Germaine Barré, who had worked for Allied intelligence and was initially sentenced to death by the Germans, confirmed that she saw Petiot verbally abuse his captors.

During the next three days, lawyers from both sides gave their summary statements. Mostly long and often boring, they were punctuated with a few highlights. One such moment came when *Maître* Véron offered an analogy of Petiot's actions:

> There is a legend that you all know well: the story of the ship-wreckers. Cruel men placed lanterns on the cliffs to lure ashore ships in distress. The sailors, confident, never suspecting that such evil deceit could exist, sailed onto the reefs and died, and those who had pretended to lead them to safety filled their coffers with the spoils of their foul deeds. Petiot is just that: the false savior, the false refuge. He lured the desperate, the frightened, the hunted, and he killed them by turning their instincts for self-preservation against them.
>
> It was not for a Petiot, that Gabriel Peri, Brossolette, Colonel Marchal, and many others [*maquis* heroes] laid down their lives. I do not know for sure if Petiot was, in fact, connected with the Gestapo or the *Abwehr* [German Intelligence Service], but one thing is certain, namely, that the

smoke from the chimney of rue Le Sueur will join in the skies of Europe with the smoke that came from the crematories of Auschwitz and the other Nazi camps.

No, Petiot was never connected with the French Resistance and he has placed himself beyond human society. He must be eliminated forever by being condemned to death. He tried to fool us into believing he was a resistant. We are not that foolish. Death must be his finish!

In his summary, *Avocat Général* Pierre Dupin, the prosecutor, also asked for the death penalty:

> Never in a hundred years . . . has such a monster appeared before a court . . . You see before you the Bluebeard of our century, a modern Gilles de Rais. It was with horror that I undertook this case. Petiot indiscriminately murdered men, women, and children simply to rob them of their few earthly goods . . .
>
> Petiot's perversity is equaled only by his skill as an actor in a self-created role. The man you see before you is the star performer in a fictional drama of the Resistance. It is a play that has grown within his imagination, and which contains not a single shred of real life.

Petiot's lawyer, René Floriot, thundered through his 6½-hour summation with such skill that he received a standing ovation when he finished at 9:30 P.M. While a guard took Petiot into an adjacent room, the three judges and the jury retired to deliberate on their verdict.

The courtroom was so packed that day that, had someone fainted, there would have been no room to fall down. Afraid of losing their place, no one moved during the recess, which was expected to last at least all night. Only three hours later, the judges and the jury returned. Bailiffs had to awaken Petiot to return to court; he was sleeping peacefully. With 135 counts to decide, they had spent only about 90 seconds on each one—including the time it took to read them and to vote. Petiot was convicted of 126 of the charges; he was found innocent only of the death of one obscure victim and of murdering Van Bever and Mme. Khaït for profit.

Judge Leser announced the penalty: death by guillotine. As the courtroom erupted and flashbulbs popped, only one person remained placid: Dr. Marcel Petiot, the 49-year-old physician-murderer. As he was led from the courtroom, he continued to play out his internal drama, shouting, "I must be avenged!"

The judges also awarded various survivors F1,970,000 in civil damages and assessed court costs of F312,611.50 (totalling about $175,000 in 2002). The total amount was less than one half of one percent of the amount that

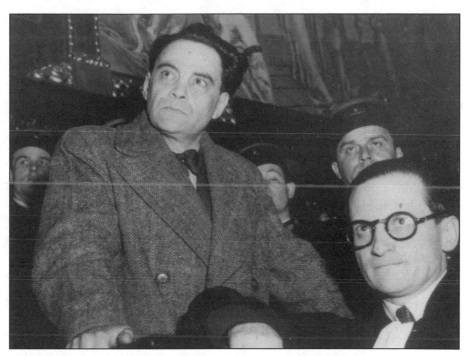

Petiot and *Maître* René Floriot at the moment he was sentenced to death.
(AP/Wide World Photos)

Petiot had obtained from his victims. Georgette Petiot eventually paid about half of this assessment.

Throughout the trial, Petiot remained an enigma: eerily perceptive yet often bizarrely inappropriate. As Thomas Maeder wrote in *The Unspeakable Crimes of Dr. Petiot*:

> No image of a human personality emerged, no motive surfaced . . . Petiot had fooled the French, the Germans, the Resistants, the courts, psychiatrists, his friends, and his own wife. He had acted as a solitary enigmatic force amidst a world in which he did not participate, and which he regarded only with scorn.

Dr. Paul, the coroner of the city of Paris who had long talks with Petiot while he was in jail, later wrote:

> [Petiot was] the coldest fish and the most brilliant criminal, yet the most convincing talker that I ever met in my long career in the fields of crime and medicine . . . Besides, I never heard of a doctor-surgeon-mayor-

murderer in fact or in fiction, much less one who was also a spy, or intelligence informer, writer, cartoonist, antique expert, mathematician or who calmly claimed possibly a 150 victims . . . he had lost count . . . but all of which he tried to justify in one way or another!

Pathologist Dr. Derobert, who actually gave Petiot a tour of the *Institut Médico-Légal* in an attempt to get him to talk, provided additional insights into his murderous personality. Derobert felt that Petiot was "the greatest individual murderer in modern history," adding that if Petiot had not been so overconfident, he probably would not have been discovered. Derobert said he got goose bumps when talking to Petiot, who had an "insane quality" but also "a certain charm, was extremely persuasive, extremely intelligent, and good at repartee, with a sharp sense of humor." While Petiot refused to discuss medical issues with Dr. Derobert, he did speak of sadism, saying, "The Marquis de Sade satisfied his sex instincts by merely beating, biting, and pinching women. I fuck them."

The Execution

Petiot's lawyer appealed, but the Appellate Court rejected their argument. Petiot spent his last days chain-smoking and writing poetry, which he distributed to the guards. Each day he would ask them, "When are they going to assassinate me?" Under French law, he would learn that just before the execution.

After some haggling, executioner Henri Desfourneaux assembled his guillotine in the courtyard of Santé Prison. (Desfourneaux, the sole French executioner, had gone on strike for higher pay. He settled for F65,000 plus F10,000 for upkeep of the guillotines, which he owned.) The guillotine consisted of two 15-foot-high, grooved posts fastened to a supporting base. A 15.4-pound triangular steel blade, the *couperet,* mounted on a 100-pound weight, delivered the blow. Petiot's body would be fastened to a plank that dropped into a horizontal position, thus positioning his neck in the blade's path. There was a small basket to catch his head.

A variety of guests assembled for the semi-private execution. (Desfourneaux had performed the last public execution, badly, in 1939.) Prosecutor Dupin, accompanied by other officials, awakened Petiot in his cell. As a final request, Petiot asked to be allowed to write a letter to his wife and son. When he was asked how long it would take, Petiot replied, "I don't know, but I once remember a condemned prisoner writing letters for four hours while everyone waited." Petiot took only 20 minutes.

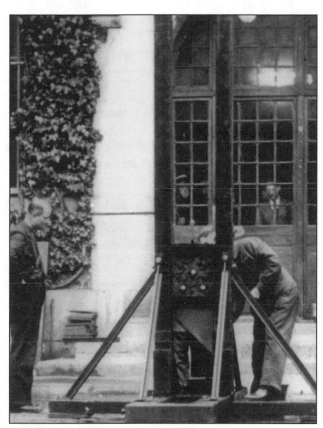

Workmen in the Santé Prison courtyard clean and dismantle a guillotine in Paris, France on May 25, 1946 after the execution of Dr. Marcel Petiot who was convicted of mass murder during World War II. (AP/Wide World Photos)

Dupin then uttered the traditional words: "Petiot, have courage. The time has come." Petiot made an obscene reply. He refused the traditional glass of rum, but puffed calmly on a cigarette. He was then led to the clerk's office, where he signed the register, and his shirt collar was cut off for his neck to be shaved. It was reported that Petiot's final words were: "*Je suis un voyageur qui emporté tous ses bagages avec lui!*" (I am a traveler who is taking all his baggage with him.) More in character, his less-frequently cited last words actually were: "Gentlemen, I ask you not to look. This will not be very pretty." Marcel Petiot, M.D., smiled, as at 5:05 A.M. on May 25, 1946, the blade fell.

Epilogue

The coroner, Dr. Paul, who had witnessed hundreds of executions, said:

> In my forty years, I never before saw a condemned man with so much scorn and indifference to death. For the first time in my life I saw a man leaving death row, if not dancing, at least showing perfect calm. Most people about to be executed do their best to be courageous, but one senses that it is a stiff and forced courage. Petiot moved with ease, as though he were walking into his office for a routine appointment.

The house at 21 rue Le Sueur was demolished in 1950, but not before treasure hunters had sifted through the rubble searching for Dr. Petiot's ill-gotten gains, most of which have never been located. Gérard Petiot emigrated to South America after his father's execution.

Marcel Petiot was buried in Ivry Cemetery, as were many executed criminals. Ironically, 860 Parisians who had been shot by Germans for Resistance activities between 1940 and 1944 were also buried there. In France, executed criminals' remains are first buried in a grave marked only with a number. After ten years, they are disinterred and, if the family claims them, reburied elsewhere. Although Georgette Petiot unsuccessfully petitioned to attend her husband's first funeral, she did not claim his body a decade later. Petiot's body was dumped in a common grave with other executed criminals. Whether his head was also buried remains a mystery.

Maître Floriot, Petiot's attorney, would later write that Dr. Petiot, known as the "Vampire of the rue Le Sueur," "the new Bluebeard," or, simply, "the monster," was the only intelligent murderer that he had known.

And Marcel André Félix Petiot was a physician.

The Guillotine

Dr. Joseph-Ignace Guillotin (1738–1814) neither invented nor improved the killing machine named in his honor. As far as anyone knows, he never even built a model of it or participated in its use. And, despite tales to the contrary, he did not die by it, but from a boil on his shoulder.

Actually, Guillotin, a physician, humanitarian, and politician, belonged to a small reform movement that sought to abolish the death penalty. But, during a debate on France's Penal Code in 1789, he suggested to the National Assembly (of which he was a member) that the country adopt an egalitarian and civilized method of execution. Up to that time, upper class criminals would often get the swifter death of decapitation (although the executioner was not always accurate), while common folk suffered through being hanged, drowned, drawn and quartered, or any number of local execution methods. Dr. Guillotin proposed:

> In all cases where the law imposes the death penalty on an accused person, the punishment shall be the same whatever the nature of the offense of which he is guilty. The criminal shall be decapitated. This will be done solely by means of a simple mechanism.

Little did he know that the French Revolution, which began the same year, would make his suggestion—and his name—infamous.

Making & Testing the Guillotine

The National Assembly approved his idea on June 3, 1791. The new law read: "Every person condemned to the death penalty shall have his head severed." But they had no machine to do this. The problem was solved when Dr. Antoine Louis, secretary of the College of Surgeons, designed one. Tobias Schmidt, a German harpsichord maker and the lowest bidder for the project, built the new device.

On April 11, 1792, Schmidt successfully tested the first machine on sheep and calves, since "the general resistance characteristics closely approach those of man." Four days later, "in a proper atmosphere of reverence and piety," he tested the machine on male and female cadavers at the prison-hospital-nursing home in Bicêtre. One well-built male cadaver presented a problem: the head continued to hang on to the trunk by some cartilage even after three attempts to sever it. On April 21, sporting an improved blade, the machine was successfully tested on three well-built, non-emaciated corpses from the military hospital. This test convinced French officials that "the machine," as it was called, was ready for action.

They didn't waste any time putting it to use. On April 25, 1792, Charles-Henri Sanson, who was the official executioner in Paris during the Revolution, used "the machine" to execute highwayman Nicolas-Jacques Pelletier.

continued . . .

The Guillotine, continued

Before the execution, Sanson supposedly said:

> Today the machine invented for the purpose of decapitating criminals sentenced to death will be put to work for the first time. Relative to the methods of execution practiced heretofore, this machine has several advantages. It is less repugnant: no man's hands will be tainted with the blood of his fellow being, and the worst of the ordeal for the condemned man will be his own fear of death, a fear more painful to him than the stroke which deprives him of life.

In May 1792, an architect named Giraud reported on the machine's functioning:

> Although well-conceived in itself, it has not been perfected to the fullest possible extent. The grooves, the tongues and the gudgeons are in wood; the first should be made in brass, the others of iron. The hooks to which are attached the cords holding up the mouton are only fixed with round-headed nails. They should be fixed with strong nuts and bolts.

Originally known simply as "the machine," the guillotine was next called "la louisette" or "le louison" for its inventor, Dr. Louis. During the French Revolution, however, the device took on its modern name, as well as many others: "Madame Guillotine," "The National Razor," "La Sainte Guillotine," "The People's Avenger," and "The Patriotic Shortener." The French underworld later dubbed it "The Widow." Dr. Guillotine and his family tried unsuccessfully to change the machine's name. Eventually, his children changed their own names instead.

The Facts

In its most common form, the guillotine blade (*couperet*) weighed more than 88 pounds. The side posts were about 15 feet high and had brass-lined grooves in which the blade, with two wheels on each side, glided. The prisoner was strapped onto the *bascule*, a board that rotated from vertical to horizontal, automatically placing the head into the *lunette*, the semi-circular depression in the wooden support which held the neck in position. Once the trigger was pressed, it took 1/30 of a second for the blade to drop. It traveled at 21 feet per second, exerting a force of 889 pounds per square inch! A basket, lined with cloth to absorb the blood, was set in place to catch the head. The body was then tipped into a waiting (sometimes short) coffin.

Between 1870 and 1872, Leon Berger, an assistant executioner and carpenter, developed an improved guillotine that included a spring system to stop the blade at the bottom of the grooves, a lock/blocking device at the *lunette*, and a new release mechanism. All subsequent guillotines were built to his specifications. In 1878, Nicolas Roch, then the Paris executioner, installed a wooden

continued . . .

The Guillotine, continued

shield to block the sight of the blade from the victim. The next year, he was replaced and the shield went with him.

The Executioners

From 1688 to 1847, the post of official executioner was hereditary, and was held by seven successive generations of the Sanson family. They trained by serving as one of an executioner's two *valets*, or assistants, and held another position when not chopping heads. At one point, seven Sanson family members were executioners in various parts of France. By 1800, however, all the positions had been abolished except for the executioner in Paris, called *Monsieur de Paris*. He served the entire country and traveled to other cities when necessary.

After 1847, anyone could qualify to hold the position, and there was no shortage of applicants. When Andre Obrecht became executioner in 1951, for example, he won out over 400 competitors.

Guillotines were the private property of the executioners, and were passed along with the position. Petiot's executioner, Desfourneaux, had two guillotines—the standard model and one for travel. Because the standard guillotine had previously been damaged, he used the traveling model on the murderous doctor.

Death by Guillotine

During France's Reign of Terror (September 1793 to July 1794), between 20,000 and 40,000 victims were executed. The guillotine claimed its most famous victim on January 21, 1793: Louis Capet (Louis XVI, King of France), at *Place de la Liberte*, now called *Place de la Concorde*. His queen, Marie Antoinette, met the same fate later that year, on October 16. Ambrose Bierce wrote in *The Devil's Dictionary* that "A Guillotine is a machine which makes a Frenchman shrug his shoulders with good reason."

Charles Dickens described a typical scene of the time in his novel, *A Tale of Two Cities*:

Along the Paris streets, the death-carts rumble, hollow and harsh. Six tumbrils carry the day's wine to La Guillotine. All the devouring and insatiate Monsters imagined since imagination could record itself, are fused in the one realization, Guillotine . . .

So used are the regular inhabitants of the houses to the spectacle, that in many windows there are no people, and in some the occupation of the hands is not so much as suspended, while, the eyes survey the faces in the tumbrils. Here and there, the inmate has visitors to see the sight; then he points his finger, with something of the complacency of a curator or authorized exponent, to this cart and to this, and seems to tell who sat here yesterday, and who there the day before.

continued . . .

The Guillotine, continued

Of the riders in the tumbrils, some observe these things, and all things on their last roadside, with an impassive stare; others, with a lingering interest in the ways of life and men. Some, seated with drooping heads, are sunk in silent despair; again, there are some so heedful of their looks that they cast upon the multitude such glances as they have seen in theatres, and in pictures. Several close their eyes, and think, or try to get their straying thoughts together.

Only one, and he a miserable creature, of a crazed aspect, is so shattered and made drunk by horror, that he sings, and tries to dance. Not one of the whole number appeals by look or gesture, to the pity of the people.

As Dr. Petiot suggested, decapitation is a gruesome spectacle. While the head drops cleanly into the waiting basket, the still-beating heart, stimulated by an adrenaline surge, pumps blood out the carotid arteries, and stomach contents may spill out through the open esophagus. When, as during the French Revolution, multiple victims were guillotined in succession, the stench became dreadful and the executioner and his assistants worked in pools of blood; rivers of blood ran down the streets.

English poet Lord Byron described the execution of three robbers he witnessed in Rome in 1817:

The day before I left Rome I saw three robbers guillotined—the ceremony—including the masqued priests—the half-naked executioners—the bandaged criminals—the black Christ & his banner—the scaffold—the soldiery—the slow procession—& the quick rattle and heavy fall of the axe—the splash of the blood—& the ghastliness of the exposed heads—is altogether more impressive than the vulgar and ungentlemanly dirty "new drop" & dog-like agony of infliction upon the sufferers of the English sentence (i.e. hanging).

The head was taken off before the eye could trace the blow—but from an attempt to draw back the head—notwithstanding it was held forward by the hair—the first head was cut off close to the ears—the other two were taken off more cleanly;—it is better than the Oriental way (i.e. with sword)—& (I should think) than the axe of our ancestors. The pain seems little—& yet the effect to the spectator—& the preparation to the criminal—is very striking & chilling. The first turned me quite hot & thirsty—& made me shake so that I could hardly hold the opera-glass (I was close—but determined to see—as one should see everything once—with attention) the second and third (which shows how dreadully soon things grow indifferent) I am ashamed to say had no effect on me—as a horror—though I would have saved them if I could.

Death by guillotine was not always swift and sure. French police records chronicle instances when the blade failed to complete its job. That horrifying

continued . . .

The Guillotine, *continued*

spectacle was imagined by Victor Hugo, an ardent death penalty opponent, in his novel, *The Last Days of the Condemned* (1840):

> The heavy triangle of iron, slowly detached itself, falling by jerks down the slides, until, horrible to relate, it wounded the man, without killing him! The poor creature uttered a frightful cry. The disconcerted executioner hauled up the axe, and let it slide down again. A second time, the neck of the malefactor was wounded, without being severed. Again, he shrieked, the crowd joining him. The executioner raised the axe a third time, but no better effect attended the third stroke.
>
> Five times the axe was raised and let fall, and after the fifth stroke, the condemned was still shrieking for mercy. The indignant populace commenced throwing missiles at the executioner, who hid himself beneath the guillotine, and crept away behind the gendarmes' horses.
>
> But I have not finished.

Experiments on Severed Heads

French physicians, especially at the beginning of the twentieth century, performed numerous experiments on the decapitated heads. Most found that the heads showed no activity or response, except for the natural post-mortem changes. The descriptions frequently quoted, however, are those that purported to demonstrate that awareness remains.

In 1907, Dr. Amirault infused dog's blood into a newly severed head and claimed that, nearly two hours later, the head stared at him momentarily in "shocked amazement." Several other physicians reported similar findings—not surprisingly, no one could ever confirm their observations. One such notorious report came from Dr. Beaurieux, who experimented with the head of the guillotined criminal Languille immediately after his decapitation in June 1905. He noted:

> the eyelids and lips of the guillotined man worked in irregularly rhythmic contractions for about five or six seconds . . . I waited for several seconds. The spasmodic movements ceased. The face relaxed, the lids half closed on the eyeballs, leaving only the white of the conjunctiva visible, exactly as in the dying whom we have occasion to see every day in the exercise of our profession, or as in those just dead. It was then that I called in a strong, sharp voice: "Languille!" I saw the eyelids slowly lift up . . . Languille's eyes very definitely fixed themselves on mine and the pupils focused themselves . . . After several seconds, the eyelids closed again, slowly and evenly, and the head took on the same appearance as it had had before I called out.

Dr. Beaurieux claimed that the eyes opened once more and gazed at him after he again called the man's name, before taking on the aspect of death after about 30 seconds.

continued . . .

The Guillotine, continued

Mechanized Decapitators

Mechanized decapitators had existed long before the French Revolution made the guillotine infamous. On April 1, 1307, one such machine was used to execute Murcod Ballagh near Merton, Ireland. A similar device was employed for centuries in Halifax, England. At first used only for cloth thieves, unfortunates were executed on market days, presumably so there would be a big crowd.

The "Halifax Gibbet" may have been used as early as 1280; it was last used in 1648. Townsmen would pull the rope together, releasing the pin that held the blade—an example of justice truly being in the people's hands. However, the punishment was used sparingly, with only 55 people ending their lives on this gibbet in its 162-year history. John Taylor's 1622 poem speaks of "the formidable Gibbet Law at Halifax":

> At Halifax, the Law so sharpe doth deale,
> That whoso more than thirteen pence doth steale,
> They have a jyn [engine] that wondrous quicke and well
> Sends Thieves all headless unto Heav'n or Hell.

The "Maiden" was used in Scotland as early as 1564. Patterned after the Halifax Gibbet, its blade was a 13-inch-long plate of iron faced with steel, with a 75-pound weight secured on top. Like the guillotine, the blade ran in copper-lined grooves cut into upright oak posts. Similar devices were used in Europe and the Mideast, primarily for condemned aristocrats. Specific examples are known to have been used in Germany, Italy (the *Mannaia*), and Persia.

The Guillotine Today

While the guillotine remains fixed in popular memory as a French tool, the Nazis guillotined at least as many people as were killed in the Reign of Terror, when up to 300 prisoners a day went to their deaths on Paris's guillotine alone.

Hitler considered the method a humiliating death, and consigned more than 20,000 political prisoners to die beneath its blade, including concentration camp prisoners and members of the German resistance movement, White Rose.

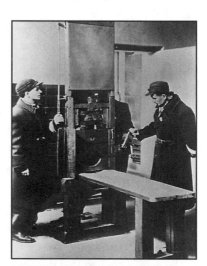

A guillotine in a Nazi death cell.
(© Sovfoto/Eastfoto/PictureQuest)

continued . . .

The Guillotine, continued

The guillotine was also used in France's colonies—and was seen as a symbol of the hated French colonialists.

Today, a guillotine sits in the War Crimes Museum in Ho Chi Minh City, Vietnam, formerly part of French Indo-China.

In April 1854, Monsieur Joseph Tussaud brought a guillotine to London to be part of the Tussaud's Waxworks, where it still resides, along with the death masks from many of the famous heads that *La Sainte Guillotine* severed from their owners' bodies.

The last person to be guillotined in France was Hamida Djandoubi, on September 10, 1977. France eliminated the death penalty in 1981.

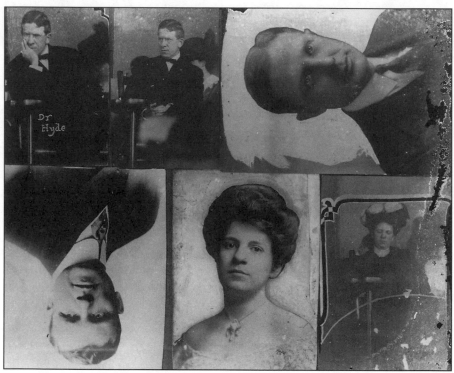

Composite photos of Bennett Clark Hyde, M.D. including images from the trial and two unidentified women. (Courtesy of the Kansas City Library Special Collections, Zeldin Collection)

7
More Doctors Who Kill

The Minor Players

This group includes physicians who killed once or twice out of professional envy, jealousy, greed, love, or other human passions. In some cases, there just isn't enough information about them to say more about their motives. Victims are often people close to them, such as their family members, colleagues, lovers, or friends. Like serial killers, they intend to get away with their crimes. Sometimes they do, and so cannot be included—yet.

Bennett Clark Hyde, M.D. — An Epidemic of Murder

"Colonel" Thomas Hunton Swope (1827–1909) combined his intelligence and luck to become one of Kansas City's leading citizens. His luck ran out, however, when he became related, through marriage, to Bennett Clark Hyde, M.D.

Swope was a tough-minded, hard-drinking man. A Yale graduate and lawyer, he settled in Kansas City in 1857 and began investing heavily in land. He made a fortune; at his death, it was valued at $3.5 million (more than $63 million in 2002). Much of his money was amassed when the railroads picked the city as the site where most trains would cross the Mississippi River. The Colonel owned the best locations for the crossing and made a killing when he sold. He then bought much of the land in what would become the city's downtown area.

Swope was also a philanthropist. He generously gave the city a tract of land at 23rd and Locust Streets on which to build the city hospital and, in

1896, he donated 1,334 acres along Blue River for Swope Park. The latter donation created such excitement that the city declared a holiday and held a huge celebration, including an impressive parade, and bestowed upon Swope the honorary title of "Colonel." Although the park was valued at $2 million in 1909 ($28 million in 2002), the donation was not as generous as it seemed, since he conditioned it on the construction of a streetcar route to the park. The Colonel, of course, owned more land along the right-of-way, which he then developed.

Colonel Swope lived quietly with several members of his extended family in a 26-room, three-story brick mansion in Independence, about 20 miles outside Kansas City. His brother, Logan A. Swope, had built the home when he moved to Kansas City to assist Thomas in his business ventures in the 1880s. It was situated on the highest ground of a 19-acre tract, surrounded by gardens and winding walks. The interior was decked out with dark wood paneling and stained glass windows. There was a freight elevator, a butler's pantry, an underground fruit cellar, a parlor, and a three-story minaret-like tower.

Following Logan's death in 1900, his widow, Margaret Swope, invited her bachelor brother-in-law, the Colonel, to come live with her and her seven children—two boys and five girls. Since there was plenty of room, she asked one of her husband's cousins and business partners, the quiet and studious James Moss Hunton, to move in as well. The Colonel and Hunton were close, and Thomas named his cousin, more than 20 years his junior, as executor of his will.

Mrs. Swope, a "large-bosomed, 54-year-old, double-chinned dowager," presided over her large loving family. When her daughter Frances wanted to marry Dr. Bennett Clark Hyde, who had an unsavory reputation with the ladies, Margaret strongly objected. Frances married him anyway. The Colonel liked Hyde, and helped the newlyweds buy and furnish a house in Kansas City, where Hyde had a profitable medical practice. Mrs. Swope finally reconciled to the marriage and frequently welcomed the couple to her home. That was where the trouble started.

Colonel Swope's will divided the bulk of his estate among his surviving heirs, meaning his sister-in-law and her children. The will stipulated that if any of them were to die, their share was to be redistributed among the remaining heirs. The heirs all knew of this stipulation and, thus, so did Dr. Hyde. There were at least nine people, including Hunton as the estate's executor, who stood between the doctor and the entire Swope fortune. (Frances Hyde was, presumably, not an obstacle, and may even have been party to her husband's misdeeds.) Dr. Hyde decided to start increasing his share of the money.

On October 1, 1909, 60-year-old James Moss Hunton suffered a stroke while eating supper with the family nurse, Ms. Keller. The family's doctor, George T. Twyman, soon arrived, followed by Dr. Hyde. They agreed that Hunton should be bled "to relieve pressure on his brain." But Hyde performed the procedure so vigorously that Dr. Twyman finally had to intervene. When the nurse measured the amount of blood removed, she found it was two quarts—equal to about four units of blood. It was no wonder that when she returned, she found Hunton dead. Hyde had eradicated his first obstacle.

After Hunton's death, Hyde tried to persuade Ms. Keller to tell the Colonel to make him the new executor of his will; she refused. The following day, they both visited the Colonel, and Hyde left a capsule "for Mr. Swope's digestion." Twenty minutes after the Colonel swallowed the pill, the nurse found him with his eyes dilated, his hands and teeth clenched, and his body trembling. Hyde then administered 1/60 grain of strychnine, a proper medication at the time, but probably also what had been in the capsule. Despite the treatment, the Colonel regained consciousness and had the lucidity to say that he should not have taken the pill.

Nurse Keller stayed with Colonel Swope during the day, and Hyde prescribed additional strychnine injections. She left the Colonel alone for only a short time while she went to dinner. Upon her return, she found Hyde and his wife, the potential heiress, in the room. "Uncle Thomas has just gone," said Francis, announcing the death—and Dr. Hyde's second murder within two days. Both corpses remained in the house.

James Moss Hunton was buried quietly on October 4, with only the family in attendance. Colonel Thomas Swope, called "Kansas City's greatest benefactor," had a more spectacular send-off: his body lay in state at the public library, where 10,000 people came to pay their respects. Kansas City's streets were packed for the funeral procession, which ended with the Colonel's burial in Swope Park.

The "Epidemic" Begins

On December 1, Margaret Swope fell ill, followed on December 2 by a daughter and, the next day, by her eldest son, 22-year-old Chrisman. The following day, three household servants also became ill. Dr. Hyde diagnosed all their ailments as typhoid. He had previously disparaged the water supply to the house and kept a separate water container for himself and his wife to use when they visited. Over the next week, Margaret's houseguest, Belle Dickson, also contracted typhoid, as did daughters Sarah and Stella. At that point, nearly the entire household was ill, so three nurses were brought in to help Ms. Keller.

Although Dr. Twyman was in charge of the family's medical care, Hyde repeatedly tried to intervene. He gave Chrisman Swope a capsule similar to the one given to his uncle and he, too, became rigid and began convulsing. The nurse could not get a pulse and Hyde, ever the great clinician, tried a number of "remedies" to restore his life. Of course, he was unsuccessful. Another "obstacle" was dead.

Away in Paris, the eldest daughter, Lucy Lee Swope, had so far escaped the plague that had struck her family. At her mother's request, she returned via New York, where Hyde met her ship and accompanied her to Kansas City. While he was absent from the mansion, all the patients improved for the first time. When he returned, the illnesses reappeared. Lucy also became ill just four days after her arrival. She later recalled that Hyde had given her a drink of foul-tasting water during their trip. (The incubation period for typhoid is from one to three weeks, although it can be as short as three days if a massive dose is administered.)

Resuming his treatments, Hyde gave Mrs. Swope another capsule. About 30 minutes later, she had an unusual type of seizure that to the nurses appeared identical to the one Chrisman experienced before he died. Luckily, Dr. Twyman entered just then and gave Margaret some injections, saving her life. The nurses had had enough and announced that they would leave if Dr. Hyde continued to treat anyone in the household. They claimed that "people are being murdered in this house." Dr. Twyman agreed to be the sole physician for the household.

That evening, one of Hyde's brothers-in-law saw Hyde drop something from his pocket and grind it under his heel. Suspicious, the man picked it up and noted that it smelled like burnt almonds. He sent it to be analyzed—it was found to contain potassium cyanide.

This was one coincidence too many; people were becoming suspicious of Dr. Hyde. Mrs. Swope mentioned her concerns to a trustee for the Colonel's estate, and he launched a series of investigations. A bacteriologist evaluated conditions within the house, but he could find no obvious reason for the typhoid outbreak and opined that someone was intentionally infecting the occupants.

On December 30, 1909, Chrisman's body was exhumed, and his organs were sent to Chicago for analysis. On January 12, Colonel Swope's body was also disinterred and autopsied. The same day, the *Kansas City Journal* ran a story that began with a question:

> Was the late Thomas H. Swope, whose benefactions to Kansas City amounted to more than a million and a half dollars, the victim of a scientific plot which had for its aim the elimination of the entire Swope family, by inoculating with typhoid germs, looking to ultimate control of the three million dollar estate?

That was just what the police and prosecutors wanted to know.

Arrest and Trial

When the report arrived from Chicago that Colonel Swope had died of strychnine poisoning, police began to collect additional evidence against Hyde. On March 6, 1910, authorities indicted the doctor for murdering Colonel Thomas H. Swope and Chrisman Swope, for manslaughter in the case of James Moss Hunton, and for poisoning the other members of the household.

It was at that point that the Swope fortune began to work against the family's interests. Mrs. Hyde, herself wealthy from her family's money—and perhaps abetting the plot to gain control of a larger share of the fortune—expressed faith in her husband and retained a lawyer, Frank P. Walsh, to represent him. Money was no object: her husband would get the best possible defense for as long as it took to clear his name.

The trial was set for April 1910. The chief prosecutor, James A. Reed, was a leader of the state bar and a prominent Missouri politician. Mrs. Swope, who wanted to see justice done to the murderer whom she had always known was dissolute and who now had destroyed much of her family, also spared no expense. Under the table, she paid expenses—and maybe more—to Reed so that he, rather than an assistant, would lead the defense team. She also paid for a slew of special investigators and experts to help prepare the case.

Before the trial began, the judge ruled that evidence could be admitted connecting all the poisonings to a single scheme designed to give Francis Swope Hyde—and thereby Dr. Hyde—a larger share of the Swope fortune. But he limited the scope of the trial to the single charge for the murder of Colonel Thomas H. Swope. This dealt a severe blow to the prosecution and was followed by more bad news: A week before the trial began, the prosecution's star witness, Dr. Twyman, died from a ruptured appendix. (Dr. Hyde was not involved in that death.)

During the first two weeks of the trial, the household's nurses testified that after each of Hyde's visits to his in-laws, their condition deteriorated. Even worse for the Hyde team, pharmacist Hugo Brecklein testified that the doctor had ordered both culture medium (in which to grow bacteria) and cyanide capsules from him. Brecklein had been particularly concerned since, in his 23 years of selling pharmaceuticals, he had never before dispensed cyanide in capsules.

A bacteriologist then testified that he had sold Dr. Hyde not only typhoid cultures but also other infectious bacteria, including anthrax and diphtheria. The scientist had second thoughts about giving Hyde the cultures and visited his offices, where he saw that all the typhoid organisms had been removed from the culture. He added, "there were enough germs taken out to inoculate the whole of Kansas City." Upon hearing this testimony, the judge revoked the doctor's bail, feeling that he was a threat to the Swope family. Dr. Hyde finally went to jail.

In subsequent days, the forensic pathologist testified that the deaths of both Thomas and Chrisman Swope were due to "some convulsing or paralyzing poison." He had found strychnine in Chrisman's liver and stomach and cyanide in the Colonel's liver. The state alleged that the Colonel was given a mixture of strychnine sulfate and potassium cyanide. They postulated that Hyde had expected that the different effects of the two poisons would prevent a diagnosis of the cause of death. Physician experts, however, testified that the Colonel's symptoms were most consistent with a death from strychnine.

The Swope mansion itself played a role in the trial. The butler's pantry had a dumbwaiter so that meals or drinks could be lifted to upper floors. Water was brought from the basement to the butler's pantry. Doctors, public health personnel, typhoid fever experts, and detectives all studied the dumbwaiter and the surrounding area to assess whether, as prosecutors alleged, this was where typhoid germs were introduced into the family's water supply. Nothing could be proven, however, and the state rested its case.

Local doctors then spoke in Hyde's defense, but they seemed unsophisticated compared to the prosecution's experts. When Hyde took the stand, he tried to explain how he had used cyanide for years to remove nitric acid stains from his fingers, but the prosecution easily demolished that story, showing him to be a blatant liar. Mrs. Hyde testified next, but did not help her husband's case.

The jury spent more than a day in deliberation before announcing that Dr. Hyde was guilty of murder and should be imprisoned for life. As a jury member later said, "Hyde was his own worst enemy. His own testimony convicted him." True enough, but the case was far from over.

In February 1911, the Hydes' attorney appealed the case to the Missouri Supreme Court. After wading through the 4,200-page trial record, as well as appeal and defense briefs of nearly 500 pages each, the court overturned the verdict, saying that the trial judge had erred in admitting evidence about Hyde's involvement in crimes other than Colonel Swope's death. They remanded the case for a new trial, with the stipulation that the prosecution could introduce evidence relating only to Colonel Swope's death, rather than to any larger plot. Dr. Hyde was released from jail.

When the next trial began, the Hydes had just returned from a Colorado holiday and seemed upbeat. James Reed, who by then had been elected to the U.S. Senate, returned to lead the prosecution, since he would not take office for several months. With the publicity from the first trial still fresh in people's minds, it took a month to select a jury.

The proceedings finally began on November 21, 1911. Hyde and his counsel had learned a lesson from the first trial; he would not take the stand this time. In response, the prosecution read his entire testimony from the first trial to the jury. However, six weeks into the trial, one of the jury members climbed through a transom and jumped 15 feet from a fire escape to flee from the hotel where they had been sequestered. He was found three days later. The judge declared that the juror was insane and ordered a mistrial, setting a new trial date of May 1912. Rumor had it that the Hydes had actually bribed some jurors.

Hyde, still out on bond, resumed his medical practice, although few patients had the courage to consult him. The trial began as scheduled, and Senator Reed returned to give the prosecution's opening statement. But, three weeks into the case, a jury member became seriously ill. Since he was a Christian Scientist, he refused medical care and his condition steadily deteriorated until, with the agreement of all parties, he was replaced. When the trial ended, four days passed before the jury declared that they were deadlocked, with the majority favoring acquittal! Dr. Hyde remained free while the prosecutors decided what to do next. (By now, Mrs. Hyde had spent $150,000 (about $3 million in 2002) on his defense. Oh, what true love—or conspiracy—will do!)

Four years later, after many delays, the court had finally had enough. Judge Porterfield dismissed the indictment against Hyde on April 9, 1917, almost seven years to the day after the first trial began. He may have been influenced by the more pressing concerns facing the nation: three days earlier, the United States had declared war on Germany.

True love can be a fleeting thing, however. Frances Swope Hyde sued for divorce in October 1920, and obtained custody of their two children. Dr. Hyde abandoned his medical practice in 1934. At age 64, he quietly died of a cerebral hemorrhage while reading a newspaper.

~

John White Webster, M.D. — The Harvard Murder

John White Webster, born in Boston on May 20, 1793, was the son of a successful apothecary who financed his son's foreign travel and Harvard education. At Harvard, Webster obtained a master's degree in 1811 and his medical degree in 1815. After a stint at London's Guy's Hospital, he visited São Miquel in the Azores in 1817. While there, he met and married Harriet Fredrica Hickling, the daughter of the local American vice consul.

When Webster returned to Harvard, he was an internationally known scientist with memberships in the American Academy of Arts and Sciences, the London Geological Society, and the St. Petersburg Mineralogical Society. He had gained some notoriety as the author of several books on geology and chemistry and as a spendthrift. He had also amassed a valuable gem and mineral collection. In 1827, Webster was appointed the Erving Professor of Chemistry and Mineralogy at Harvard University's Medical College. He had a large laboratory which occupied two floors in the medical school's new building.

By all accounts, Webster was a gregarious man with a loving family. While Webster's large circle of friends found him a pleasant social companion who spent lavishly when entertaining, the doctor was also spoiled, self-indulgent, and quick to show his anger. Webster had obtained his teaching position at Harvard only through the sponsorship of one man: Dr. George Parkman.

George Parkman had been one of Webster's classmates at Harvard, but he was from an entirely different social class. The scion of a wealthy Boston family, he increased his wealth through land investments and private moneylending. Tall and thin with a prominent lower jaw, he was something of a character, and always leaned forward with determination while walking. He was punctilious to a fault and, while generous, he did not tolerate sloth or deceit.

A major philanthropist at Harvard, Parkman had donated the land on which the new medical school building had been erected. It was this rather dreary three-story, red-brick structure on North Grove Street in which Webster worked. Parkman also endowed the Parkman Chair of Anatomy and Physiology,

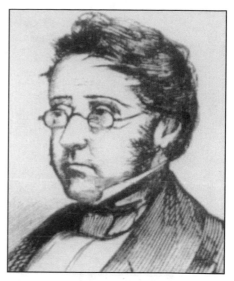

John White Webster, M.D. (Sketch for *New York Daily Globe*, 1850)

which, at mid-century, was occupied by Dr. Oliver Wendell Holmes, the medical school's dean.

By 1842, Webster had spent the fortune (worth more than $800,000 in 2002) that his father had left him less than a decade earlier. He was deeply in debt, and had only a $1,200 (less than $20,000 in 2002) university stipend plus some lecture fees to support him, his wife, and their four daughters. (Aside from the stipend, each medical school professor earned money from tickets sold to students each semester to attend their lectures.) This income was far from enough—particularly given the large sums he continued to spend on additions to his gem and mineral collection.

Because Webster counted Dr. Parkman and his family as friends, he felt free to go to his colleague for a loan. Parkman lent his friend $2,500 (more than $40,000 in 2002), accepting Webster's home and his mineral collection as collateral. In 1846, after some of the money was repaid, they renegotiated the terms.

Webster's financial situation grew worse and, in April 1848, he went to Mr. Shaw, Dr. Parkman's brother-in-law, for a $1,200 loan. Having nothing else to use to secure the loan, Webster pledged the gem collection—although it was still being used as collateral for the loans from Parkman. When Parkman found out, he was furious.

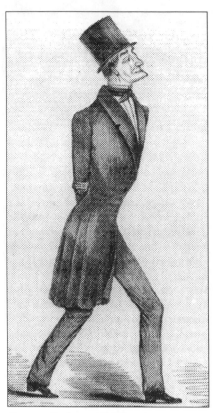

George Parkman, M.D.
(Sketch circa 1850)

On November 19, 1849, the day Webster was to receive the money from selling tickets to his lectures, Parkman came to his laboratory and demanded payment. Webster protested that he did not yet have the money to repay him, and they agreed to meet again on Friday, November 23. This encounter was witnessed by the medical school's janitor, Ephraim Littlefield, who was in the lab to assist Webster with an experiment.

On Friday, at about 2 P.M., Parkman was seen walking "very fast" toward the medical school building. That was the last time he was seen alive by someone other than Webster. Moments later, he confronted Webster in his laboratory, demanding his money and an explanation of why Webster had defrauded him by using his collection as collateral for two different debts. "Was he stupid?" Parkman yelled, according to Webster. The other lender was his brother-in-law. Didn't Webster think that he would find out? Parkman threatened to have him drummed out of the university if he didn't immediately pay his debts.

Panicked and mortified at Parkman's threats, the short-tempered Webster grabbed the nearest implement and struck Parkman in the head. Parkman dropped to the floor, probably only unconscious. Rather than going for medical help, Webster's thoughts unreasoningly turned to disposing of the body. He then began a series of actions to eliminate any trace of Dr. Parkman. Over the next week, he became a very busy man.

At first, Webster intended to hide the body, but, even though his laboratory was adjacent to the anatomy lab, he couldn't find a suitable place. He then tried to dissolve the body with potash, boring a hole in the chest to facilitate its entry. To successfully dissolve the body with this method, however, Webster needed about 70 pounds of potash and a kettle large enough to dissolve the substance before using it on the body, neither of which he had. He then used a

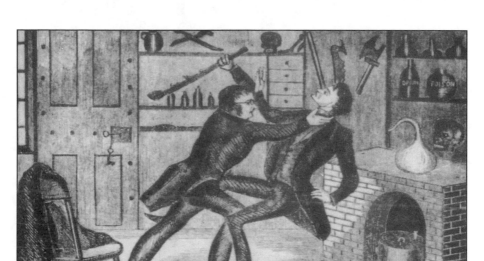

Dr. Webster and Dr. Parkman struggling. (Sketch circa 1850)

saw to cut up the corpse, washing the blood away in his sink. He eventually put some pieces of the body in a tea chest and others in his private lavatory until he could dispose of them.

The Investigation

When the habitual Dr. Parkman didn't show up on time that Friday evening, his family knew they had reason to worry. They became increasingly frantic after he failed to appear during the night, so they went to the police the next day with their concerns. Throughout the week that followed, the police extended their search to all of western Boston, where Parkman had real estate holdings—and perhaps delinquent debtors. Police even dredged the Charles River and made inquiries in a 60-mile radius around the city. The family distributed handbills offering a reward of $3,000 if the doctor was returned alive or $1,000 for his body.

The police were having no success locating the errant doctor, but Littlefield, who lived at the school, was fairing somewhat better. Littlefield's rooms were adjacent to Webster's laboratory and he was becoming suspicious of the professor. Not only had he witnessed the angry exchange between Drs. Webster and Parkman the prior week, but he was also the last person to see

Parkman approach the medical school building on the day he disappeared. Now, he wondered whether Professor Webster was involved and decided to conduct his own investigation.

First, Littlefield tried to enter Webster's laboratory, as he routinely did on Friday evenings, but found it locked from the inside long after the time the professor normally left school. Even after the doctor finally left, Littlefield still found Webster's laboratory locked—again, quite unusual. The next day, Webster came in early and spent all day in his laboratory with the doors locked. Sometime during the day, the doctor slipped out to deposit the check that was to have gone to Parkman into his own account at Charles River Bank. Later that evening, Littlefield was able to enter the professor's lecture hall, but found the adjacent back room locked, which also was peculiar.

On Sunday, Webster visited his friend and sometimes pastor, Reverend Francis Parkman, the brother of the missing doctor. Without showing any concern for his friend, Webster admitted meeting with Dr. Parkman on Friday and blurted out that he had given him $483.60 and thus the mortgage should be canceled. That evening, Webster appeared at the medical school and asked the janitor if he had seen Dr. Parkman the prior week. When Littlefield acknowledged that he had seen him the previous Friday, Webster said, "That is the very time I paid him $483.60." This was an unusual conversation for the doctor to initiate with Littlefield, whom he routinely treated as his inferior.

Although the following week was a holiday and the medical school was closed, the janitor again found Webster's doors bolted on Monday morning. Tuesday, Littlefield was present as police inspected Professor Webster's laboratory. Dr. Parkman's business agent, Charles Kingsley, and some police officers had arrived to search for Dr. Parkman's body in the vault where the remains of dissection cadavers were stored. They also persuaded a reluctant Webster to let them into his laboratory, which appeared to have been recently cleaned.

Webster continued to act in a suspicious manner. The laboratory's furnaces were found ablaze—and remained so all week—but Webster, uncharacteristically, would not let the janitor near them; rather, he tended them himself. Tuesday afternoon, Webster, again uncharacteristically, gave Littlefield a turkey for Thanksgiving. In retrospect, lawyers suggested that this gift may have been an attempt to silence the janitor, or at least to stop his investigation.

Wednesday, Littlefield began trying to cut a hole in the laboratory door, but, fearful that the professor would hear him, he gave up. He noted that the walls of the laboratory had become so hot that he feared that the building itself might catch fire. Climbing through the laboratory's unlatched window, he found the kindling and water supplies were nearly depleted. On the stairs, he discovered some spots of a substance which tasted like acid. Also unusual, the professor's private lavatory was sealed shut and the large key that normally hung beside the door was missing.

On Thursday, Thanksgiving Day, Littlefield began digging a hole to access the lavatory, which had been locked when the police investigated. Indeed, the professor seemed to have intentionally steered them away from it as soon as an officer expressed interest in the room. Littlefield worked for over an hour using a hatchet and chisel, but did not make much progress, so he went off for a night of revelry.

On Friday, Littlefield revealed his suspicions about Webster to two other medical school professors, who encouraged him to keep looking for answers. Borrowing a crowbar, hammer, and chisel from a foundry worker, he broke into the lavatory and made a grisly discovery: a man's pelvis and two parts of a human leg. He quickly notified a professor who lived nearby and they both went to summon the city marshal.

Arrest and Trial

Three policemen immediately went to Dr. Webster's home in Cambridge and asked him to accompany them to his laboratory for a search. As they entered Boston, Webster commented that their cab was not going toward the college. Indeed it was not, and soon they stopped in front of the Leverett Street jail. There, police notified Webster that he was in custody for Dr. Parkman's murder. At that, the normally staid professor decompensated and began babbling, "You might tell me something about it. Where did they find him? Did they find the whole of the body? How came they to suspect me? Oh! My children! What will they do? What will they think of me! Where did you get the information?"

Dr. Webster then took something out of his pocket, put it into his mouth, and immediately had spasms. The police suspected that he had poisoned himself. Indeed, he had ingested strychnine, which he had been carrying ever since he murdered Parkman, although it was not enough to kill him. Despite his rigid limbs and the sweat pouring down his cheeks, with his teeth chattering so hard that they broke a water glass, the police dragged Webster to his laboratory. There they found additional grisly items, presumably some of Dr. Parkman's remains.

On further examination of the laboratory's seldom-used assay furnace, designed to test metals, police discovered human bone fragments and false teeth. In the tea chest tucked into a corner of the lab, they discovered a human thorax and a left thigh, as well as Webster's hunting knife imbedded in tanning materials and covered with minerals. Dr. Webster was then returned to jail, where he lay immobile until the next afternoon, when his limbs regained enough flexibility to allow him to sit.

The trial, the first in the United States to use medical and scientific experimental evidence, began on March 17, 1850, before Chief Justice Lemuel Shaw of the Supreme Court of Massachusetts. They were all Harvard men, the cream of the American crop: the judge, 25 of the expert witnesses, the prosecution and defense lawyers, the victim—and the killer. There was so much interest in the trial that nearly 60,000 spectators were admitted at ten-minute intervals.

During the trial, Dr. Oliver Wendell Holmes, one of the first American physicians to use a microscope (he had brought Harvard's first instrument from Europe in 1835), identified the mysterious stains that Littlefield had seen in Webster's laboratory as human blood. Webster had tried to dissolve them with copper nitrate, which explained the acidic taste. This was the first time that blood was identified using a microscope and the first time such evidence was admitted at a trial.

Dr. Nathan Cooley Keep, who had been Dr. Parkman's dentist for 25 years, testified, in the first-ever use of forensic dentistry evidence in court, that the teeth found in Webster's laboratory furnace were part of Parkman's dentures. Dr. Keep had fashioned the appliance, an unusual and elaborate set of false teeth, from molds taken of Parkman's mandible, which protruded about six inches beyond his upper jaw. The dentures included "mineral" (porcelain) teeth, which Keep had pioneered. According to the *New York Globe*, Keep testified:

> There was shown to me . . . a block of mineral teeth . . . I recognized them to be the teeth made by me for Dr. P. in 1846; there was a great peculiarity in Dr. P.'s jaw and the peculiar structure of it left an impression on my mind; when I made the teeth for Dr. P., he was in a great hurry for them; he said that he was going to speak at the opening of the Medical College in N. Grove Street, and that there was but two days intervening before the day on which the College would be opened . . .
>
> He ordered that the utmost skill that could be employed should be exercised in the construction of the teeth . . . I went to work in the usual manner, to take an impression of each jaw . . . I got them done just 30 minutes before the ceremonies of opening the Medical College commenced . . . I was satisfied that the right upper teeth which were put into my hands by Dr. Lewis, were Dr. P.'s. There could be no mistake about them.

Dr. Keep, who began a dentistry practice after a stint as a jeweler's apprentice, obtained his M.D. from Harvard in 1827. He later became famous as the first doctor to use anesthesia for childbirth (for Henry Wadsworth Longfellow's wife), and was the first dean of Harvard's School of Dental Medicine.

Dr. Jefferies Wyman, a Harvard anatomy professor who examined the remains, determined that the decedent was 5'10½" tall, exactly the height of Dr. Parkman. This was one of the first instances of testimony based on forensic anthropology. The "medical committee" assigned to autopsy the remains determined that the head had been sawn off at the seventh vertebra and that the sternum had been removed by someone with anatomical knowledge. They also noted that, unlike the bodies used for anatomical dissection, this one had not been injected with antiseptics or wax.

Webster, through his two well-known lawyers, lashed out at the janitor and accused him of the murder. Unfortunately for Webster, his lawyers had little criminal experience. Edward D. Sohier, the lead attorney, had practiced primarily civil law, while Pliny Merrick was a Court of Common Pleas judge who had, for a short time, served as district attorney. Although Webster had prepared 194 pages of notes to help in his defense, his lawyers ignored them. When they were discovered 120 years after the trial, legal scholars suggested that had the notes been used, they might have gained him an acquittal—or at least a better defense.

The Parkman family donated $1,150 to Attorney General Bemis to assist in Webster's prosecution, but there was a seemingly insurmountable problem: there was no corpse. According to the standard legal principles of the time, there could be no conviction for murder unless the *corpus delicti* could be established; that is, until the dead body was found. This was to avoid executing alleged criminals only to have the "victim" reappear alive. Judge Shaw dealt with that problem when he instructed the jury:

> It has sometimes been said by judges that a jury never ought to convict in a capital case unless the dead body is found. That, as a general proposition, is true. It sometimes happens, however, that it cannot be found, where the proof of death is clear. Sometimes, in a case of murder at sea, the body is thrown overboard on a stormy night. Because the body is not found, can anybody deny that the author of that crime is a murderer?

After an 11-day trial, the jury deliberated for fewer than three hours before finding Dr. Webster "guilty of wilful murder." The following morning, Justice Shaw sentenced him to death.

After all his appeals were denied, Dr. Webster, to the dismay of his family who had steadfastly supported him, filed a full confession to the murder with the Massachusetts Executive Council's Committee on Pardons. He said that in a wild moment of rage induced by violent taunts and threats, he had struck Dr. Parkman on the head. Ironically, if he had used this confession as a defense, he probably would have been convicted of a lesser charge, or even acquitted.

On August 30, 1850, Dr. Webster was hanged. The *Boston Evening Transcript* described the event:

> The number of tickets issued for the admission of witnesses within the jailyard was about two hundred and fifty. Professor Webster slept until six o'clock and awoke calm and refreshed. He ate a hearty breakfast, drank two mugs of tea, smoked a cigar and passed the balance of his supply of cigars to the officers in attendance, with whom he conversed cheerfully and freely . . .
>
> The gallows was surrounded by some one hundred and fifty persons . . . but only a few members of the bar or the medical profession were present . . . the tops of the adjacent houses, sheds, outhouses and every available point of view were occupied . . . [Webster] was dressed in a black frock coat, buttoned up in front, black pants and shoes, without any neckcloth and only a portion of the shirt front visible. He entered into conversation with his spiritual adviser . . . the rope was drawn down and adjusted around his neck. The knot was placed a little behind the right ear . . . The black cap was drawn over his head, thus shutting out the beautiful sunlight and blue sky of the fair summer day . . .
>
> Sheriff Eveleth announced that in the name of the Commonwealth he would now proceed to carry into effect the sentence of the law. As he placed his foot on the trigger of the drop, the prisoner fell some seven-and-a-half feet and his mortal career was at an end. The body swayed slightly to and fro . . . After hanging 30 minutes the body was examined by Dr. Henry C. Clark, city physician, and Dr. Charles H. Stedman of the Lunatic Hospital, and they informed the sheriff that life was extinct.

Littlefield collected a substantial reward for his efforts. Mrs. Parkman later raised funds to help support Dr. Webster's wife and children. The Harvard Medical School building in which Professor Webster killed and then tried to eliminate traces of Dr. Parkman became the School of Dental Sciences and, later, a medical/dental museum. The building was later razed; today, the site is near the main entrance to Massachusetts General Hospital.

Hawley Harvey Crippen, M.D. — Love & Death

On July 20, 1910, the 5,500-ton Canadian Pacific liner *Montrose*, with 280 passengers on board, sailed from Antwerp, Belgium, to Canada, as she had many times before. But this voyage would be very different. Shortly after leaving port, Captain Henry George Kendall received a message from the police via the newly installed Marconi wireless aerial machine: "Watch out for Dr. Hawley Harvey Crippen and his mistress, probably dressed as father and son." They were being sought for the murder of Crippen's wife.

As it turned out, Captain Kendall had a copy of the local newspaper containing photos of the wanted Dr. Crippen and Ethel Le Neve on the front page. After close inspection, the captain found that "Mr. Robinson" perfectly matched the description of the fugitive Dr. Crippen, aside from a mustache and the spectacles—both easily discarded. The "Robinsons" were never seen apart and, although polite, would speak to others only when the situation required it. The captain noted that the "boy," who appeared to be in his mid-teens, was a shy, delicate youth with distinctly feminine features and mannerisms. "Mr. Robinson" was constantly solicitous of his charge, holding his son's hand and fondling him in a very non-paternal way.

On July 22, Captain Kendall made history when he wired back that he believed that the couple was aboard his ship. Sent from a point 120 miles west of Cornwall, England, to the White Star Company in Liverpool, the wire read:

> Have strong suspicion that Crippen London Cellar Murderer and accomplice are among saloon passengers. Mustache taken off growing beard. Accomplice dressed as boy. Voice manner and build undoubtedly a girl. Both traveling as Mr. and Master Robinson. Kendall.

The message was forwarded to Scotland Yard, making it the first wireless communication that resulted in a criminal's capture. Inspector Walter C. Dew wired back that he was on his way. On July 23, Dew boarded the White Star liner *Laurentic*, a faster ship and, accompanied by a horde of reporters, he followed the *Montrose* and Crippen in hot pursuit.

The world followed the suspenseful chase as Dew's ship closed in on the *Montrose*. As soon as he neared Canada, Captain Kendall began wiring reports about what the unsuspecting pair was doing on board. At Father Point on the St. Lawrence River in Canada, which Dew later described as a "lonely little place . . . with scarcely more than a dozen cottages and a Marconi [telegraph] station to it," the two ships finally met.

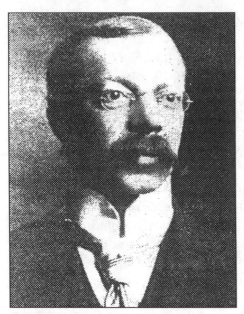

Hawley Harvey Crippen, M.D.
(Circa 1898)

Dew, in a borrowed pilot's uniform, and two Canadian police officers boarded a tender to reach the *Montrose*. As he came on board, he "saw Crippen pacing the deck about two yards away. I sent Mr. McCarthy and Denis (the officers) to bring him in. I said, 'Good morning Dr. Crippen,' and he replied, 'Good morning.' He made no attempt to dispute his identity." Crippen and Ethel le Neve had been captured.

Early Years

Hawley Harvey Crippen, born near the Coldwater River in Michigan in 1862, grew up admiring his Uncle Bradley, the town physician. After graduating from the University of Michigan, he obtained his M.D. degree in 1883 from a private homeopathic medical school in Cleveland, Ohio. He was only 21 when he graduated, but that was not unusual at a school that had low standards and a minimal educational program.

In 1885, Crippen acquired another diploma, as an eye and ear specialist, from Hahnemann (homeopathic) Hospital in Manhattan, New York. While there, Crippen met and married an Irish nurse, Charlotte Bell. Crippen also spent a short time at a hospital in London, England, although it did not qualify him to practice medicine in that country. The Crippens then wandered about the United States as Hawley practiced in a number of cities. The couple soon had a son, Otto. However, while in Utah in 1891, Charlotte died, and Crippen sent his three-year-old son to live with a grandmother in California. Crippen, now 30, then traveled to Brooklyn, New York, where he met Cora Turner.

Born Kunigunde Mackamotzki, Cora Turner was an attractive blonde of Russian-Polish descent and just 17 when Crippen first met her. She had left home the prior year to become the mistress of a prosperous industrialist who, in the spirit of *Pygmalion*, had hired teachers in a futile attempt to transform her into a lady. After meeting Crippen, she abandoned her lover and, in September 1892, the two married. Cora was enamored more by the doctor's profession and the possibility of wealth than by the bespectacled, erudite Crippen himself. She saw him as a means to achieve her goal of stardom on the musical stage.

After his marriage, Dr. Crippen practiced homeopathy, but the populus preferred traditional medicine, and his medical practice dwindled. As the money disappeared, the couple's relationship soured. Crippen briefly, and unsuccessfully, practiced dentistry from his apart-

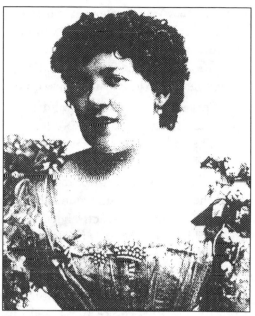

Cora Crippen, aka Belle Elmore.
(From a theatrical ad, circa 1899)

ment. He soon found a position as a "consultant" with Munyon's Homeopathic Remedies, a successful patent-medicine company selling cheap and generally ineffective mail-order nostrums to those who could not afford doctor visits or regular medication.

The company's owner, Professor Horace Munyon, immediately liked the bright, hard-working Crippen, and later told the *New York Times* that he "was one of the most intelligent men I ever knew." In 1895, Munyon made Crippen general manager of the main office in Philadelphia, where he increased the company's sales. Munyon then felt that Crippen was ready for major assignments, first opening the company's new office in Canada, and then, in 1897, doing the same in London, England, where he earned a guaranteed salary of $10,000 a year (more than $150,000 in 2002).

Meanwhile, the well-endowed and ostentatious Cora remained in Philadelphia, traveling to New York to take acting and singing lessons and conducting a number of amorous dalliances with attractive men. She attempted to break into New York's music scene, but her voice was described as matching her personality: loud, vulgar, unsubtle, and without feminine charm. Her lack of success was partially due to the worldwide financial depression. Many marginal New York theaters, in which the untalented Cora might have found a niche, had closed. After about six months, Mrs. Crippen decided to join her husband in London and, once there, she tried her luck at the local music halls, using the name "Belle Elmore." Dr. Crippen was ecstatic and believed that life in their new luxurious apartment would restore their relationship; it didn't.

Cora still harbored the grandiose and naive ambition of becoming an opera star. She debuted in a libretto, *The Unknown Quantity*, at Old Marylebone Theatre but, in her first performance, Cora demonstrated that she barely qualified as a chorus girl. Not unexpectedly, the audience detested her and she subsequently performed only intermittently in out-of-the-way theaters. Nevertheless, Cora continued to consider herself an integral part of London's theater community and actively participated in the Music Hall Ladies Guild. The Guild, composed of not only theater veterans but also the wives of stage performers, raised money and clothing for needy "artistes" who had fallen on hard times.

In November 1899, the doctor, in an attempt to support Cora in her unfortunate career choice, purchased a full-page ad promoting her theatrical efforts and listing himself as her business manager. Although Crippen meant well, Professor Munyon believed that the doctor was spending too much time on activities outside of his business, and he immediately fired him. With a spendthrift wife and no job, Crippen was in trouble.

He then worked for a series of failing patent medicine companies and even tried, without success, to market his own remedy, the nerve tonic "Amorette." Cora became even more unhappy when they were forced to move out of their fine apartment and into inexpensive dwellings.

Ethel Clara Le Neve

In December 1901, two years after he was dismissed from Munyon's, Dr. Crippen found a full-time position at Drouet's Institute for the Deaf. Despite its name, Drouet's was just another mail-order house selling plasters, drops, gargles, and snuff that were supposed to cure disorders of the ears and throat. In reality, they were the stuff of patent medicine quackery. Crippen served as one of several "consulting physicians" who diagnosed disorders by mail and prescribed the most appropriate of the company's products. While Crippen's income was far below what he had earned at Munyon's, the job did have its benefits. Not only did he have a beautiful office overlooking Hyde Park and a modern consulting room for walk-in patients, but he also had the pretty and poised Ethel Le Neve as his typist.

Born in Diss, Norfolk, in 1883, Ethel Clara Le Neve was one of six "Neve" children. She changed her name to the more glamorous sounding "Le Neve" after leaving home. When she met Dr. Crippen in 1901, he was 39 years old; she was 18 and still living with her parents. Ethel had just graduated from Pitman's Secretarial College in London and had obtained a shorthand-typist job at Drouet's through the graces of her younger sister, Nina, the head secretary. When Nina left Drouet's, Ethel became Crippen's private secretary and bookkeeper. To Crippen, Ethel had everything Cora lacked—she was sweet, sympathetic, genteel, and educated. Within a year, they had become intimate.

Crippen wasn't much of a catch for a young woman. The doctor was a small pale man, only 5′5″ tall, whose most striking features were his gray eyes, which were slightly magnified by gold-rimmed spectacles. He had an unkempt sandy mustache above a receding chin, and tried to cover a bald spot with his light brown hair. He spent every night with Cora, but spent afternoons with Ethel. Eventually, the pair grew less careful, inciting talk among their associates, but most did not believe the rumors until Dr. Crippen left Drouet's for another position and took his secretary with him.

Troublesome Cora

In 1902, Crippen returned to New York on business. While he was away, Cora began a relationship with Bruce Miller, a former Chicago prizefighter who had become a showman and purported ladies' man. Although Miller left for America before Crippen returned to London, Crippen eventually found his amorous letters to Cora and the intensity of their arguing increased.

In September 1905, Cora pestered him to move into better lodgings. They leased a three-story brick townhouse at 39 Hilldrop Crescent, an address that would become infamous throughout Britain. The townhouse, in a block-long row of similarly dull detached structures, was larger than their old apartment and, at £52 per year, much more expensive than the couple could really afford. Cora decorated her home in her favorite color, pink. By this time, Crippen had learned to ignore her gaudy taste.

The house had several extra bedrooms and, in November 1906, they rented the third-floor rooms to three exchange students from Heidelberg University. Cora insisted that her husband fix them breakfast, do their laundry, and shine their boots each morning before going to work while she remained in bed. On December 6, Crippen came home from his office earlier than usual and found one of the students in bed with Cora. That ended their stint with boarders.

This episode, however, didn't end Mrs. Crippen's extramarital affairs. She continued to supplement her income through the good graces of her paramours, buying fox furs and jewelry and saving substantial amounts of money—mostly in her own name.

Crippen had long wanted to return to medical practice, although he was not eligible for a British medical license. Knowing that he had once practiced dentistry, Ethel persuaded him to begin a dental practice in a fashionable locale. In 1909, Crippen opened Yale Tooth Specialists in partnership with Dr. Gilbert Rylance. Coincidentally, the office was housed in the same building as Munyon's Homeopathic Remedies, Crippen's old firm. If Cora hadn't known the identity of her husband's "other woman" by that time, she figured it out when Ethel followed him to his dental practice as his assistant.

At the end of 1909, the Crippens' life together fell apart. The couple fought constantly and Cora threatened to leave and take her jewelry and their bank deposits with her, leaving her husband destitute. Cora hoped to either scare Crippen out of the house, which would allow her to file for divorce on grounds of abandonment, or enrage him so that he would file for divorce first. Cora may have gone too far, driving Crippen to desperation: what she didn't know was that Ethel had become pregnant. Although Ethel miscarried, this apparently motivated Crippen to make a fateful decision.

Crippen Kills Cora

On January 17, 1910, Crippen ordered five grains (300 mg) of hyoscine, or scopolamine, from a chemist. With a therapeutic dose of less than one milligram, the drug causes drowsiness, euphoria, amnesia, and fatigue; administration of a large amount causes death. Just prior to this, a new law was enacted in Britain that required physicians to register when they purchased potentially poisonous substances, including hyoscine.

During the investigation after Cora's death, police reviewed chemists' records and found that on January 19, Dr. Crippen had personally picked up the drug, which he apparently had not used before. Crippen would later claim that, while in England, he had dispensed this drug in several hundred homeopathic doses sent to mail-order customers. He could not, however, produce even one customer's name or address. The state's toxicologist determined that Cora's body contained at least 30 milligrams of hyoscine—many times the lethal dose.

On January 31, 1910, Cora disappeared. Surprisingly, her jewelry, furs, and money remained behind. London coroner and barrister S. Ingleby Oddie postulated that Crippen mixed a hot toddy laced with hyoscine for his wife before bedtime. However he did it, Crippen gave his wife the drug. He planned to wait until her body was cold and then, feigning shock, call a personal friend and well-respected colleague, Dr. John S. Burroughs, to tell him that he had found his wife dead. But Cora did not react as he expected—first she babbled, then she screamed. Crippen realized that the drug had caused the agitation and, although the drug would have eventually killed her, he feared that her shouting would rouse the neighbors. Panicking, he grabbed his .45-caliber revolver and shot his wife in the head. Neighbors remembered hearing shrieks "and a loud noise like a pistol shot" from his house that night.

To dispose of the corpse, Crippen turned to dissection, a skill he had learned in medical school. Using his enameled bathtub to reduce the mess, he filleted the flesh off her bones. Wrapping the bones in an oilcloth, he took them to the kitchen hearth and burned them, planning to pulverize any remnants in the morning. He then wrapped her limbs, head, and organs in a heavy cloth, which he stored in a crate in the garbage can for later disposal. He foolishly wrapped the remaining body parts in a pair of his own pajamas and buried the bundle under the stone blocks in the cellar, just below the back staircase.

After throwing his bloodied clothes into the fire, he took a short nap before going to his dental office as usual at 9 A.M. That evening, after dinner, he lugged the sack of body parts a few blocks to the Holloway Sanitation Canal. Weighting the sack with bricks from his garden, he dropped it into the murky waters. His work done, he then went home to bed.

Dr. Crippen announced to Cora's friends that she had gone to California on business. To allay suspicion, he wrote a letter from Cora stating that she resigned from her beloved Guild and that she was returning to America to tend to a sick relative. On February 2, when Cora should have attended the Guild's weekly meeting, Ethel went instead, carrying two letters that were signed by Cora, but that were not in her handwriting. One read:

> Dear Friends, Please forgive me a hasty letter and any inconvenience I may cause you, but I have just had news of the illness of a near relative and at only a few hours notice I am obliged to go to America. Under the circumstances, I cannot return for several months and, therefore, ask you to accept this as a form letter resigning from this date my hon. treasureship.

The Guild ladies were suspicious: Cora would have called one of them before leaving, rather than writing a letter. As time passed, Cora's friends thought it strange that they had not heard from her.

Twice in February, Crippen pawned some of his wife's jewelry. He gave Ethel four of Cora's diamond-and-ruby rings and what Cora used to refer to as her "rising-sun brooch," a pendant whose central black stone was cut with a cluster of diamonds from which extended a ray-beam design of smaller inlaid diamonds. On February 20, when Crippen and Ethel attended the Guild's dinner dance, Ethel was wearing Cora's distinctive brooch as well as some of her clothes.

Ethel openly became Crippen's companion and, on March 12, she moved into 39 Hilldrop Crescent. Calling themselves "Mr. and Mrs. Crippen," they went to Dieppe, France, for five days on their "honeymoon." On the day they left for France, Clara Martinetti, Cora's friend from the music hall, received a telegram from Crippen that read, "Cora died yesterday at six o'clock . . . Shall be away a week." He later explained that there would be no funeral, as she had been cremated in America.

But Cora's Guild friends were confused: She had been a Catholic and, at that time, Catholics did not accept cremation. They went to Scotland Yard with their suspicions and talked to Chief Inspector Walter C. Dew, who had earned his promotion to detective in 1887 in the midst of the Jack the Ripper crisis. Dew, already inundated with other missing person reports, was unimpressed.

Cora's friends became increasingly uncomfortable with the tale of her death. They found that the *La Touraine*, the only ship scheduled to go to America at the time Crippen claimed that Cora left, had not sailed because it was undergoing repairs at Le Havre. Guild president Isabel Ginnett contacted California authorities and learned that no person named Cora Crippen or Belle Elmore (Cora's stage name, which she preferred) had died recently in that state. A friend of Cora's, John Edward Nash, confirmed this while on a business trip to California.

Upon returning to England on June 30, 1910, Nash and his wife met with Inspector Dew at Scotland Yard's Criminal Investigation Department. According to Nash, Crippen could not recall in what town his wife had died—San Francisco, Los Angeles, or Alameda. Nor could he remember the name or location of the crematorium.

Now intrigued, Dew agreed to speak with Crippen and, a few days later, he visited 39 Hilldrop Crescent. The doctor admitted that his wife had not died after all; he had fabricated the tale to avoid the scandal of being left for another man. This made sense to Dew. He persuaded Crippen to place a newspaper notice addressed to Belle Elmore. It read:

Communicate with H.H.C. or authorities at once. Serious trouble through your absence. Twenty-five dollars reward for anyone communicating her whereabouts to Box Number 7, New Scotland Yard.

The inspector also made a routine search of the Crippen home, but found nothing suspicious. Crippen explained that a .45-caliber ball-cap revolver lying in the armoire was only for protection. To Dr. Crippen, all this activity was ominous. He and Ethel Le Neve immediately fled London, sailing first to Rotterdam and then to Antwerp to board the Canadian-bound ship *Montrose*.

At the Ladies' Guild's insistence, Inspector Dew went to talk with Crippen one more time. On Monday, July 11, he stopped at Yale Tooth Specialists, where the clerk told him that Crippen, apparently accompanied by Miss Le Neve, had suddenly taken a trip and was not expected back for some time. The clerk did not know their destination.

Rushing to Crippen's house, Inspector Dew found only the maid, whose employment was to be terminated once she closed the house. She did not know where the pair had gone. Dew again searched the house, but found nothing. Doggedly, he returned to continue his search the next day. On the following day, July 13, while probing the bricks in the cellar floor, he discovered that one of them could be raised. Removing a few, he began to dig and soon discovered lime-permeated human internal organs, removed *en bloc* just as a pathologist would have done, wrapped in pajamas. There was also a portion of a thigh and a piece of skin with muscle and hair. Although the forensic findings were later disputed, this piece of skin from the lower abdomen contained a scar similar to the one Cora had from an oophorectomy (removal of her ovaries).

The famous forensic pathologist Sir Bernard Spillsbury's notes on the case read:

Human remains found 13 July ... Medical organs of chest and abdomen removed in one mass. Four large pieces of skin and muscle, one from lower abdomen with old operation scar 4 inches long—broader at lower end. Impossible to identify sex. Hyoscine found 2.7 grains. Hair in Hinde's curler—roots present. Hair 6 inches long. Man's pyjama jacket label reads Jones Bros., Holloway, and odd pair of pyjama trousers.

Inspector Dew, who had found one of Jack the Ripper's mutilated victims (Mary Kelly, in 1888), believed that Crippen's work was a close second to that monster's.

Arrest and Trial

The Metropolitan Police immediately issued arrest warrants for Dr. Hawley Harvey Crippen and Miss Ethel Le Neve. Police were able to track the couple to Belgium where, with Le Neve posing as Crippen's son, they had boarded a steamer for Canada. After Captain Kendall wired that the pair was on board the *Montrose,* Inspector Dew gave chase. He boarded the *Laurentic* and arrived in Quebec a day earlier than Crippen and Le Neve.

Wireless messages allowed the public to stay abreast of the chase and the capture of the culprits in what became known as the "North London Cellar Murder." The music halls even developed a popular tune about the chase:

> Oh Miss Le Neve, oh Miss Le Neve,
> Is it true that you are sittin'
> On the lap of Dr. Crippen
> In your boy's clothes
> On the Montrose,
> Miss La Neve?

On July 31, the "Robinsons" were arrested and officially extradited from Quebec; they arrived in England on August 28. On October 18, 1910, Dr. Crippen went on trial before Lord Chief Justice Lord Alverstone in the No. 1 Court of London's Central Criminal Court (Old Bailey) for murdering his wife. There was so much public interest and so many requests for seats that half-day tickets were issued.

Bruce Miller, Cora's her ex-lover, traveled with her sister from the United States to testify for the prosecution. The defense's case was weak. On the stand, Crippen denied having killed anyone, although he admitted that he had lied when he said that Cora had died in America. He claimed that he had concocted the story to avoid the embarrassment of Cora's flight to America to join her lover. He could not explain, however, why she would have left her money, jewelry, and furs behind—especially in mid-winter. Although he seemed to be indifferent to his own fate throughout the trial, he continually insisted that Ethel Le Neve knew nothing of Cora's murder. How Cora's body came to be buried in his cellar he could not say; he had left England because he hadn't understood that he was expected to remain. The doctor would not allow Ethel to be called in his defense.

The trial lasted five days. Lord Chief Justice Alverstone then instructed the jury: "If the evidence points to the fact that he, and he alone, is responsible for the death of his wife, Cora Crippen, you will not hesitate to do your duty."

Twenty-seven minutes later, at 2:45 P.M. on October 22, 1910, the jury returned their verdict finding the doctor "guilty of willful murder."

When Dr. Crippen was asked if he had anything to say about why the judgment of death should not be passed upon him, Crippen murmured, "I still protest my innocence." Lord Chief Justice Alverstone, having placed a black scarf over his white wig, solemnly pronounced:

> Harvey Hawley Crippen, you have been convicted, upon evidence . . . that you cruelly poisoned your wife, that you concealed your crime, you mutilated her body, and disposed piece-meal of her remains; you possessed yourself of her property, and used it for your own purposes. It was further established that as soon as suspicion was aroused, you fled from justice . . . I implore you to make your peace with Almighty God. I have now to pass upon you the sentence of the Court, which is that you be taken from hence to a lawful prison, and from thence to a place of execution, and that you be there hanged by the neck until you are dead . . . And may the Lord have mercy on your soul!

Two weeks later, Crippen's appeal was denied. His only hope was for a reprieve from Home Secretary Winston Churchill—but, perhaps because of political considerations, it never came. Four days after his trial ended, Ethel Le Neve stood trial for murder as an accessory after the fact, and for being a fugitive from justice. Public sentiment weighed heavily in her favor. After 20 minutes of deliberation, the jury found her "not guilty."

Ethel visited her lover daily in jail. They followed each visitation with a letter. But, at 8 A.M. on Wednesday, November 23, 1910, the love affair ended when 48-year-old Harvey Hawley Crippen, M.D., dropped to the end of the hangman's noose at Pentonville Prison. Ethel's letters were buried with Crippen and, per his last request, her photograph was also included.

Epilogue

Number 39 Hilldrop Crescent remained vacant for the next 30 years. In the decade following Crippen's execution, a Scottish comedian attempted to turn it into a museum devoted to the Crippen case; he was unsuccessful. The house met an appropriate end when German bombs destroyed it during World War II. Cora Crippen's remains were reburied in Finchley Cemetery a week before the start of her husband's trial. Scotland Yard's Walter C. Dew, who was 47 years old, retired from active duty three weeks before Crippen was hanged. It was said that he had come to like Dr. Crippen and was distraught over the final outcome.

On the day of Crippen's execution, Ethel le Neve boarded the *Majestic* and sailed for New York under the name "Miss Allen." She moved to Toronto, where she started calling herself "Ethel Harvey." She worked as a secretary in Canada for five years, while writing her memoirs. In 1916, she returned to London, changed her name to "Nelson," and married an accountant, Stanley Smith. The couple settled down to married life, her husband seemingly unaware of her past, and they had several children. Ethel died in bed in 1967, at age 84.

Alfred Hitchcock's movies *Rear Window* and *Vertigo*, Francis Isles's (pseudonym of Anthony Berkely Cox) 1931 novel *Malice Aforethought*, and Frederick Knott's play and subsequent movie *Dial M for Murder*, all had elements based on the Crippen case.

But the eeriest aftermath involves Captain Henry George Kendall and the *Montrose*. The *Montreal Daily Star* reported that as Crippen was led from the *Montrose*, he turned and cursed Captain Kendall, saying: "You shall pay for this treachery, sir!" On May 29, 1914, "Crippen's Curse" would come true. Kendall had by then been appointed captain of the CPR liner *Empress of Ireland*. On a voyage from Quebec to Liverpool, with 1,477 passengers and crew on board, the *Empress* had just passed Father Point at 1:38 A.M. (the scene of Crippen's capture four years earlier), when the lookout spotted the Norwegian ship *Storstad*.

A bank of fog rolled from the shore and reduced visibility to zero. Less than 20 minutes later, the *Storstad*, loaded with 10,400 tons of coal, emerged from the fog and cut into the *Empress*. Within 14 minutes, the mighty *Empress* had, in the words of a survivor, "rolled over like a hog in a ditch" and disappeared in the St. Lawrence River. One thousand twelve people died—almost as many died as on the *Titanic* or the *Lusitania*. The same year, the *Montrose* sank off Dover, England. Captain Kendall, however, survived and lived to be 91.

John Kappler, M.D. — The Crazy Killer

John Kappler, M.D., was an anesthesiologist for most of his medical career and an unstable psychiatric patient most of his adult life. He was also a murderer,

> a terribly angry man [whose] rage had fueled his repeated acts of violence. He had never been able to tolerate the critical eyes of others, instinctively turning any anxiety or fear or embarrassment he felt into fury.

Even though they knew of his mental illness, medical licensing agencies, colleagues, and prestigious medical institutions continued to support Kappler until the truth could no longer be hidden. Then they abandoned him—and he killed again.

When he finally stood trial for murder in Massachusetts Superior Court in December 1990, Kappler was a 60-year-old "wiry little man gone gray." Standing 5'10" tall and weighing barely more than 150 pounds, he was a shadow of what he had once been—but his green eyes reflected madness rather than the rationality of his chosen profession.

Early Years

For a physician of his generation, Kappler followed an unremarkable route into medicine. His early performance in school was mediocre, despite having above-average intelligence and an excellent memory. He was bullied by his classmates and beaten by his parents, who were heavy drinkers. His Protestant father detested his mother's Roman Catholicism, and they had open conflicts over religion. After serving in the U.S. Army, including a combat tour in Korea, Kappler returned home, and married Tommie, a psychiatric nurse. They eventually had several children, one of whom became a lawyer.

Kappler graduated from North Carolina's Leonard Medical School in 1960, at the age of 31. Following his general internship in Charleston, South Carolina, he briefly entered general practice. About this time he began suffering bouts of severe depression and sought psychiatric assistance. This forced him to stop practicing clinical medicine and to take a less demanding (and probably more lucrative) position promoting a pharmaceutical company's new medications. His mental illness worsened, and he began having paranoid delusions. He believed that the CIA was stalking him, that his house was bugged, and that his wife was trying to poison him. He was hospitalized several times and, after a short period, his psychiatrists thought he had improved enough to be released.

The tranquilizers and antipsychotic medications prescribed for him seemed to help, although he took them intermittently. In 1966, two months after being released from the psychiatric ward, he stopped taking all his medications, ended his psychiatric counseling sessions, and began training as an anesthesiologist at the University of Southern California. He spent the rest of his professional life in Los Angeles.

Psychotic Years

Over the next 20 years, Kappler was admitted to psychiatric hospitals multiple times. He believed that people were after him or that he was hearing voices commanding him to commit violent acts. After each committal, he returned to his medical practice. For example, in 1975, he heard voices demanding that he give a pregnant patient the wrong anesthetic, then he called a "code" saying that she had suffered a cardiac arrest (she hadn't). When he called a "code" on two other stable patients that day, the operating room team demanded that he leave. He did, only to crash into a vehicle that he then stole and crashed as well. He was jailed until his wife and some hospital doctors bailed him out. Despite their knowledge of these events, his colleagues at the hospital allowed him to continue practicing medicine.

In 1980, still working as an anesthesiologist, he stopped a patient's heart by injecting excess lidocaine. The patient lived and Kappler continued to practice. In 1985, he was finally charged with attempted murder after he unplugged a quadriplegic patient's ventilator. The case was dismissed for lack of evidence, although Kappler's wife later admitted knowing that voices had told her husband to do this.

Shortly thereafter, in part because of the adverse publicity surrounding the attempted murder case, and after again being diagnosed with depression, Kappler retired. Despite repeated legal and psychiatric difficulties, he was allowed to keep his California, North Carolina, and Georgia medical licenses.

In 1990, he drove to the East Coast to visit his family. At that point, he was taking both antidepressants and antipsychotics intermittently. While driving through Cambridge, Massachusetts, he suddenly veered onto a jogging path and hit 32-year-old Paul Mendelsohn. Mendelsohn was thrown into Kappler's windshield and lay on the moving car's hood for several hundred feet before falling off. He sustained an ultimately fatal head injury. Ironically, Mendelsohn, who was on the jogging path to train for a marathon, was a psychiatric resident at New England Medical Center.

(In a macabre episode, reported elsewhere as medical folklore, Dr. Mendelsohn initially was unidentified, since he carried only his pager with him when he jogged. While he was a still-unidentified patient in Massachusetts General Hospital's intensive care unit, his pager went off. When the staff called the number to answer the page, a junior psychiatry resident at New England Medical Center answered and explained that he was trying to reach Dr. Mendelsohn—thus identifying the patient.)

Accelerating his car, Kappler then struck 32-year-old Deborah Brunet-Tuttle as she returned from the grocery store with Easter eggs for her church. After being dragged for hundreds of feet, she was left in critical condition with multiple broken bones. He then abandoned his car and hitched a ride with a young woman. Kappler's plan was to enter her house under the ruse of needing to use the phone and then strangle her. Wisely, she refused his request and lived.

Following the voices' commands, Kappler then wandered the streets, rode the subway, and considered suicide. At midnight, he took a bus to New York City where he met his son and tried to strangle him. He was locked in a psychiatric clinic and, eventually, turned over to the police.

A Massachusetts jury convicted him of second-degree murder, armed assault with intent to murder, and assault and battery by means of a dangerous weapon. He was given the mandatory life sentence and sent to the Massachusetts Correctional Institute at Cedar Junction. The Massachusetts Supreme Court later denied his request for a new trial.

~

Buck Ruxton, M.B. — Bits & Pieces

Although torrential rains had fallen during the past week, the small Scottish village of Moffat, only 32 miles north of the English border, was a beautiful spot for a vacation. The bridge over Gardenholme Linn, a stream running to the River Annan, provided a quiet and picturesque place to stroll. That is exactly what Susan Johnson was doing on September 19, 1935, when she paused to look at the stream below. What she saw—a human arm emerging from some type of package—would forever change her life.

Racing back to her hotel, she told her brother, Alfred, what she had seen. After giving his sister a shot of "medicinal" whiskey, Alfred ran to the bridge to confirm that Susan had not gone mad; she had not. Scrambling down the embankment, Alfred saw not one, but two packages. Gingerly opening the second, wrapped with newspaper and bed sheets, he found pieces of human flesh and bone. That was more than enough for him to get the police.

Sergeant Robert Sloan, from the Dufriesshire Constabulary, soon arrived and examined the grisly scene. He quickly discovered two more parcels containing hands with mutilated fingertips and thumbs, two heads so disfigured that they could not be identified, and parts of legs, trunks, and other flesh.

Sloan carefully marked each package's position on the ground and then took them to the local mortuary. The gruesome find eventually led area residents to name the stream "Devil's Beef Tub."

Forensic experts from Edinburgh and Glasgow descended on the scene. One of them was Dr. John Glaister, the University of Glasgow's professor of forensic medicine, who was following in his famous father's footsteps. He took the "bits and pieces" to his anatomy department for further study.

Over the next two weeks, additional parcels were discovered in the area; the farthest was nine miles from Moffat. Most were found where the recently raging streams would have deposited them after the water receded. When the pathologists, an anatomist, and a dentist began trying to piece together the 70 human parts into what they termed two "jigsaw puzzles," they found a formaldehyde-preserved, malformed "Cyclops eye" of an animal among the grisly collection. They surmised that someone with an interest in ophthalmology was involved in what appeared to be two murders.

Although wrappings for the dismembered heads included a blouse and a child's playsuit, most body parts had been wrapped in newspapers, one of which contained a limited-circulation advertisement. Inserted into the September 15, 1935, *Sunday Graphic*, the ad had been placed into only 3,700 papers around Morecambe and Lancaster. This limited the search area.

Lancaster, England, lies 105 miles south of the bridge at Moffat. It is an ancient city of about 50,000 people on an offshoot of Morecambe Bay, an inlet of the Irish Sea. Police soon discovered that, in mid-September, 22-year-old Mary Jane Rogerson had disappeared. She had been the nanny for the children of Buck Ruxton, a general practitioner in Lancaster.

Rumors abounded that his wife had left Ruxton about the time that the nanny was last seen. Police visited Ms. Rogerson's stepmother, who immediately recognized the recovered blouse as one she had given to her daughter. She suggested that the landlady where her daughter and the Ruxton children had spent a vacation might know about the playsuit. The woman did. Indeed, after putting in a new elastic band—tied with a knot only she used—the landlady had given the playsuit to Rogerson for her small charges. After hearing this, police considered Dr. Ruxton to be their primary suspect.

Early Years

Born in 1899 as Bukhtyar (or Bukhtar) Rustomji Hakim in Bombay, India, Hakim legally changed his name to Buck Ruxton around 1929. Although the area was predominantly Hindu, he adamantly referred to himself as a Parsee, a member of a religious sect descended from the Aryans in pre-Islamic Iran. Interestingly, Parsees, or Zoroastrians, traditionally use carnivorous birds to dispose of their dead on "Towers of Silence." In England, though, Parsees use cremation—not dismemberment and exposure.

Ruxton received two medical degrees from the University of Bombay, after which he served three years in the Indian Medical Corps. At that time, India's military was a part of the British Army, and colonial India (now India, Pakistan, and Bangladesh) was a British colony. After his military service, Ruxton moved to London and worked sporadically while he obtained a British medical degree (MB) from the University of London. He then took the entrance examination for the Royal College of Surgeons in Edinburgh, but failed.

About the same time, he fell in love with a waitress who worked in a restaurant he frequented. Isabella Van Ess, two years younger than Ruxton, was a sharp-nosed plain woman who was estranged from her Dutch husband. Believing that she would not take his advances seriously, Ruxton initially courted her in the guise of "Captain Hakim," a decorated army officer. In 1928, the doctor returned to London and the now-divorced Isabella followed. Between 1929 and 1933, they produced three children, although they never married.

After their first child, Elizabeth, was born, the family moved to Lancaster, where Ruxton set up practice on the ground floor of their three-story, nineteenth-century home. He soon had a large number of patients, both because of the physician shortage in Lancaster and because his practice included dentistry and ophthalmology.

Over time, the relationship became increasingly rancorous. Ruxton's jealousy and bad temper often flared. At one point, Isabella had him dragged to the police station where, in the detective's words, Ruxton "flew into a violent passion and said, 'My wife has been unfaithful. I would be justified in murdering her.' " Several months later, the same detective went to the Ruxton home to help settle yet another domestic dispute.

After both Isabella and the children's nanny disappeared, Ruxton alternately claimed that they had gone on vacation, that they were traveling, that the nanny had run off with a lover, or that she was pregnant and Isabella had taken her to get an abortion. When newspapers incorrectly described the Moffat bodies as being those of a man and a woman, Ruxton was so overjoyed that he made his housekeeper listen while he ranted, "So you see, Mrs. Oxley, it is a man and a woman—not our two," at which point he began laughing hysterically.

The Investigation

A week later, the newspapers had it right and were suggesting that the doctor was a key player in the gruesome murders. Ruxton sped to police head-quarters, where he demanded that they issue a statement exonerating him; he said that the notoriety was ruining his practice. Ironically, the officers had just discussed arresting him on murder charges. The next evening, Saturday, October 12, Dr. Ruxton was invited back to headquarters. After ten hours of questioning, he was charged with Mary Rogerson's murder. On November 5, they added the charge of killing Isabella, his children's mother.

The police had compiled damning evidence against the doctor. Soon after the disappearances, Ruxton had hired one of his patients as a cleaning lady to scrub blood from his staircase. He claimed that he had cut himself opening a can. But the stairs were covered with straw and all the carpets had been removed and rolled up—most still blood-stained. Suits, which he had offered to the cleaning lady as a gift (she refused), other clothing, and more carpets lay in the backyard, all covered in blood and partially burned. Also, two bedrooms were locked and had straw protruding from under the doors, which police speculated had been used to soak up more blood.

Forensic experts slowly pieced together the bodies, initially labeled "Number 1" and "Number 2." The team's anatomist, Dr. James Couper Brash, used anatomical formulae and radiographs to identify pieces as belonging to one "puzzle" or the other and to align adjacent parts. Soon, they could pre-sumptively label "Number 1" as Mary Rogerson and "Number 2" as Isabella. The manner in which the dismembered parts were mutilated actually helped solidify these identities. In each case, tissues had been removed exactly where the decedents had uniquely identifying marks or features, such as a birthmark, a scar, the teeth, and even Isabella's lower legs, which were remarkably stout.

Forensics, including several never-before-used techniques, played a large part in the investigation. The experts determined that the bodies had been dissected by someone with surgical skill and anatomical knowledge: A surgical knife, rather than a saw, had been used and there was little damage to adjacent body parts. In a forensic first, experts superimposed enlarged photographs of the women's faces over the skulls, a process pioneered in 1883 to identify Im-manuel Kant's skull. They matched. Using another revolutionary method, offi-cers from Glasgow City's fingerprint department took fingerprints from the mutilated fingers and matched them to fingerprints found at Ruxton's house.

In a landmark event for forensic entomology, investigators collected a group of maggots feeding on the decomposing body parts. They were sent to

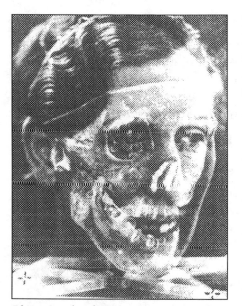

Photograph of Mrs. Ruxton superimposed on photograph of her skull.

Professor A. G. Mearns's University of Edinburgh laboratory. He identified them as maggots (third instar larvae) of a blowfly, *Calliphora vicina*. He estimated that, when collected, the maggots were between 12 and 14 days old. Since these maggots developed from eggs that adult flies laid, the bodies had to have been near the stream for at least that long. This, then, was the minimum time between the deaths and the discovery of the bodies.

When police examined Ruxton's residence, they found an unusual bedsheet that exactly matched some of the recovered wrappings. They also identified the bathtub in which Ruxton had dissected the bodies. (According to the *Manchester Evening News* of January 14, 1983, after spending many years in the Lancaster forensic laboratory's "black museum," the notorious bathtub found its way to the police stables at Longton where it served as a horse trough.)

The Trial

Ruxton's eight-day trial began at Manchester Assize Court on March 2, 1936. His defense was led by the tall, bespectacled, velvet-voiced Norman Birkett, who was often called "the courtroom magician" or "the murderer's best friend" for his abilities. J. C. Jackson, a well-known prosecutor, led the Crown's team. More than a hundred witnesses testified for the prosecution. It appeared that Ruxton strangled his wife in a fit of rage and then, when the nanny suddenly entered the room, he suffocated her to keep her from testifying.

The defense called only one witness—Dr. Ruxton himself. He was warned to remain calm, to carefully listen to each question, and to only answer what had been asked. He didn't. Describing his relationship with Isabella, Ruxton said, "I can honestly say we were the kind of people who could not live with each other and could not live without each other . . . Who loves most chastises most." The jury, as expected, delivered a guilty verdict.

Asked if he had anything to say before sentencing, Ruxton raised his right palm to the judge and uttered some incomprehensible words. He was sentenced to hang. His appeals failed and, probably due to his sympathetic portrayal in the media, tens of thousands of people signed petitions for a reprieve—6,000 in Lancaster alone. Nevertheless, he was hanged at Strangeways Prison in Manchester on Tuesday morning, May 12, 1936.

The following Sunday, a local newspaper printed Ruxton's confession to both murders, written the day after his arrest. A rhyme (which can be sung to the tune "Red Sails in the Sunset") then became popular:

> Red stains on the carpet, red stains on your knife,
> Oh Dr. Buck Ruxton, you murdered your wife.
> The nursemaid saw you, and threatened to tell,
> Oh Dr. Ruxton, you killed her as well.

Drs. Tei-Sabro Takahashi & Mitsuru Suzuki — Private Bacteriological Wars

Dr. Tei-Sabro Takahashi

Ironically, while the Japanese Army's medical team was testing biological warfare agents on Chinese civilians in Manchuria (see Chapter 8, *Japan's Inhuman Experiments*), Japanese police arrested a civilian physician for doing the same thing to his compatriots on the home island. On May 8, 1937, Saitama Prefecture police arrested Dr. Tei-Sabro Takahashi on charges of intentionally infecting 17 people, three of whom died, with *Salmonella typhi* using contaminated food.

The doctor had graduated from Chiba University of Medicine in 1928, and then worked as an otorhinolaryngologist in Tokyo. While there, he learned about clinical microbiology and eventually obtained a strain of *S. typhi* from a colleague. He conducted his own research until 1933, when he opened his own practice.

Takahashi began his killing spree in March 1935, when he gave *S. typhi*-laced pastries to another physician, Dr. Tokio Hojo. Although Dr. Hojo did not eat the tainted food, other members of his household did and they became extremely ill. In October 1936, Takahashi again sent confectioneries to a physician, Dr. Chiyo-Saburo Sato, but they went uneaten.

When prosecutors began to investigate Takahashi, they had insufficient evidence to charge him in those two instances. But they did charge him in five other incidents involving food contaminated with *S. typhi*. The first of these involved a competing physician, Dr. Kazukichi Tsukada. Takahashi was jealous of Tsukada and, apparently, hoped to undermine his practice. On March 7, 1936, Takahashi purchased some cakes, contaminated them with *S. typhi*, and, on that same day, took the contaminated cakes to Tsukada's office as a gift for his rival's children. The four children ate the cakes; afterwards, at least one was diagnosed with typhoid.

The second incident was in June 1936. Takahashi took *S. typhi*-contaminated pastries to Dr. Tadanobu Ono, another rival. Again, the motive apparently was to undermine his rival's medical practice. Three of Ono's staff became infected and one died.

The third incident involved a concerted effort to disable or kill his wife, Sekiko, who was unable to conceive a child. Takahashi wanted to divorce his wife and thought that it would be easier to accomplish this if she were disabled. Using his now-established method, he gave Sekiko some *S. typhi*-contaminated pastry while she was preparing to undergo an operation to improve her fertility. Sekiko ate the pastry and became ill on October 23. Six days later, she was admitted to the hospital, where Takahashi tried to murder her by injecting her with morphine. She survived due to the efforts of the medical team.

The fourth incident involved Sekiko's physician, Dr. Masao Yanagida. Takahashi resented not only Yanagida's prosperity but also his role in saving Sekiko's life. On November 22, 1936, he asked a department store to deliver some pastries that he had contaminated to Yanagida's house. Six members of Yanagida's family became ill, including his wife, four of his daughters, and one of his sons. The wife died from typhoid on January 3, 1937, and one of his daughters died a month later from pneumonia, her strength having been sapped by the typhoid infection.

The final incident occurred on November 23, 1936. Takahashi tried to infect Dr. Ei-ichiro Sato, a staff member at Tokyo's Do-Ai Hospital whom he disliked. At a party given to honor another physician, Takahashi tried to get Sato to eat some *S. typhi*-contaminated salmon eggs. Sato refused, but three other physicians ate them. All three became ill, and one died.

Dr. Yanagida uncovered Takahashi's activities after discovering that everyone in his family had become ill after eating some of Takahashi's pastries. He took the remaining pastries to the Ministry of the Interior's Hygienic

Laboratory, where they determined that the food was laced with *S. typhi*. The laboratory notified the local authorities.

When officials investigated, they found that the pastries' producer could not have accidentally infected them with *S. typhi*. Police then concentrated on Dr. Takahashi. On July 4, 1938, a judge found Takahashi guilty in all five incidents and condemned him to death. An appeals court upheld the sentence the following year and he was executed.

Takahashi told authorities that he thought his use of *S. typhi* would go unnoticed for several reasons. He believed that it would be difficult to identify the source of the infection, given that *S. typhi* has a lengthy incubation period and people might forget what they had eaten by the time they got sick. He also thought that other physicians might misdiagnose the disease. Finally, he believed that since there was considerable typhoid in Japan at that time, the cases would not be considered unusual.

Dr. Mitsuru Suzuki

Many physicians get frustrated with the medical system in which they work. Few take revenge by sickening or killing their co-workers, friends, patients, and family. But Dr. Mitsuru Suzuki, a physician with training in bacteriology, did just that. He used *Salmonella typhi* and *Shigella* to infect up to 120 people, and killed four of them. On April 7, 1966, Japanese police arrested Dr. Suzuki for infecting four of his colleagues using a sponge cake contaminated with dysentery. Subsequent investigations linked the doctor to a series of typhoid and dysentery outbreaks between December 1964 and March 1966.

Angry about the treatment he was receiving in his medical training as a resident, Suzuki retaliated by infecting other health care providers and patients. His motivations were further complicated by suggestions that he may have created clinical cases to further his academic research into *S. typhi*.

On December 26, 1964, in what came to be known as the "sponge cake incident," Dr. Suzuki purchased a sponge cake from a store near Chiba University Hospital. That night, after lacing the cake with dysentery, he offered it to four of his hospital colleagues. All four became ill and were hospitalized.

Although Suzuki laid low for a while, Chiba Hospital officials had discovered his nefarious activities. Rather than reporting him, however, they suppressed their findings to avoid embarrassment to the university. Only after the Ministry of Health and Welfare received an anonymous tip, nearly a year later, did an official investigation start.

Unaware that anyone had discovered his activities, Suzuki's personal bacteriological war accelerated in mid-1965. Suzuki was working part-time in the clinic of Kawasaki Steel Corporation's Chiba City factory. On August 6, he laced bottles of a milk-based Japanese soft drink with typhoid and gave the contaminated drinks to 16 co-workers, who all became sick. But the doctor was not finished. Under the guise of giving them something "good for curing this kind of disease," he injected four of them with additional dysentery bacteria. Prosecutors charged that he also used a nasogastric tube to force dysentery-contaminated water into a patient at the Kawasaki Steel plant's clinic.

Ten days later, Suzuki made anonymous phone calls to three Chiba City hospitals warning them to report anyone with typhoid symptoms "because they are acute and infectious typhoid cases." Police surmised that he made these calls to determine how well his method of spreading the disease had worked.

On September 4, Suzuki gave an *S. typhi*-contaminated cake to an internist at Chiba University Hospital. The man shared the cake with two members of his family, and all three became sick with typhoid. That same day, ten nurses and doctors who ate typhoid-contaminated bananas they received from Suzuki also fell ill. The following day, Suzuki purchased another ten bananas from a shop near the hospital and immediately took them to his laboratory. There, he inoculated six of them with typhoid and distributed them among five hospital nurses, all of whom became infected, as did two of their relatives.

Suzuki immediately left to visit his uncle's family in Gotemba, Shizouka Prefecture. On September 9, eight of the nine family members developed typhoid after Suzuki gave them contaminated bananas. Dr. Suzuki returned to Chiba University Hospital, where 13 patients developed typhoid after eating contaminated bananas.

On December 27, Suzuki gave typhoid-contaminated bananas to a nurse at Mishima Social Insurance Hospital in Shizuoka Prefecture. The nurse, in turn, gave one to the hospital's deputy director, Dr. Masahisa Matsuda—he died from typhoid within the month. Over a several-month period starting in December 1965, Suzuki gave typhoid-laced medicines to Mishima Social Insurance Hospital patients; 42 of them developed typhoid, and three died.

On January 1, 1966, Lt. Col. Toshikazu Yokoto became ill after Suzuki gave him typhoid-contaminated clams. In what was labeled the "barium incident," Dr. Suzuki put *S. typhi* into a barium solution that was distributed to two of Mishima Social Insurance Hospital's outpatient clinics in Shizuoka. The same day, February 28, he used a typhoid-contaminated tongue depressor on a patient. On March 15, three hospital nurses became sick after eating mandarin oranges left in their dressing room. The oranges were later shown to be infected with the same D2 strain of typhoid as in the other cases. That same month, Suzuki's brother and sister-in-law and five of his parent's friends, all of whom lived in Koyama, developed typhoid.

Originally, Suzuki told police that he gave the dysentery-contaminated cake to his colleagues as an experiment to test a new theory he had developed. He eventually told police that he was actually motivated by revenge:

> It is true I wanted to see how a mass outbreak of disease would develop from the planted bacilli, but I spread the germs out of my deep antagonism to the seniority system which prevails in [Japanese] medical circles... I was unpaid and my status was unstable... I thought I was being discriminated against as I am not a graduate of Chiba University.

He said that he infected his relatives because they refused to provide him with financial support for his research. Prosecutors claimed that Suzuki actually caused the typhoid cases so he could complete his dissertation thesis, which involved studies of *S. typhi* organisms recovered from numerous patients.

But how did Suzuki obtain the typhoid organisms? His bacteriology work provided him with several opportunities. He cultured typhoid from a patient whom he treated. He also illicitly obtained typhoid cultures from Japan's National Institute of Health when he worked there as a trainee in September 1965. The typhoid strain he used was later found to match those in his laboratory. It is unclear where he obtained the *Shigella*.

The Chiba District public prosecutor ultimately charged Suzuki with 13 separate cases involving 66 infected people. (He was not charged with any of the deaths.) Suzuki had confessed to all 13 cases within a week after his arrest, but he recanted after the trial began. He was acquitted. Unhappy with the verdict, prosecutors took the case to Tokyo's Court of Appeal, which, on May 25, 1982, overturned the original verdict, sentenced him to six years in prison, and revoked his medical license. After completing his sentence, Suzuki continued to maintain that the cases were all natural outbreaks. It is not known whether his license to practice medicine was reinstated.

Dr. Levi Weil & His Apple Dumpling Gang

Levi Weil emigrated from Holland to London, England, in the 1760s, after studying medicine at the University of Leyden. He anticipated opening a busy practice in a city consumed by disease and lacking trained practitioners. The combination of his Dutch accent and a prejudice against Jewish physicians, however, kept his practice small and him destitute. That, however, was about to change.

One day, a local merchant asked Dr. Weil if he would make a house call on his elderly sister, since her regular doctor was ill. Traveling with the merchant to Enfield, he treated the woman (apparently with some success), ate dinner with the brother, and then returned with him to London. As soon as they parted company, however, Weil returned to the wealthy patient's home in Enfield, where he stole £90 (about $13,500 in 2002). The heist was so easy, he vowed to repeat it.

And so he did, casing the homes of wealthy patients when he made house calls. Seeing the potential for even greater wealth, he wrote to friends in Amsterdam and suggested that they come to London to help his burglary operation. His brother Asher and a group of five others soon arrived. Dr. Weil gave his inside information to his brother, who ran the gang of thieves under Levi's direction, while other gang members surveyed the exterior. Ironically, Dr. Weil's medical practice boomed as his thefts began generating enormous sums of up to £500 a month (about $75,000 in 2002). Despite his new wealth, he continued to practice medicine, both as a cover for his activities and to find new prospects to rob.

One of his biggest windfalls came when Weil heard of an old caretaker who lived near St. Paul's Cathedral and who supposedly had his life's savings stored in his room. The cache was a well-known secret among London's thieves; many had previously broken into the room and torn up the floor and the walls, all to no avail. The next time the old man became ill, Dr. Weil arranged to care for him. Weil tried to send him to the hospital so he could explore the room without hindrance, but the old man adamantly refused to leave, solidifying Weil's belief that the money was in the room.

After giving the man a soporific to make him sleep, the doctor investigated the only place left, the ceiling. There he found a cavity in a large beam, from which he extracted £3,000 (about $450,000 in 2002). The old man never discovered the theft: he died—or possibly was killed—as he slept.

The gang by now had eight members. One, a German Jew named Isaacs, was kicked out of the group after he tried to swindle the others. That turned out to be a major mistake.

In the fall of 1771, the gang, including Dr. Weil, robbed a house in Chelsea. They waited until 10 P.M. when everyone had gone to sleep—except for Mrs. Hutchings, the lady of the house, and her maids. The gang pounded on the door and, when the maid opened it, demanded to be let in. She refused. The *Complete Newgate Calendar* described what happened next:

> [The men] rushed in, seized the terrified females, and threatened them with instant death in the event of their offering any resistance. Mrs Hutchings, being a woman of considerable muscular strength, for a time opposed them; but her antagonists soon overpowered her, tied her petticoats over her head, and proceeded to secure the servants. The girls having been tied back to back, five of the fellows proceeded to ransack the house, while the remainder of the gang remained below to guard the prisoners.

The gang then rushed from room to room, searching for loot. They finally entered the room in which two farm laborers, John Slow and William Stone, lay sleeping, unaware of the commotion. The *Complete Newgate Calendar* continued:

> It was soon determined that these men were likely to prove mischievous, and that they must be murdered; and Levi Weil, a Jewish physician, who was one of the party, and was the most sanguinary villain of his gang, aimed a blow at the breast of Stone, intended for his death, but which only stunned him. Slow started up, and the villains cried: "Shoot him! Shoot him!" A pistol was instantly fired at him, and he fell, exclaiming: "Lord have mercy on me! I am murdered!"
>
> They dragged the wounded man out of the room to the head of the stairs; but in the meantime Stone, recovering his senses, jumped out of bed and escaped to the roof of the house, through the window.

The gang stole all the silver they could find and, after some serious persuading, got Mrs. Hutchings to turn over her watch and £65. It was not a big haul for so much trouble, but time had run out, and the thieves fled. The women then went searching for John Slow. When they found him, he muttered, "I'm dying," and slumped unconscious to the floor. He died the following afternoon.

At that point, Isaacs, the erstwhile and now destitute gang member, reappeared to exact his revenge. He knew that if he identified the gang and then testified against them, he would receive not only a monetary reward, but also leniency regarding his other crimes.

Arrest and Trial

The Bow Street Runners, the forerunner of Scotland Yard, arrested Dr. Weil and his gang, thus aborting the next robbery, the heist of a consignment of jewels to a diamond merchant worth £40,000 (about $6 million in 2002). Six members of the gang were tried at the Old Bailey in December 1771. Two were acquitted for lack of evidence. The four who were convicted, including Dr. Levi Weil and his brother, were sentenced to death and "anathematised in the synagogue." [sic] The *Complete Newgate Calendar* described the scene:

> They were attended to Tyburn, the place of execution, by immense crowds of people, who were anxious to witness the exit of wretches whose crimes had been so much the object of public notice. Having prayed together, and sung a hymn in the Hebrew language, they were launched into eternity, on the 9th of December 1771.

Debora Green, M.D. — Fire & Ricin

The windswept fire raged out of control, racing through the luxurious six-bedroom Tudor-style home in Prairie Village, Kansas. Fire trucks raced to the scene, but arrived too late to save the house—or the two children, Tim Farrar, age 13, and his 6-year-old sister Kelly, who both died trapped upstairs amidst the black smoke and searing flames. The fire on October 24, 1995, exposed a tale of adultery, murder, poisonings, and psychosis that would rock the upscale Kansas City suburb.

As fire consumed her home and siblings, a third child, 10-year-old Kate, climbed out of a second-story window to the garage roof and jumped to safety in the arms of her mother, who was calmly standing outside the house. Investigators soon came to believe that the fire had been deliberately set: they found flammable liquid had been poured in several areas of the home. They honed in on the children's mother, a furiously defiant Debora Green, when neighbors noted that she had serenely stood by and watched as the fire consumed her house and her children. Investigators also decided to take a closer look at the fire that had ruined the family's previous home, as well as the mysterious disease attacking her estranged husband.

That night's blaze punctuated the destruction of Michael Farrar and Debora Green's deteriorating 18-year marriage. Just the night before, Dr. Farrar had informed his wife, whom he was planning to divorce, that he was seeking custody of their three children. Characteristically, Green was furious.

Early Years

Born Debora Jones on February 28, 1951, Green had been a brilliant but lazy student. She first attended the University of Illinois and then the University of Kansas Medical School, where she graduated in only three years. After divorcing her first husband, she met Michael Farrar, a physician four years her junior, whom she married on May 26, 1979.

Although Debora and Michael seemed content, their marriage was rocky. Debora deeply resented giving up her oncology practice to stay home with their three children while Michael, a well-liked cardiologist, built a thriving medical practice. Her violent temper was triggered by even the smallest slight, and she often became cruel and vindictive.

A psychologist who examined Green determined that "she is immature and quite unable to handle emotion. She has the emotional processing capacity, the ability to handle emotion, like that of a young child, even younger than a toddler perhaps." With the help of pills and alcohol, she held herself together well enough to fool the outside world. Although her family knew her to be volatile and often nasty, they continued to defend her against her detractors— that is, until the second fire.

Burning and Poisoning

In July 1986, the family moved into an upscale Kansas City neighborhood. Soon afterwards, Mike and Debora separated; mysteriously, their house burned to the ground. After the fire, the couple reunited "for the children's sake," and moved to Prairie Village, Kansas, to begin anew.

By 1995, Mike had had enough of their pathological relationship. When he and Debora traveled to Peru with their son on a school-related trip, he felt it would be their final act as a couple; it was. While on the trip, Mike met beautiful Celeste Walker, Debora's old friend and the wife of a successful but unhappy doctor. After their return, Mike and Celeste began having an affair, which Debora soon discovered.

Mike suddenly began to suffer extremely severe stomach problems, causing him to be hospitalized three times in the weeks before the fire. His doctors thought that he had a strange type of typhoid from his trip to Peru, but they couldn't be sure. The first time Mike fell ill, he was hospitalized and nearly died. He returned home, but the illness recurred. The night of the fire, he had been hospitalized again for an infection believed to be related to his previous illness.

On September 25, police answered a domestic disturbance call at the Farrar house. Mike had called police after Debora had become extremely abusive during an argument. Her aberrant behavior made him try to have her committed, but she was released after voluntarily spending four days at the Menninger Institute. Informing Debora that he was getting a divorce, Mike moved out of the house and immediately began to recover.

During a routine search of Debora's handbag, police had confiscated eight packets of beans, some empty. They turned out to be castor beans. Debora had read in an Agatha Christie novel that the beans are the source of a deadly poison, ricin. Only a few days before, a garden store had sold her ten identical packages of castor beans. The assistant manager remembered the transaction because he had special ordered the beans from the store's main office. It had probably been her second castor bean purchase.

Ricin

Michael Farrar was lucky that his wife did not completely understand how ricin works or he most likely would have died. The FBI laboratory, with technical advice from the Naval Medical Research Institute in Bethesda, Maryland, later found antibodies in Michael's blood that proved he had been poisoned with ricin. In retrospect, police determined that he was probably poisoned when Green served him meals three times during August and September; Farrar had been hospitalized after each meal. The ricin perforated his gastrointestinal tract, resulting in an infection of the heart (endocarditis) and brain abscesses, both of which required surgery. Complications resulted in additional hospitalizations during the following months.

No one knows how Green prepared the beans prior to contaminating Farrar's food. Despite pleading guilty, she refused to describe how she poisoned Michael. Intact castor beans are not poisonous because the digestive tract does not break down the shell to expose the ricin. Thus, Green must have either prepared the beans in a way that exposed the ricin or extracted the ricin from the beans and added it to the food. Without medical intervention, the lethal dose for an adult may be 15 to 20 beans. Any evidence of her activities, however, was destroyed when she set her house on fire. She has subsequently blamed the poisonings on her dead son.

Actually, ricin is rarely fatal when taken orally. However, as in Michael Farrar's case, ricin can cause serious ulceration and bleeding in the stomach and intestines, sometimes causing perforations. Without aggressive modern medical intervention, Michael would have died. The poison is much more lethal in other forms, such as when inhaled or injected, and has been investigated as a military biowarfare agent. During the Cold War, ricin was used in the assassination of Bulgarian defector Georgi Markov, who died from a secret injection of a poison pellet.

Arrest and Trial

Nearly a month after the second fire, the police finally filed charges against 44-year-old Dr. Debora Green, charging her with two counts of murder and aggravated arson as well as the attempted murders of her surviving daughter, Kate, and of her husband. She was arrested at a Kansas City theater where she had taken Kate to practice for her role as Clara, the heroine in "The Nutcracker." Her other daughter, Kelly, was to have played an angel in the same production. The next day Michael Farrar filed for divorce and sought custody of Kate.

The news that an affluent woman physician could commit such heinous crimes stunned the community, made national headlines, and became the subject of a book by Ann Rule. Dr. Green spent months in the Johnson County jail, under a $3 million bond, awaiting trial. Her lawyer, former district attorney (and future U.S. Congressman) Dennis Moore, said his client claimed she was innocent and was grieving for her children. This was a surprising statement, given that everyone who saw her said she showed absolutely no emotion.

While she had earlier pleaded "not guilty" to all the pending charges, she changed her mind after Johnson County Prosecutor Paul Morrison stated he would seek the death penalty. At that point, she negotiated a plea bargain taking the death sentence "off the table." On April 17, 1996, Dr. Debora Green waived her right to a trial and pleaded no contest to all the charges.

Although Dr. Green never wept for her children during her months of incarceration, she broke down as she read a statement to the court at her sentencing hearing on May 30, 1996. She sobbed that

alcohol, psychiatric illness and even more basic communication failures within our family set the stage for this tragedy ... I do not seek to use that fact to escape my personal responsibility. I do hope, however, that the recognition of these problems, and the fact that signs of these problems

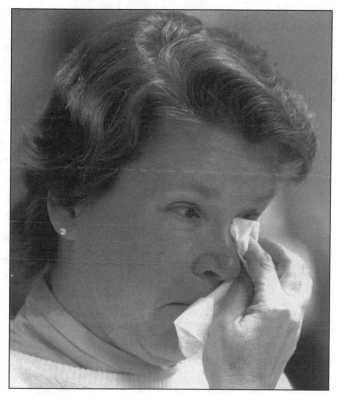

Dr. Debora Green wipes away tears during her preliminary hearing in Olathe, Kansas, in 1996. (AP/Wide World Photos)

could have led to earlier intervention, will be a lesson learned from their tragic deaths.

The judge sentenced her to two concurrent terms of life imprisonment for murder, specifying that she would not be eligible for parole for 40 years. She also received to two eight-year terms for attempted murder and four years for arson. All the terms are being served concurrently at the Topeka Correctional Facility's maximum-security unit, where she still resides.

Epilogue

The story, however, was not over. In a July 13, 1996, letter to *New York Times* reporter Jill Musick, Dr. Green announced her remorse at the loss of her children and for accepting the plea agreement:

I'm sorry my children are dead. I'm sorry I'm here and not with Kate. But what I'm sorry "for" (my fault) is that I took a plea bargain for something I didn't do and didn't fight for my rights and my innocence through the legal system. I'm sorry I put my parents through all this—they knew I was making a big mistake with the plea, but I was so scared I didn't know what else to do.

On August 27, Green wrote again, claiming that her attorneys wanted to avoid a trial, and so did not advise her properly. She singled out Sean O'Brien, a specialist in death penalty cases, saying he wanted to "avoid the death penalty at all costs." Green later wrote that she wasn't able to make any reasonable decisions until she was taken off Prozac when she got to prison.

In yet another letter to Musick, Green played the "woman card," writing on February 5, 1997:

My honest opinion is that I'm here because the legal system is largely geared against women right now. If I had committed a crime, I would own up to it—I am an honest person. I did not. My situation in the county jail— overmedication, fear, and isolation—prompted me to want things to be over with, and I would have done nearly anything to have that happen. I didn't receive very good advice. I allowed myself to be frightened and bullied into pleading to something I didn't do. Maybe God wanted me to be here to teach or tell me something. I cannot believe this is His plan for the rest of my life.

On June 1, 2000, Green went before District Judge Peter Ruddick in a hearing to try to rescind her original plea agreement and to be released on bail until a new trial. She claimed that medication and mental problems made her unable to understand the original agreement and that she was "unduly influenced" by her attorney's advice. Green's new attorney, Kurt Kerns, said, "The new evidence is essentially evidence that was there that no one discovered at the time—the fact that she was on four different types of medications . . . there are some concerns with regard to whether she was even competent to make the decision or not."

District Attorney Paul Morrison, who prosecuted Green, dismissed her motion as "without merit," saying:

The plea bargain was an opportunity to escape execution, and she accepted the bargain. It's very common for prisoners to do this after they've been in prison for a while. They seek to escape their responsibility for the decision they made and get out. That's what she's doing.

Morrison added that the chance of Green getting a new trial was "not very good." Morrison also affirmed that, in the unlikely event Green should be granted a new trial, he would ask for the death penalty.

Primarily because of the potential for the death sentence if she were retried, Dr. Green voluntarily withdrew her motion. She remains in prison and will be eligible for parole consideration in 2035. Green's former husband, Dr. Michael Farrar, has since remarried, and is doing well with his surviving daughter.

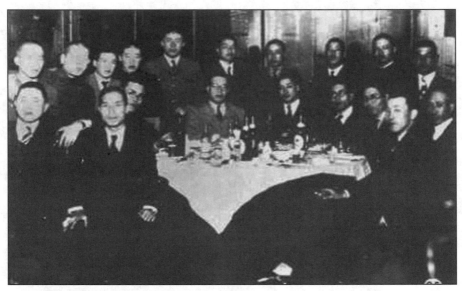

Top scientists of Japan's secret Unit 73, 1939.

8
Viruses & Vivisections

Japan's Inhuman Experiments

*M*anchuria, 1941.

Lin Minga and Tamara Kazursky shrank in fear, petrified by the sight before them. They stood at the entrance to an operating room with two tables, wearing only flimsy gowns. Neither of them needed an operation.

Seventeen-year-old Lin Minga had been living with her parents and working in the local factory when the dreaded kenpeitai, *the Japanese military police, had taken her to their headquarters for interrogation. Her brother was in the communist-led anti-Japanese resistance, but she did not know anything about it. After three days of torture, she was bound hand and foot to another woman, put in the back of a closed van, and driven to a prison. A virgin, she had been forced to have sex with numerous men, all of whom, she later discovered, had venereal diseases. Not surprisingly, she became pregnant. During her pregnancy, the Japanese doctors repeatedly examined her and took blood, urine, and vaginal tests. She had given birth to a beautiful son two days ago. Now she had been dragged to this death laboratory.*

Nineteen-year-old Tamara Kazursky, a beautiful White Russian whose family had lived in Harbin for more than 20 years, worked at her parents' bakery and was engaged to be married. She had been walking home when she was caught in a "sweep" by the local militia. The soldiers had been told to obtain subjects for experiments, and she had been in the wrong place at the wrong time. Bundled into a tight "package," she was thrown onto a sealed boxcar and brought to this place of horrors. She, too, had been forced to have sex with many men, and had contracted a venereal disease that was causing her severe lower abdominal pain. The Japanese doctors had taken a special interest in her once the pain developed.

313

"Get up on the table and take off your gown," said the Japanese nurse in broken Chinese. "This is a medical procedure, and won't hurt a bit." Orderlies and doctors stripped the two women and pushed them back onto the tables, securing their arms, legs, and torsos. Eight men in white clustered around the tables. One doctor, apparently in charge, said "No anesthesia; it might compromise our findings."

At each table, a doctor took a scalpel and quickly cut open the abdomen. The girls let out nightmarish screams as their bellies were ripped open and their entrails exposed. Lin Minga had enough composure to yell, "Kill me, but not my baby," before she lapsed into unconsciousness. Tamara's body continued to twitch as her uterus and ovaries were removed; blood sprayed the ceiling. The doctors had the samples they wanted.

Eventually, the women's hearts stopped beating and their agony ended. Their bodies were dragged to the incinerator and their identities were lost forever. None of the doctors felt any guilt. They had done this countless times and, besides, these were only worthless maruta *[logs].*

~

Dr. Ishii Shiro

The story of Japanese biological warfare is actually that of a military physician-researcher and mass-murderer, Dr. Ishii Shiro. With the support of his government and the willing assistance of other physicians, researchers, and military personnel, Dr. Ishii carried out a methodical, gruesome killing spree in the name of science. On the strength of his intellectual gifts, political connections, and hard work, he developed the horrendous and macabre killing machine that was Japan's venture into the field of biological warfare (BW). Dr. Ishii set this terrible story in motion through his driving ambition, lack of morality, and persistent efforts to stimulate Japan's development of biological weaponry. Over little more than a decade, he and his colleagues were responsible for hundreds of thousands of deaths.

Writing about Ishii, historian Sheldon Harris said, "He was a monster . . . Dr. Mengele could have taken lessons in evil from Ishii." Ishii also knew when to lie. While being interrogated in February 1946, then General Ishii Shiro stated, "Biological warfare is inhumane and advocating such a method of warfare would defile the virtue and benevolence of the Emperor." His thousands of experimental victims who suffered prolonged and agonizing deaths would certainly have agreed.

Ishii Shiro was born on June 25, 1892, in the Japanese village of Chiyoda Mura, in the Kamo district, Chiba prefecture. He was the fourth son of a wealthy family that was the largest landowner in the area southeast of Tokyo that now lies near Narita airport. As a child, Ishii received a traditional primary and secondary education at the local schools. Early on, he was noted to have an extraordinary gift for memorizing long and complex texts. His classmates, however, regarded him—as would others later in his life—as brash, abrasive, and arrogant.

In April 1916, Ishii entered the Medical Department of Kyoto Imperial University, where, due to his intelligence and abilities, professors gave him advanced research assignments. The school's curriculum was based on Western medicine, which the Japanese medical establishment had recently embraced. With an emphasis on clinical instruction and an assumption that graduates would behave morally, no medical ethics courses were included in his curriculum. Ishii graduated from medical school in December 1920, at age 28.

Ishii stood out from his compatriots. He was taller than most Japanese, occasionally wore glasses, and spoke with a sharp, booming voice. He also was said to have extraordinary—almost superhuman—physical energy.

Typical of his generation's elite, Ishii was fanatically loyal to his country and emperor. Combining this with his interest in medicine, he decided to become an Imperial Japanese Army physician. So, less than a month after graduation, he began military training as a probationary officer with the Third Regiment of the Imperial Guard Division. On April 9, 1921, he was commissioned as surgeon-first lieutenant.

To pursue his research interests, he arranged to be transferred to First Army Hospital in Tokyo on August 1, 1922. While in Tokyo, Ishii became known as a big-spending womanizer, night owl, and heavy drinker. His preferences ran to apprentice geishas no more than 16 years old and his drunken binges became legendary. Nevertheless, because of his obvious intellectual talents, his superiors decided to send him back to Kyoto Imperial University in 1924 for advanced training.

At Kyoto, Ishii studied and did research in bacteriology, serology, pathology, and preventive medicine. During this time, he helped identify the viral source of a new epidemic illness, Japanese B encephalitis. By ingratiating himself with the powerful university president and later marrying his daughter, Ishii solidified his connection to Japan's medical and scientific elite. Yet Ishii demonstrated a pushy indifference, if not contempt, for his colleagues. A scientist who worked with him later said:

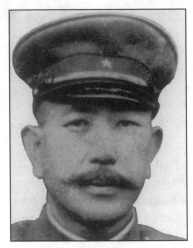

Dr. Ishii Shiro, circa 1940.

[Ishii] is very clever and a hard worker. However, he is not a scholarly minded person. He is very ambitious and likes to do big things (in a way he is a boaster). He is very eager about promoting himself to a higher position by achieving meritorious deeds . . . He takes [a] haughty attitude toward his senior fellows.

His supervising professor, Ren Kimua, remembered Ishii as being flamboyant and often inconsiderate. For example, when Ishii was at Kyoto, 30 to 40 research students needed to share the limited supply of laboratory test tubes and other glass apparatus. Cleaning them was a laborious, time-consuming procedure that was done each evening. However, Ishii would steal into the labs at night, use the clean glassware, and leave the problem of cleaning up to the other students when they arrived at dawn.

In 1927, now-Captain Ishii graduated from Kyoto with a doctorate in microbiology. He then worked at Kyoto Army Medical Hospital, publishing scientific papers, and gaining respect as a medical scholar. During this time, he began to associate with ultra-nationalists who espoused anti-capitalist, anti-bourgeois, anti-liberal, and pro-National Socialist (Nazi) views. Throughout his life, neither his work nor his family (which eventually included seven children) ever detracted from his raucous nightlife. For example, when he later directed the biowarfare unit at Ping Fan, he would hold planning meetings at 3 A.M., after he returned from carousing.

Ishii apparently had an epiphany when he reviewed a report from Dr. Harada, who had attended the 1925 Geneva Disarmament Convention for the War Ministry. Although the Convention had banned biological weapons, Ishii believed that Japan's army should develop them anyway. Stressing that they were cheap and effective, he struggled to get his superiors to see the usefulness of having biological weapons within Japan's military arsenal. His efforts were only partly successful.

In April 1928, Ishii was sent on a two-year worldwide inspection tour of foreign research establishments to investigate the state of international BW activity. Visiting 26 countries in Europe, Asia, and North America, Ishii met with many microbiologists and toured countless laboratories. He came to the (incorrect and self-serving) conclusion that all major powers were secretly researching BW.

Returning to Japan, Major Ishii was named professor of immunology at Tokyo Army Medical School and, later, chairman of the new Immunology Department at the Army Medical College. In these posts, he was positioned to advocate for biological weaponry. He argued that biological weapons cost very little compared to conventional weapons and "must possess distinct possibilities, otherwise it would not have been outlawed," therefore, he concluded that the Japanese should employ the "silent enemy" of microbiology as a "silent ally."

The Beginning of Japanese Biological Warfare

By the early twentieth century, Japanese medicine and the Japanese Army had established their expertise in microbiology and sanitation. Dr. Shiga Kiyoshi had discovered the *Shiga* bacillus that caused the devastating diarrheal illness, shigellosis. Researchers had also discovered the cause of the nutritional deficiency illness, beri-beri. Because of their expertise during the Russo-Japanese War, just over 1 percent of Japanese soldiers died of disease and only 1.5 percent died of gunshot wounds, although 24 percent were wounded. No other army had ever had such medical success.

In this setting, Ishii convinced Japan's leading military physician, Dr. Koizumi Chikahiko, to support his ideas. Called the "father of Japan's chemical warfare program," Koizumi served both as the army's surgeon general and as Japan's minister of health. An ultra-nationalist, he often quoted the Chinese proverb, "Great doctors tend their country, good doctors tend people, and lesser doctors heal the illnesses." As dean of the Army Medical College and Ishii's boss, Koizumi once wrote, "Ishii is a strange one, but I think he is good at his work." Koizumi had a large building erected behind his office in which Ishii could begin his biological warfare research.

Some of the appalling residua from this work reappeared in 1989, when construction workers uncovered a cache of more than 100 non-Japanese human remains just steps away from the site of Ishii's former laboratory. Ironically, the workers were building the new Ministry of Health facility in Shinjuku, Tokyo's prestigious new administrative center. The remains all showed signs that surgeons had practiced on the bodies. Said one person who worked at the complex, "I think that there are more bones there than were found. If someone looked, they would discover more."

The Japanese government wanted to cremate this reminder of their grisly past, but protesters demanded that they be held pending further investigation—which has so far not been concluded. As historian Hal Gold wrote, "In what could seem like a pathetically small act of revenge from the grave, the victims may be thought of as having returned, years after they were put to their agonizing deaths, to create minor torture for Japan's political elite."

While he had some successes in his laboratory experiments, Ishii was convinced that he needed to perform large-scale human tests. He often said:

> There are two types of bacteriological warfare research, A and B. [Type] A is assault (Angriff) research, and [Type] B is defense research. Vaccine research is of the B type, and this can be done in Japan. However, A type research can only be done abroad.

To accomplish his Type A research, Ishii obtained an assignment with the Kwantung Army in Manchuria.

In 1919, Japan's military established the Kwantung Army to protect its investment in Manchuria against the Russians, whom they had decisively defeated more than a decade earlier in the Russo-Japanese War. In 1933, Manchuria was a de facto Japanese colony with a puppet Chinese government. The area (now the northeastern part of Mainland China that borders Russia) is still rich in resources and has a small population. The Kwantung Army's commander, appointed by the Tokyo High Command, was totally independent of either Japanese or Manchurian civilian (Chinese) authority, and so had broad powers. Ishii had found the perfect setting for his human research.

The Kwantung Army's leadership was very receptive to Ishii's ideas about biological weapons. They believed that Japan's future success depended on controlling Northern China and Siberia and that the Russians would eventually attack their smaller forces. Bioweapons could provide an important advantage. General Umezu Yoshijiro, who was Japan's chief of staff at the end of World War II, said later when he was interrogated:

> Under the supposition that biological weapons could be employed in modern warfare, the Japanese military made a considerable study and research in BW in order that it might be able to cope with it in the event that it was used. I may say that in this connection, I have received no report on the use of BW by the U.S., Britain, or China. But neither did I receive reports that this weapon would NOT be used. Therefore the Japanese Army had to extend itself to study BW and to obtain knowledge in this field. As to the Soviets . . . reports were received concerning their intentions to use BW in the eventuality of war . . . This was considered one of the principal motives of the Japanese study in BW.

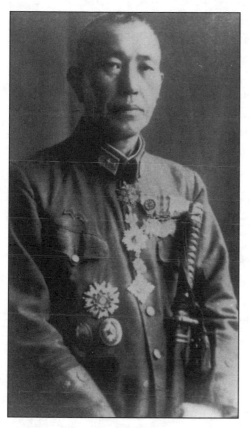

Dr. Ishii Shiro in military uniform, 1946.

The army initially supplied Ishii with 300 men to work in what he code-named the "Togo Unit," but which later became known as the "Ishii Unit." He set up shop in the industrial sector (Nan Gang District) of Harbin, the capital of Heilongsiang Province in northern Manchuria. It was a thriving city built near a major railway hub, with a population mix of 30 different ethnic groups, including Han Chinese, Koreans, Mongols, Russians, and Europeans. Because the facility was in the middle of a large city, any human experiments Ishii's unit did could be exposed— something that neither he nor the Japanese Army wanted.

So, in August 1932, Dr. Ishii Shiro, whom the Chinese called *Zhijiang Silang*, established a secret experimental site in Beiyinhe, an isolated but accessible village 60 miles south of Harbin. He ordered everyone living in Beiyinhe to leave within three days and his men burned all the buildings except one, a large market that had contained 100 Chinese shops, which he used as administrative offices. Using coerced Chinese peasant labor, they then cordoned off about 124 acres (1/2 a Chinese *li*) to build a prison-experimental laboratory complex consisting of about 100 buildings. It became known locally as the Zhong Ma Prison Camp. Security was assured by a three-meter-high brick wall topped with both barbed and high-voltage wires, as well as around-the-clock patrols.

The largest building, situated in the center of the camp, was known as the "Zhong Ma Castle." The "Castle" consisted of two wings: the first held offices, barracks, warehouses, a canteen, and parking for military vehicles. The second wing, off-limits to all Chinese, had nearly 6,500 square feet of laboratory space, a crematorium, a munitions dump, and a prison.

The prison generally housed 500 to 600 prisoner-experimental subjects in tiny cells, although the structure was built to hold 1,000. Prisoners included common criminals, captured members of the anti-Japanese underground or guerrilla fighters, and innocent civilians caught in the frequent roundups of "suspicious persons." Handcuffed and shackled most of the time, they were kept healthy with frequent exercise and a diet far superior to that which they would have had on the outside. Once they became experimental subjects, however, few prisoners lived longer than a month before being "sacrificed."

The pathogens that Ishii's unit tested at Beiyinhe included anthrax (*Bacillus anthracis*), plague (*Yersinia pestis*), and glanders (*Pseudomonas mallei*). Anthrax and plague are still deadly components of biological warfare; glanders is a disease that is usually deadly to horses, but is also communicable to humans. Once their human guinea pigs were infected with a disease, doctors withdrew about one unit (500 ml) of blood from them every three to five days for testing. When the prisoners were no longer useful as research subjects, physicians either injected them with deadly poison or had them shot. Pathologists then performed autopsies to analyze the effects of their experiments.

Although the written records of these research trials were supposedly destroyed, U.S. military interrogators later obtained significant information about them. The following examples typify the physician-directed tests at Zhong Ma. In one instance, three communist guerrillas were captured and injected with plague bacteria. All three victims soon became delirious with fevers to 104°F. While they were still alive, but unconscious, unit pathologists executed them by performing autopsies. Dr. Endo Saburo, who eventually would become a lieutenant general, wrote dispassionately about the brutal experiments he witnessed when he visited the Unit on November 16, 1933:

> The Second Squad, [which] was responsible for poison gas, liquid poison; [and] the First Squad, [which was responsible for] electrical experiments. Two bandits were used [by each squad for the experiments].
>
> 1. Phosgene gas—5 minute injection of gas into a brick-lined room; the subject was still alive one day after inhalation of gas; critically ill with pneumonia.
> 2. Potassium cyanide—the subject was injected with 15 mg of it; [subject] lost consciousness approximately 20 minutes later.
> 3. 20,000 volts—several jolts of that voltage not enough to kill the subject; injection [of poison] required to kill the subject.
> 4. 5,000 volts—several jolts not enough; after several minutes of continuous currents, [subject] was burned to death.

More than 1,000 prisoners were "sacrificed" for human experimentation at the Zhong Ma Camp from late 1932 until the prisoner rebellion in the fall of 1934, when 12 captives escaped and told their tale to partisan guerrillas. Although the lethal human experiments continued, the work at Zhong Ma was scaled back until it was abandoned and the evidence of its existence was eradicated in 1937. The operation was then shifted to other, larger sites.

Ping Fan — The Devil's Laboratory

Undeterred, Lt. Col. Ishii moved and enlarged his biological warfare organization. On August 1, 1936, he was appointed chief of the Kwantung Army Water Purification Bureau (*Boeki Kyusui Boeki Kyusui Bu*, literally meaning Anti-Epidemic Water Supply and Purification Bureau). The unit was supposedly established to provide the Japanese troops with clean water after they had experienced a major cholera epidemic. Intelligence sources claimed that the epidemic was due to either Chinese or Russian BW activity, but it may really have been due to the soldiers' living conditions. Ishii was chosen not only because of his experience in BW, but also because he had developed a filtration pump. He subsequently sold the pump to the army through a monopoly and received large "consultant" fees. Ishii's innocuous sounding unit became the nucleus of further, extended human biological warfare experiments.

Ishii based his network at what became known as the "Ping Fan complex," a cluster of 10 villages covering about 1,500 acres located about 15 miles south of Harbin. He initially ordered three of the villages, covering about 144 acres, to be evacuated in autumn 1936; the others were appropriated over the next two years. Ishii, always a meticulous and expansive planner, constructed an enormous complex at Ping Fan. Centered around an immense administrative building, the compound included laboratories, state-of-the-art dormitories for Japanese civilian workers, barracks, an arms magazine, barns and stables for test animals, an autopsy-dissecting building, a laboratory for frostbite experiments, a prison for test subjects, a power plant, three crematoria, an airfield, and a farm used both to grow consumables and to test BW agents.

Comforts for the Japanese workers were not omitted. These included a 1,000-seat auditorium with a library and bar, swimming pools, gardens, small bars and restaurants, athletic fields, a special brothel, and four fully equipped medical facilities—which treated only Japanese. The compound also had primary and secondary schools for Japanese children and a large Shinto temple.

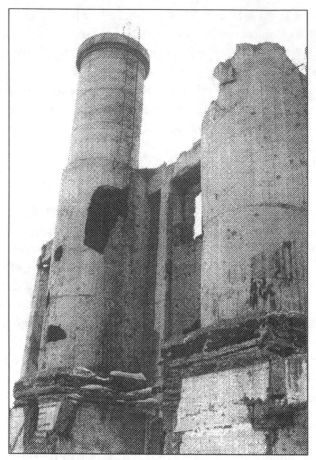

The chimneys at Ping Fan. (Photo reproduced from *Unit 731: Testimony* by Hal Gold.)

Dr. Ishii and his family lived in Harbin at a Russian mansion appropriated for their use. His daughter later described it as being "a graceful mansion indeed, like something out of a romantic movie such as *Gone With the Wind.*" Ishii commuted to Ping Fan in an armored limousine. On occasion, his family lived with him at Ping Fan—supposedly unaware of what was happening around them.

The complex was honeycombed with tunnels that were 60 feet wide and 10 feet high. Some ran from the prison to the experimental laboratories and the crematoriums. A secret tunnel ran from the administrative center, known as "The Square Building" where future victims arrived, to the heavily guarded, massive prison facilities in Buildings 7 (*Ro*) and 8 (*Ha*). These buildings housed future human fodder for the BW experiments; each was only two stories high so it would be hidden by the surrounding three- to five-story administrative structures. They were so solidly built of reinforced concrete that, at the war's end, Japanese Army engineers were unable to destroy them as they did the other Ping Fan buildings.

Building 7 housed male inmates, while Building 8 held both men and women. Together, they were built to house up to 400 prisoners, although they usually held only 200 at any one time. The prison was a vision of hell. Spy holes in each cell's steel door allowed guards and researchers to constantly monitor the chained prisoners' condition. Depending upon the tests, the subjects were bloated, emaciated, blistered, or had open wounds. Some had rotting limbs or bone protruding through necrosis-blackened skin from frostbite experiments. Others sweated with high fevers, writhed in agony, or moaned in pain as they suffered from physician-induced infections. Those with respiratory infections coughed incessantly.

The area was so secret that the army designated it a "Special Military Region." As such, extraordinary permission was required for any civilian to enter and civilian aircraft were barred from flying overhead. Three types of police (the dreaded *kenpeitai*, the Kwantung Army, and the local force) guarded the perimeter. Japanese Army aircraft constantly patrolled the skies, and trains that passed by had to close their window shades. A moat, 16-foot brick wall, guard towers, and a barbed wire-electrified fence surrounded the headquarters complex.

Local Chinese citizens were drafted to build and staff the complex. As many as 15,000 were forced into servitude from the camp's inception until August 1945, when the Japanese destroyed it. Of these, more than one-third died from mistreatment. As one guard said, "there are lots of Chinese; it does not matter if one or two died." The Japanese at first provided coffins for these casualties, but the numbers became too great to squander valuable resources. Eventually, clothes and valuables belonging to the dead were given to other workers, and the corpses were dropped into a common grave. Superstitious Japanese officers claimed to hear strange noises from the "laborers' graveyard," so, to appease their souls and placate vengeful spirits, they offered sacrifices to these dead once each year.

Organization

Ping Fan was divided into eight sections, each with its own responsibilities. Section I was responsible for research and also maintained the prison.

Outfitted with the best equipment, they used the "shotgun approach" to investigate the potential military use for organisms that caused the following:

- anthrax
- botulism
- brucellosis
- cholera
- diphtheria
- dysentery
- gas gangrene
- glanders
- hemorrhagic fever
- hepatitis
- influenza
- meningitis
- paratyphoid
- plague
- pneumonia
- scarlet fever
- smallpox
- tetanus
- tick encephalitis
- tuberculosis
- tularemia
- typhoid
- typhus
- undulant fever
- venereal diseases
- whooping cough

All organisms were tested on human captives. They also tried to develop vaccines against the most probable BW agents. In their spare time, Section I personnel investigated the effects of frostbite on their prisoners.

At full capacity, the massive bacterial cultivators could produce about *70 pounds* of disease-causing bacteria at a time. General Kawashima Kiyoshi later boasted they could:

> manufacture as much as 300 kilograms [661 pounds] of plague bacteria monthly ... 500–600 kilograms of anthrax germs, or 800–900 kilograms of typhoid, paratyphoid or dysentery germs, or as much as 1,000 kilograms of cholera germs.

Section II developed and tested bombs, as well as other BW delivery methods. Eventually, they tested two types of artillery shells, both of which proved unworkable. Of the nine types of bombs they developed, the two that were produced in large numbers were the 40-kilogram *Ha* bomb filled with a mixture of shrapnel and anthrax spores and the 25-kilogram *UJI* porcelain bomb, also filled with anthrax spores. Over 1,600 of these BW bombs were made.

The Mother-Daughters bomb, in which cluster-bomb "daughters" were detonated by a radio transmitter in the "mother," proved too difficult and expensive to construct. A method to create bacterial clouds showed initial promise: both U.S. and Soviet BW researchers continued this line of investigation when they obtained Japanese data after the war. Most of these tests were carried out at Anda, a nearby field research site, using Section II's own fleet— navy usually.

Section III managed the hospital and water-purification operations. During the last two years of the war, this group also constructed the BW bombs in conjunction with Section VII. Section IV maintained the bacteria-growing machinery and stored the bacteria and viruses that were produced. Section V trained newly assigned personnel, including the many medical students who spent time at the facility. Section VI handled business affairs, and Section VIII cared for the Japanese personnel's medical problems.

The massive BW operation that Lieutenant Colonel Ishii controlled in 1936 had an annual budget of more than 10 million yen (equivalent to more than $62 million in 2002)! According to Lt. Gen. Kajitsuka Ryuji, former chief of the Kwantung Army's Medical Administration, Ishii was directed to begin his Ping Fan experiments and was funded at this extraordinary level by "command of the Emperor." This contention is supported by the identity of the staff officer commanding Ishii's Operations Division, Lieutenant Colonel Miyata, who was also known as Imperial Prince Takeda no Miya, Emperor Hirohito's cousin. Indeed, at Ping Fan's first conference in 1938, the just-promoted Colonel Ishii bragged:

> This unit which is referred to as the "remote island" is completely iso-
> lated from our surroundings and we have no complaints on the research
> environment. Compared with the research laboratories with which you
> are familiar in the universities in the large cities, this facility is inferior to
> none, and we can be rather proud of the fact that we have several times
> the equipment . . . On top of this, we have no worry whatsoever about the
> availability of research funds.

Although the Japanese were aware that the 1925 League of Nations Convention banned biochemical weaponry, they expected to win the war and, as Col. Hojo Enryo, Japan's science attaché to Berlin, said in a 1941 speech, "In the case of a victorious enemy such a moral agreement might possibly be only a dead letter." Yet, just to be careful—including avoiding any hostility from their own citizenry stemming from their activities—Ishii had his people operate under various pseudonyms. In 1941, to further hide its activities, Ishii's BW group was code-named "Unit 731."

During his service in Manchuria, Ishii spent at least three months each year in Japan, lecturing at the army medical schools, Tokyo Imperial University, Kyoto Imperial University, and other prestigious medical colleges. As part of his talks, he showed movies of his BW experiments using human subjects.

Ishii remained in command of the major BW facilities until August 1942, when, as a surgeon-major general, he was transferred to Nanking to become chief of the First Army Medical Department. He continued, however, to pursue his BW laboratory and field experiments.

Major General (later Lt. Gen.) Kitano Masaji assumed Ishii's position at Ping Fan. Dr. Kitano had followed a career path remarkably similar to Ishii's. About the same age as Ishii, Kitano had studied at Tokyo Imperial University at the same time that Ishii had been at Kyoto Imperial University. Kitano graduated from medical school in 1922, two years before Ishii. Both immediately entered the Army after medical school, rose through the ranks at about the same rate, and went to Manchuria in 1932 as majors in the Medical Corps. Kitano had the unusual dual positions of professor at the Manchurian (Army) Medical College in Mukden and active-duty army officer. Over a ten-year period, he killed thousands of prisoners, dissecting most of them alive (vivisection) for his work.

Described as wily and self-effacing, Kitano was an excellent scientific researcher and published scores of scientific papers—many more than Ishii. Kitano served as Unit 731's "acting" commander for 22 months, expanded the human BW testing, and improved the system for producing pathogenic bacteria.

As the war ended, Unit 731 members were issued vials of poison. Ishii, who directed the closing of the BW units, had wanted all personnel in Unit 731 and the associated units to commit suicide with their families. Several men did this. However, Maj. Gen. Hitoshi Kikuchi, Unit 731's research chief, vehemently disagreed with this plan, so Ishii made them swear to a "life in the shadows." He ordered them to "take this secret to the grave," to never again take official positions, and to never contact each other. All these prohibitions have since been broken and, for decades, surviving personnel held annual reunions. As the Russians approached, records and equipment were sent to Korea and Japan. Most high-ranking staff members escaped on August 13, 1945, via the ever-efficient South Manchuria Railway using a special train; Ishii fled in an airplane.

Ping Fan's Human "Logs"

To conceal the nature of their operation, Japanese administrators circulated the story that Ping Fan was a lumber mill. They called their human subjects *maruta*, meaning "wooden logs," a derogatory term symptomatic of a longstanding feeling of racial superiority and suggesting that their victims were subhuman. The victims were chiefly Han Chinese from nearby Harbin who were anti-Japanese underground workers, Communist Party members, and prisoners of war (POW). However, they also included random civilians lured off the street, sometimes with bogus employment offers. Some were stateless White Russians (including many Jews who had lived there for generations), Soviet prisoners captured in border skirmishes, Mongolians, Koreans, and various Europeans.

Before being sent to Ping Fan to be used as "experimental material," the Japanese formally sentenced all the *maruta* to death. It was often said, "there is no shortage of living wood" on which to experiment. The prisoners were delivered in a bizarre and callous fashion from processing points near Harbin, either in camouflaged freight cars or sealed paneled trucks. As Sheldon Harris relates in his book, *Factories of Death: Japanese Biological Warfare, 1932–45, and the American Cover-Up*, one Ping Fan worker described the process:

> Several Japanese technicians, their white coats flapping in the ever-present Manchurian breeze, ran from the great square building hauling flatbed carts to the train. Tenderly, large objects wrapped in straw were passed from the train to the Ping Fan technicians. They handled the parcels with the care that museum specialists devoted to transporting priceless artifacts from ancient cultures. Instead of marble statues, Fang was shocked to see that two live humans were inside each bag. The bags were so tightly bound that the prisoners head and feet touched each other.

Each prisoner was given a number to be used for their specimens during the experiments. No personal data about them was ever recorded. Since the numbering system was reused whenever it reached 1,500, the exact number of victims remains unknown. To keep their human guinea pigs in the best possible condition for the experiments, the Japanese gave them excellent medical care and at least as good a diet as the guards received. This continued nearly to the end of the war, even when Japanese troops and civilians were on short rations. However, each prisoner received such treatment only until he or she was "sacrificed" in a medical experiment. Major General Kawashima Kiyoshi described the fate of the *maruta* at Unit 731:

> From 500 to 600 prisoners were consigned to Detachment 731 annually. If a prisoner survived the inoculation of lethal bacteria, this did not save him from a repetition of the experiment that continued until death from infection supervened. The infected people were given medical treatment in order to test various methods of cure, they were fed normally, and after they had fully recovered were used for the next experiment, but infected with another kind of germ. At any rate, no one ever left this factory alive. Following anatomical study, the bodies of the dead were burned in the detachment's incinerator.

When Soviet tanks crossed the Siberia-Manchuria border at midnight on August 8, 1945 (Russia having belatedly declared war on Japan), about 400 prisoners remained alive at Unit 731. During the next week, before the Russians arrived at the complex, unit personnel killed some prisoners by throwing Erlenmeyer flasks of toxic chemicals into their cells to gas them. Others died after potassium cyanide was put in their food. Six hundred Chinese laborers who had been forced to work for the Japanese were machine-gunned. According to reports, "It took 30 hours to lay them in ashes."

Experiments on Prisoners

Thousands of prisoners were "sacrificed" in experiments that included testing new vaccines and a wide variety of BW agents. The cholera test conducted on 20 "logs" in mid-1940 was a typical vaccine experiment. Eight healthy prisoners, 20 to 30 years old, were given cholera vaccine developed using a new method. Eight others received an older type of vaccine, while the remaining four were not vaccinated. Three weeks later, all 20 were forced to drink cholera-laced milk. The four not vaccinated and some of those given the old vaccine died. A similar test was then conducted using plague vaccines. Each year the unit produced more than 20 million doses of vaccine.

The physician-researchers also routinely dissected living prisoners both for research and for surgical practice. For a 1995 *New York Times* article, Nicholas Kristof interviewed a cheerful 72-year-old farmer who had been a medical assistant in Unit 731:

> He switches easily to explaining what it is like to cut open a 30-year-old man who is tied naked to a bed and dissect him alive, without anesthetic. "The fellow knew that it was over for him and so he didn't struggle when they led him into the room and tied him down ... I cut him open from the chest to the stomach and he screamed terribly and his face was all twisted in agony. He made this unimaginable sound, he was screaming so horribly. But then finally he stopped. This was all in a day's work for the surgeons, but it really left an impression on me because it was my first time ..."
>
> The old man, who insisted on anonymity, explained the reason for the vivisection: "The prisoner, who was Chinese, had been deliberately infected with the plague as part of a research project ... After infecting him, the researchers decided to cut him open to see what the disease does to man's insides."

Anesthesia was not normally used for vivisections—researchers wanted to examine the body under "normal circumstances."

Dr. Masakuni Kurumizawa, deputy head of the vivisection team, became a farmer after the war, giving up on the world in which he had done "at least one thousand vivisections." A former surgical technician, Naoji Uezono, recalled, "Sometimes there were no anesthetics. They screamed and screamed. But we didn't regard the logs as human beings. They were lumps of meat on a chopping block."

Tamura Yoshio, another member of Unit 731, had a similar experience:

> One morning a Chinese, whom I sprayed with antiseptic, was sched-uled to be anatomized, no matter if he was dead or alive ...
>
> Holding that Chinese's neck, Hosojima used his right hand to cut onto the neck's vein with a knife. Blood gushed out. Due to the pain of the plague and the cut, that Chinese swayed his head left and right. Hosojima used the knife's blunt end to pound on the victim's heart and shouted: "Two doses of camphor!"
>
> Then he cut through the victim's vein. That Chinese left a word full of hatred, "Son of a Devil," lost his color and then his breath. Hosojima cut from the upper abdomen to the lower abdomen, and then through the chest ... The victim's body was completely dissected after 20 minutes.

Part of Unit 731's responsibility was to develop methods of delivering their biological devastation. They used *maruta* to test various fomites (disease-carrying objects such as food, clothes, and tools) to see which were most effec-tive. Prisoners were forced to ingest anthrax-laden chocolates, plague-filled cookies, and bacteria-contaminated drinks. They also tested the effectiveness of the human flea, *Pulex irritans*, to distribute plague—and found it to be an especially lethal method.

For their large-scale open-air tests on humans, they used a mountain site at Anda, 87 miles north of Harbin. They had their own squadron of planes to drop the weaponry they developed. Dr. Tabei Kanau, who used several hun-dred prisoners while assisting with typhoid experiments at Anda from 1938 to 1943, reported:

> One subject was exposed to a bomb burst containing buckshot mixed with 10 mg bacilli and 10 gm of clay. The buckshot had grooves, which were impregnated with the bacteria-clay mixture. Bomb burst one meter from the rear of the subject. He developed symptoms of typhoid fever with positive laboratory signs.

Some of the *maruta* were in such agony, Kanau said, that they committed suicide.

Other experiments that Unit 731 performed at Anda included tying pris-oners to stakes and setting off shrapnel bombs at varying distances. In one instance it was to test the effects of shrapnel on the human body. In another, as Nishi Toshihide, chief of the Training Division, testified:

> In January 1945 . . . I saw experiments in inducing gas gangrene, conducted under the direction of the Chief of the 2nd Division, Colonel (Dr.) Ikari, and researcher Futaki. Ten prisoners . . . were tied facing stakes, 5 to 10 meters apart . . . The prisoners' heads were covered with metal helmets, and their bodies with screens . . . only the naked buttocks being exposed. At about 100 meters away a fragmentation bomb was exploded by electricity . . . All ten men were wounded . . . and sent back to the prison . . . I later asked Ikari and researcher Futaki what the results had been. They told me that all ten men had . . . died of gas gangrene.

Kashi Sadao, a former Unit 731 member, described a typical Anda field experiment for dispersing the plague bacteria:

> At one corner of the airfield, there was a warehouse-like wooden structure enclosed in tin sheets. This was the test laboratory for germ bombs. Each time about 30 *maruta* in chains would be put into it. A fuse was used to detonate the bomb. The sound of the explosion could hardly be heard from outside. Inside, after the explosion, numerous fleas would jump on the *maruta*. They had nowhere to hide but to get infested by the plague-carrying fleas. One hour later, *maruta* were retrieved from the room and fully sterilized before sent to the laboratory . . .
>
> Soon the *maruta* would start to develop symptoms such as high fever or septicemia. Dead *maruta* would be autopsied. Blood would be withdrawn from the living ones for making serum. Un-infested *maruta* would be saved for the next round of experiments. As the experiment material, the bodies of the *maruta* were fully used, not wasted at all.

Researchers took precautions to avoid being infected themselves. They covered their bodies with a glycerin and phenol concoction, dressed in rubber clothing, and wore face masks.

According to Kashi Sadao, during one experiment at Anda, 40 *maruta* attempted to escape. They had been bound to crosses that were secured in the ground with ice in the –40°C to –50°C weather. Before the BW bombs could be set off, several freed themselves and then freed others. Japanese soldiers hunted them down in trucks. Those who were not run over were returned to headquarters and dissected. On occasion, Imperial Prince Takeda no Miya observed the Anda field tests. He later became the chairman of the Japan Olympic Committee.

Experiments Using American POWs

Since World War II, the question of how many Allied POWs were used in biological experiments has repeatedly arisen. The answer is still unknown.

Enough evidence existed in 1944 for the U.S. Navy to prosecute 19 Japanese on Truk for a series of medical experiments they conducted in Micronesia. These researchers injected some American POWs with streptococcal bacteria and placed tourniquets on others' arms and legs for extended periods; two of the POWs died. Anecdotal and circumstantial evidence suggest that such experiments may have occurred in Japanese occupied China. For example, only 4 percent of American and British POWs held by Germany and Italy died during the war, compared with 27 percent of those held by Japan.

At the Khabarovsk Military Trial, held in Russia in 1949, one witness claimed that as early as 1943, a Unit 731 researcher was sent to POW camps to test Anglo-Saxons, especially Americans, for immunity and susceptibility to infectious diseases. In July 1947, a U.S. official advised that the story about American prisoners should be covered up, even though the Soviets had discovered evidence that "American prisoners of war were used for experimental purposes of a BW nature and that they lost their lives as a result of these experiments."

One Japanese surgeon, Dr. Toshio Tono, recently confessed to having participated in vivisecting U.S. POWs in Japan: "I could never again wear a white smock. It's because the prisoners thought that we were doctors, since they could see the white smocks, that they didn't struggle. They never dreamed they would be dissected." He was speaking about eight American airmen whose B-29 bomber was rammed by a Japanese fighter on May 5, 1945, after bombing Tachiaral Air Base in southwestern Japan. Of the 13 crew members, one died when another Japanese fighter tore his parachute, and another killed himself with his last bullet after being attacked by villagers. Two more were killed on landing. Of the nine others, only Capt. Marvin Watkins would survive—because the Japanese took him to Tokyo for interrogation. The eight remaining airmen were taken to Kyushu University in Fukuoka, midway between Hiroshima and Nagasaki.

The first victim, Teddy Ponczka, had been wounded, and he assumed that he was being taken to the operating room to be treated. Instead, to test surgery's effect on respiration, his chest was opened and his lung removed. According to Dr. Toshio, he was then given intravenous injections of sea water to determine if it could be substituted for sterile saline solution. Ponczka bled to death—apparently without anesthesia. The others had parts of their livers, brains, or stomachs altered or removed to perform bizarre medical tests. Dr. Toshio noted "there was no debate among the doctors about whether to do the operations . . . that is what made it so strange."

Other Biological Warfare Units

Unit 100

Unit 100, like its counterpart Unit 731, was also established in 1936. It was located in the small village of Mokotan, less than four miles south of Changchun and 150 miles south of Harbin and Ping Fan. It, too, had an innocuous-sounding name, the Kwan Tung Army Horse Epidemic Prevention Department (Wakamatsu Unit). It received its code name of Unit 100 in 1941.

Changchun, with a population of 500,000, was a strategic railway hub with a large film industry. In the mid-1930s, it became the capital of the Japanese puppet state of Manchukuo. The city was dominated by "Chief Executive" Pu Yi's palatial complex—appropriately located next to Kwantung Army headquarters, where the real power lay. (Pu Yi had abdicated his throne as China's last Manchu emperor in 1912.)

Unit 100 was laid out similarly to Ping Fan, with a large concrete head-quarters building containing laboratories, prison cells, offices, and underground tunnels to other laboratory sites. Several dozen other buildings included barns for large animals, autopsy rooms, and three crematoriums. A ten-foot-high electric fence surrounded the complex. Major Wakamatsu Yujiro, a veterinarian, commanded Unit 100 throughout its existence.

The unit's original task was to research animal and plant diseases and preventive agents. Researchers initially worked on anthrax, glanders, sheep and cattle plagues, and red rust and other plant diseases. Eventually, they performed thousands of brutal human BW experiments. In September 1941, Unit 100 began mass-producing pathogenic bacteria. Although the unit never reached its full production capacity, it was targeted to produce 1,000 kilograms of anthrax, 500 kilograms of glanders, 100 kilograms of *Brucella abortus*, and 100 kilograms of red rust bacteria each year.

In mid-1942, the unit began spreading animal diseases along the Siberia-Manchuria border. The doctors also performed gruesome medical experiments. Unit 100 eventually became the most prolific Japanese BW research unit (after Unit 731) in the scope of its activities and the number of prisoners killed during experiments. There were at least ten subsidiary branches throughout China and they also conducted field tests at Anda with Unit 731 personnel.

A senior sergeant later described a typical Unit 100 "experiment":

> I put as much as a gram of heroin into some porridge and gave this porridge to an arrested Chinese citizen who ate it; about 20 minutes later

he lost consciousness and remained in that state until he died 15 to 16 hours later. We knew that such a dose of heroin is fatal, but it did not make any difference to us whether he died or lived … One of the prisoners of Russian nationality became so exhausted from the experiments that no more could be performed on him, and Matsui ordered me to kill that Russian by giving him an injection of potassium cyanide. After the injection, the man died at once. Bodies were buried in the unit's cattle cemetery.

The doctors limited prisoners to one pathogen or chemical each, and then killed them because, as the doctors explained, "the materials were no longer worth keeping for further experiments." Days before the war ended, Unit 100 personnel used potassium cyanide to kill all their remaining prisoners, along with nearly all the Chinese workers at the complex. They also killed most of their experimental animals, saving only 60 glanders-infected horses and thousands of plague-infected rats that they released into the surrounding communities. The Changchun area suffered plague, glanders, and anthrax epidemics in 1946, 1947, and 1951. In 1949, farmers planting crops in the area discovered a huge burial site, which seemed to be limitless: "Even after digging 2–5 meters [more than 16 feet] deep, we found that there were still human bodies."

Unit Ei 1644

Unit Ei 1644 was located inside Nanking (Nanjing). Unlike the other BW operations that were situated in relatively new and remote Manchurian cities, this unit was in a major city that had served as China's capital several times. In what the world has come to know as the "Rape of Nanking," Japanese troops ran amok in the city from December 14, 1937, until February 7, 1938, raping more than 20,000 women, killing more than 200,000 civilian men, and looting at will. On April 18, 1939, the city became the site for a branch of the Central China Anti-Epidemic Water Supply Unit, which became known publicly as the "Tama Unit" and secretly as Unit Ei 1644. Its primary mission was to perform BW experiments on prisoners that they called *zaimoku* (lumber), a play on Unit 731's term, *maruta*.

Unit Ei 1644 was run by Dr. Masuda Tomosada, a talented physician-scientist who was Ishii's friend and protégé. The eldest son of a retired army physician, he was intelligent, handsome, and ambitious—but he had no moral compass. After graduating from Kyoto Imperial University Medical School in the early 1920s, he married and joined the army reserve. After serving as a medical officer in the 4th Regiment of the Imperial Guards, he returned to Kyoto Imperial University where he received a Ph.D. in microbiology in 1931.

He next joined the faculty of Tokyo's Army Medical College, where he and Professor Ishii became close friends. In 1932, they traveled on a secret mission to scout locations for Manchurian BW installations. In September 1937, Dr. Masuda was named acting director of Darien Anti-Epidemic Center, a branch of Unit 731. He also served as Ishii's associate at the main unit in Harbin, spending most of his time there. Masuda lived well beyond his means while in Manchuria and may have received kickbacks from contractors. In 1939, Ishii picked him to direct the new BW unit in Nanking.

Dr. Masuda was openly callous about the use of BW. In a lecture at the Army Medical College in 1942, he said:

> BW can be used not only against the enemy personnel but all living matter within the enemy territory, including the people, livestock, domestic animals, grains, and vegetables . . . It can be also employed against the neutral countries which manifest signs of becoming the allies of the enemy country . . .
>
> Regardless of the results, to disseminate bacteria among the civilized people will affect their morale . . . The outbreaks of epidemics at various places will necessitate the country to expend much of its manpower and materials in bringing the epidemics under control and will greatly hinder the nation in carrying out its war . . .
>
> The offensive tactics can be carried out in forms of bacterial rain or dropping bombs or firing shells filled with bacteria or through spies . . . It can be used against the enemy not in direct contact with the friendly troops, especially against their navy by contaminating their foodstuffs with typhoid bacteria just prior to their ships leaving port.

The Tama Unit was based in a Chinese hospital in the heart of Nanking. (The building reverted to a hospital after the war.) At any time, there were about 1,500 Japanese employees. An adjacent annex housed research facilities and a 100-person prison for experimental subjects. Mazmodo, a prison guard at Unit Ei 1644, recalled:

> On the fourth floor of the prison, there were iron cages. The height of the cage was about the height of a sitting person. The prisoner could not move freely in it. In experiments, live germs were injected into the *zaimoku's* body. Blood tests were performed afterwards. Prisoners could not sleep and were constantly moaning. In one instance, a *zaimoku's* main artery in the thigh was cut open to draw blood, and he bled to death.

A ten-foot-high brick wall topped by electrified fencing surrounded the entire complex. For added security, the large camp incinerator, which was used only between 11 P.M. and 2 A.M., was surrounded by its own locked fence. A

Tama Unit member was told that "prisoners killed in experiments were incinerated using the oil burner, then the bones were crushed and buried on the grounds." The prisoners used for Unit Ei 1644's experiments were mostly Chinese, but also included White Russians and other nationalities. Proportionately more women and children were sacrificed in the name of science at this site than at any other.

In addition to testing the same organisms as Unit 731, Dr. Masuda also tested snake (cobra, habu, and amagasa) venoms, blowfish poisons, and arsenic on his unwilling subjects. The unit had a massive capability for producing pathogenic organisms and plague-infected fleas. They also used their BW agents in the field, as Kozawa, a former Unit Ei 1644 worker, recalled: "They put plague-infected fleas in bottles and placed them near the camp of the Chinese Army at night. They poured germs into the wells and rivers to poison civilians."

In 1942, Col. (Dr.) Ota Kiyoshi, another Ishii protégé, replaced Dr. Masuda as unit director. Yet, the routines of testing and killing *zaimoku* did not change. As with the other BW units, the entire complex was leveled by Japanese Army sappers in the last week of the war. All *zaimoku* were killed and the researchers escaped to Japan with their data.

Other BW facilities included Nami Unit 8604, with headquarters at Zhongshan Medical University near Guangzhou, the capital of Guangdong Province. Researchers used human subjects to test typhus, observe the effects of starvation, and perform daily vivisections. Since they did not have an incinerator, a chemical pond within the University compound was used to dissolve their victims' bodies. In 1997, torrential rains uncovered waist-high lidded urns, each with the bones of two or three people who had presumably died in Tama Unit's grotesque experiments.

The Deployment of Biological Warfare

The Japanese first used specially trained saboteurs to disperse BW agents in the so-called Nomonhan Incident on July 13, 1939, after the Russians had defeated the Japanese Army in a nearby battle on the Manchuria-Mongolia border. Unit 731 personnel tried to contaminate the Halha River; it was probably ineffective. Under the direction of Dr. Kakizoe Shinobu, a Japanese Army physician, cholera-causing bacteria were then dumped into the Wei River, ultimately causing the death of more than 25,000 Chinese civilians. During the same period, the army fired at least 2,000 bacteria-filled shells at the Russians, with uncertain effect.

Many field tests occurred in the Chinese villages surrounding Harbin, with devastating results. It is estimated that more than 200,000 Chinese were killed in germ warfare field experiments. Cities reportedly used for field tests of plague included Ning Bo, Chang teh, and Congshan.

In July 1940, the Japanese launched a BW attack on Ning Bo, a resort community near Shanghai and the birthplace of Chiang Kai Shek, China's wartime leader. Over a five-month period, using several methods, Dr. Ishii's Unit 731, in conjunction with Dr. Masuda's Unit Ei 1644, distributed 70 kilograms of typhoid bacteria, 50 kilograms of cholera bacteria, and 5 kilograms of plague-infected fleas. More than 1,000 residents became ill, and at least 500 people died from these illnesses. So proud was the Japanese Army Command of these "successes" that they made a documentary film of the raids and their outcomes. The result, however, was even more far-reaching: plague was introduced into the local rat population, resulting in lethal outbreaks in 1941, 1946, and 1947.

Unit 731 personnel also released tens of thousands of plague-infected rats, causing widespread plague in 22 counties of Heilongsiang and Kirin Provinces and taking more than 20,000 lives. But it was only in June 1942, after the Japanese dropped bacteriological bombs on Chang teh, that President Franklin D. Roosevelt, based on limited evidence, warned Japan that if they continued to use poison gases or other forms of inhuman warfare, their actions would invite comparable U.S. retaliation. In a belated response to the Japanese threat, the secret U.S. biological warfare program began in September 1943 at Camp (now Fort) Detrick, Maryland.

A classified message sent from U.S. Headquarters in Tokyo on June 22, 1947, subsequently confirmed Japan's BW attacks:

> Strong circumstantial evidence exists of use of bacteria warfare at Chuhsien, Kinghwa and Chang teh. At Chuhsien, Japanese planes scattered rice and wheat grains mixed with fleas on 4th October 1940. Bubonic plague appeared in same area on 12th November. Plague never occurred in Chuhsien before occurrence . . .
>
> At Kinghwa, located between Ningpo and Chupuien, 3 Japanese planes dropped a large quantity of small granules on 28th November 1940. Microscopic examination revealed presence of numerous gram-negative bacilli possessing [deleted when declassified].

The Russians also publicized Japan's use of BW agents during the Khabarovsk Military Trial, which began on December 25, 1949. For example, Gen. Tamurai Tadashi, who had been the Japanese Imperial Army's commander in China, said, "General [Ishii] Shiro openly pointed out to me that his Unit [731] was preparing germ warfare against Russia . . . Their effectiveness had already been proved in laboratories and humans."

In July 1942, Dr. Ishii led another BW excursion in Nanking, again with Dr. Masuda's local Unit Ei 1644. He took 130 kilograms of paratyphoid "A" and anthrax bacteria, as well as a large amount of typhoid bacteria. They laced wells, marshes, and citizens' homes with the deadly agents. They also distrib uted typhoid- or paratyphoid-laced dumplings (dumplings were a favorite holiday treat) to 3,000 POWs. Japanese soldiers left about 400 bacteria-infested cakes near fences and trees, to be found and eaten by starving locals who probably thought that the soldiers had forgotten their food. They also distributed anthrax-laden chocolates to hundreds of Nanking children. The expected epidemics broke out shortly thereafter, delighting the physician-researchers.

Similarly, in August 1942, a Japanese plane flew over Congshan in Zhejiang Province, spraying "a kind of smoke from its butt." Two weeks later, rats in that area began dying en masse, a plague epidemic followed, and, over a two-month period, 392 out of 1,200 residents died. After some of these tests, Dr. Ishii's pathologists, dressed in protective clothing, conducted dissections on farmer-victims in the fields where they died.

Patrick Tyler, of the *New York Times*, interviewed local survivors:

> At its peak that terrible November, the plague here was killing 20 Chinese a day, all of them civilians. Their screams sundered the night from behind shuttered windows and bolted doors, and some of the most delirious victims ran or crawled down the narrow alleys to gulp putrid water from open sewers in vain attempts to vanquish the septic fire that was consuming them. They died excruciating deaths.
>
> "You buried the dead knowing that the next day you would be buried" said Wang Peigen, who was ten when the horror began . . .
>
> "The thing I remember most is the fear," said Wang Da, another survivor." People closed their doors, and all you could hear through the night was people dying and people crying for the dead."

A 15-year-old survivor of this attack poignantly recalled:

> My mother and father—in all, eight people in my family—died. I was the only one in my family left. My mother had a high fever all day. She was crying for water, and clawing at her throat. Then, she let out a roar like a lion, and died before my eyes.

In 1944, a plan to disperse plague on Saipan, which the Americans had just captured, failed when the team's ship was torpedoed. Ishii then worked on plans to deliver these pathogens to the continental United States. One method was to use giant unmanned balloons; up to 9,000 such balloons with explosives on board had already been successfully used. Ishii was later asked why he had not used his bioweapons in December 1944, when 200 of the balloon bombs landed in the United States. The U.S. contact with Ishii, Lt. Col. Murray Sanders, said: "The only explanation I had, and still have, is that Ishii wasn't ready to deliver what he was making in Ping Fan; that he hadn't worked out the technology. If they had been, we were at Ishii's mercy."

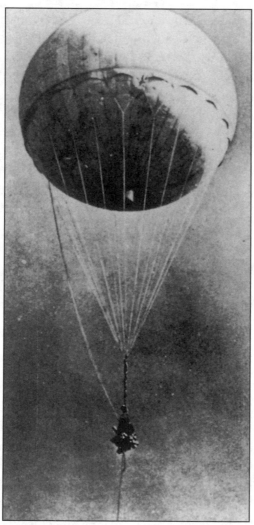

Japanese balloon bomb.

Before Japan surrendered, a kamikaze mission had been planned to rain plague on San Diego, California. Using an I-400 submarine, nicknamed "underwater aircraft carriers," the Japanese intended to attack with plague, cholera, and other BW weapons by air and ground on September 22, 1945. The submarine could carry up to three seaplanes, with their wings folded, on launch catapults inside watertight compartments under the conning tower. The submarine's crew was to carry out the ground attack as a suicide mission. Code-named "Cherry Blossoms at Night" or "Operation PX," the planned attack became irrelevant when Japan surrendered in August 1945. Ultimately, and despite vigorous opposition from the BW team, Gen. Yoshijiro Umezu, chief of the General Staff, canceled the project, believing both that Roosevelt meant to retaliate in kind and that such actions would bring disgrace on the emperor. General Umezu was later found guilty of war crimes and died in prison.

Other Medical Experiments

Japanese doctors also used prisoners as subjects in their sadistic, pseudo-scientific experiments with poisons, tuberculosis, venereal diseases, cold, deprivation, pressure, and conventional weapons.

Early in the war, the Japanese Army sought a poison that would be fatal several minutes after it was ingested. At Noborito Army Research Center in Kawasaki, a unit that worked closely with Ishii's project, doctors found what they were seeking: acetone cyanohydrin. When tested on Chinese prisoners, it killed them within five to six minutes after they ate it.

Dr. Hideo Futagi headed a tuberculosis research group at Unit 731. Tuberculosis acts too slowly to be used as a BW agent; it was tested solely for academic reasons. Using local adults and children as for his experiments, Hideo tested C1 *Tuberculosis hominis* and "all doses produced miliary [widespread] tuberculosis, which was fatal within one month in those injected with 10.0 and 1.0 mg. The others [who received other doses] were severely ill, lived longer but probably died later." In a similar test, he reported that "death at one month occurred following a stormy course with fever immediately post-injection."

Venereal diseases were rampant in the Japanese Army, so Unit 731 and Dr. Hideo were assigned to investigate them. A unit member told historian Hal Gold:

At first we infected women with syphilis by injection. But this method did not produce real research results. Syphilis is normally transmitted through direct contact... And so we followed a system of direct infection through sexual contact.

They did this by forcing male and female prisoners, one of whom had syphilis, to repeatedly have sex with each other until the partner contracted the disease. Then researchers monitored the progress of the disease by both observing external signs and, at different stages, dissecting different parts of the body to observe the physical findings.

One doctor involved with the venereal disease experiments participated in vivisections on six women, sometimes using chloroform and sometimes with the woman wide awake. After the war, he felt that he no longer had the moral standing to practice medicine. He related one incident in which a Chinese woman, although she had been given some chloroform, woke up with her abdomen cut open. She tried to get up, screaming, "Go ahead and kill me, but please don't kill my child!"

"There were four or five of us working on the vivisection," said the doctor. "We held her down, applied more anesthesia, and continued." The typical anesthetic, if used, was applied by covering the prisoner's nose and mouth with a medication-soaked cloth. They then quickly cut the victim from the neck to the groin, just as in an autopsy—which it actually was, even though the person still lived.

Dr. Yoshimura Hisato, from Kyoto University Medical School, was one of the researchers testing treatments for frostbite, a problem threatening the Kwantung Army during the extremely cold Manchurian winters. The standard therapy at the time was to rub frozen extremities until they thawed. Dr. Yoshimura, using unwilling human subjects, found otherwise. According to Gen. Okamura Yasutsugu, deputy commander-in-chief of the Kwantung Army from August 1932 to November 1934, "The best treatment for frozen limbs is soaking in water 37 degrees Celsius ... [This was] based on invaluable data from in vivo experiments with humans who repeatedly were frozen and then defrosted."

In a process similar to that of the notorious Nazi, Dr. Josef Mengele, naked prisoners had their limbs frozen by either exposing them to −30°C temperatures for up to one hour or "their arms were bared and made to freeze with the help of an artificial current of air. This was done until their frozen arms, when struck with a short stick, emitted a sound resembling that which a board gives out when it is struck." They were then immersed in waterbaths at various temperatures to see how well they warmed.

Filmed for "educational purposes," most of these subjects died or lost limbs. Those who survived often ended up having rotting hands with protruding bones and then became fodder for poison gas experiments. General Yasutsugu later said, "I did not know the details of the medical advances he made, but after the war, Ishii told me that his work produced more than 200 patents." In one notorious test, a three-day-old baby, who was born to a prisoner impregnated through forced sex during venereal disease experiments, had a temperature-monitoring needle inserted in its hand while it was immersed in ice water.

Unit 731 occasionally combined biological warfare and freezing experiments, as described by Col. Toshihide Nishi:

> An experiment in which I participated was performed by infecting ten Chinese war prisoners with [the bacteria causing] gas gangrene. The object of the experiment was to ascertain whether it was possible to infect people with gas gangrene at a temperature of 20°C below zero.
>
> This experiment was performed in the following way: ten Chinese war prisoners were tied to stakes at a distance of 10–20 meters from a shrapnel bomb that was charged with gas gangrene. To prevent the men from being killed outright, their heads and backs were protected with special metal shields and thick quilted blankets, but their legs and buttocks were left unprotected.
>
> The bomb was exploded by means of an electric switch and the shrapnel, bearing gas gangrene germs, scattered all over the spot where the experimentees were bound. All the experimentees were wounded in the legs or buttocks, and seven days later they died in great torment.

Sadao Kashi, a former Unit 731 member, described poison gas tests performed primarily on *maruta* who had survived the freezing or BW tests. These subjects were often deformed and severely ill before the experiments began:

> There was a square building, covered with boards ...This was the poison gas generating room. Inside there was a poison gas experiment chamber with glass walls on three sides. The motor and the fan started to rattle after we put three to five *maruta* into the chamber. Odorless and invisible gas started filling the room. Through the glass windows, we observed the painful expression of the *maruta*. Because different types of poison gas were used, the reactions of the *maruta* were different. Some threw out foam, some vomited blood, and others spilled liquid through their noses.

About ten people were busy working outside the chamber, some using stopwatches, some using cameras, and some taking records. About 20 minutes later the *maruta* were dragged out of the chamber and placed on straw bags for an hour of observation.

Unit 731 also carried out deprivation and slow starvation tests in which their prisoners were denied food and water for varying lengths of time. In some cases they had to subsist on army biscuits and water while doing hard labor. None lasted more than two months on this regimen. Others were dehydrated under hot lamps.

Supposedly on behalf of the Japanese Air Force, physicians also performed experiments in pressure chambers that tested human survivability at extremely low atmospheric pressures with minimal oxygen, such as would be found at high altitudes. Multiple sensors were attached to prisoners' bodies and they were exposed to the equivalent of thousands of feet of elevation. Researchers filmed them as they slowly asphyxiated; their eyes bulged, their eardrums ruptured, and they finally died as their blood vessels burst.

Ping Fan doctors performed other gruesome tests on prisoners: replacing human blood with animal blood (inevitably fatal), studying the result of electrocution on human tissues, testing the effect of high-dose x-rays on the human liver, shooting prisoners in the head at various angles to evaluate the effect on the brain, and burning prisoners by various methods, including with hot water and fire bombs. Doctors also hung the "logs" upside down to determine how long it would take a person to choke to death, injected them with air to test the amount needed for an air embolism, injected horse urine into their kidneys, and gave intentional heroin overdoses to observe their deaths.

Experimenting on prisoners was not confined to research units; it also occurred in Japanese Army hospitals throughout China. Dr. Kanisawa, who worked as a military physician at Lu-An Japanese Army Hospital in China's Shang Xi Province, testified he first performed live, unanesthetized dissections as a medical student:

> When I studied surgical operation at that medical facility, I killed 14 Chinese alive. At that time, to me it was like killing a dog. That type of killing was routine . . . During vivisection, we brutally performed spinal block or general anesthesia. After victims became unconscious, I practiced appendectomy, arms and legs amputation, and bronchial opening and feather insertion for cleaning a chest with bullet. After the operation, we threw dead bodies into nearby ditches. If a victim was still alive, we injected 5 mm. of ether and thus killed the victim after half a minute.

Sometimes organs obtained from anatomy were sent to Japan's drug manufacturing factory for making drugs. Another time, we practiced surgery of bullet-shot victims at the surgery table without using any anesthesia . . . The first time I was very hesitant to do what I was told to do. The second time you get used to it. The third time you more or less volunteered . . .

There are times when I look at my hands and remember what I have done with these hands. What is really scary is that I don't have any nightmares of what I have done . . . We did not treat Chinese as living human beings. Probably youngsters may not understand why we committed such atrocities. This was caused by an education of militarism and contempt of other ethnicities.

Unit 516, primarily a chemical warfare research unit, carried out joint experiments with Unit 731 at Ping Fan and at Hailar. Prisoners were forced to drink liquid mustard gas, producing vomiting and bloody diarrhea. Normally, mustard gas is dispersed as a spray, causing long-lasting debilitating effects on the eyes and skin. Unit 516 doctors also tested hydrogen cyanide, acetone cyanide, and potassium cyanide on prisoners. Prisoners who were given large doses of hydrogen cyanide became confused and dizzy within a few seconds. Unable to hold their breath, they rarely survived the test, even when physicians administered experimental medical aid to test its efficacy. As did the other units at the end of the war, Unit 516 personnel killed all the prisoners and local Chinese laborers to destroy evidence of their research.

Dr. Ken Yuasa, born into a doctor's family, served as a Japanese Imperial Army surgeon in China beginning in 1942. After the war, he practiced medicine in a Tokyo clinic until 1995, when he began lecturing about his war experiences in an attempt at redemption. Although not a member of Unit 731, as an army physician specializing in infectious diseases he drilled holes into prisoners' brains to take tissue samples. When he arrived in China, he was asked if he wanted to "practice surgery" on prisoners:

About half the Army doctors did not know how to use a scalpel . . . One function of the Army hospital was training doctors. Vivisection was used to practice for performing operations at the front lines. I operated on living Chinese for whom I had no hatred whatsoever to gain surgical ability in order to win the war . . . Living persons are good for scalpel practice, so people were brought in to the hospital by the *kenpeitai* [military police] to get cut up just like the *maruta* in Unit 731.

In his first experience, two Chinese prisoners were brought in, stripped naked, laid on the operating table, and given an anesthetic. One looked like a farmer, the other like a soldier. When one resisted lying on the operating table, a nurse said, in broken Chinese:

> "We're using ether; it won't hurt, so lie down." She gave me a wry smile when she said that . . . She was handling so many vivisections it was routine. People who repeat evil acts do not remember them. There is no sense of doing wrong . . .
>
> Surgery began. The man was given ether and dissected. His appendix was so small that it was like looking for a burrowing worm. I had to cut and search repeatedly. The blood flow was stopped, nerves were cut, bones were cut with a saw, and a tracheotomy was performed. Blood and air escaped from his body, and blood came foaming up. Practice time was two hours.
>
> The man died, and his body was thrown into a hole and buried. The burial area near the operating room was full, so we had to dig a hole farther away. We had received a request from a Japanese pharmaceutical manufacturer; I scraped samples from the outer covering of his brain, placed them into ten 500 cc bottles with alcohol, and sent them to the company for rheumatism research.
>
> The other man, the soldier, was still panting. The hospital head used him for hypodermic practice and injected air into him. Then, to kill him, he injected the same liquid used for anesthesia. That was my first crime. After that, it was easy. Eventually I dissected 14 Chinese.

Dr. Yuasa was put in charge of the local clinic and, when he felt he or his staff needed dissection or surgical practice, he asked the police to send over a Communist—which they obligingly did. He also witnessed surgery on un-anesthetized prisoners:

> Once, at Shanxi First Army Headquarters, there were some forty army doctors gathered from base and field hospitals. There was a lecture on military medicine, and afterward we were led to the prison cells. There were two Chinese in a cell. The jailer took out his pistol and fired two shots into each of their bellies. One of them was vivisected right there in the room. There was no anesthesia. While this was going on, I heard four more shots fired. That meant two more people. Our object was to keep the person alive until the bullets were removed. Since we neither tried to administer ether nor stop the flow of blood, the men died soon.

Subsequently, according to Yuasa, "a secret order came to the hospitals in northern China: 'The war is not going well. Perform vivisections!' Thousands, or tens of thousands, of doctors used live subjects for dissection practice and research. What are those people doing now? . . . There may be some feeling of shame, but most have forgotten."

The U.S. Government's Cover-Up

Since World War II, both the Japanese and U.S. governments have tried to suppress information about the monstrous physician-led experiments on prisoners. The Japanese supposedly destroyed all records of their BW experiments in 1945. However, apparently this story was concocted to keep secret both their results and the methods used to obtain them. Clearly, both U.S. and Soviet researchers acquired significant information about biological warfare from the Japanese. They used this data in their own research, and then tried to cover up these facts.

When the U.S. government put 16 Japanese citizens on the "Watch List" in December 1996, and barred them from entering the United States because of World War II war crimes, activists found the action too little too late. Since the U.S. Justice Department created the Office of Special Investigations (OSI) in 1979, they have put more than 60,000 people on the Watch List, yet these were the first Japanese citizens to make the list.

According to Eli M. Rosenbaum, director of the OSI, some of the men put on the list were members of Unit 731. He stated: "The top leaders of Unit 731 are no longer alive. Clearly they deserved trial and the most severe punishment. But the failure to prosecute them can't be undone." Professor John Dower, a Massachusetts Institute of Technology specialist on U.S.-Japan relations, pointed out the hypocrisy involved in this action:

> At the end of World War II, the U.S. occupying force was aware of the information about Unit 731, but deliberately exonerated the men in return for their agreement to be debriefed on the findings of their atrocious experiments. We agreed to cover up their crimes.

In fact, a documented report of Japanese attempts at inducing plague in the Chinese population appeared in the U.S. medical literature as early as August 1942. The article cited four instances that medical and epidemiological professionals had investigated. In 1943, the U.S. government again acknowledged that Japan had used both biological and chemical weapons. President Roosevelt issued a warning:

> I desire to make it unmistakably clear that if Japan persists in his inhuman form of warfare against China or against any other of the United Nations, such action will be regarded by this government as though taken against the United States and retaliation in kind and in full measure will be meted out . . . We shall be prepared to enforce complete retribution. Upon [Japan] will rest the responsibility.

After Japan surrendered, the United States and its allies investigated the BW research being done by Dr. Ishii. The Japanese doctors and scientists involved appointed Dr. Naito Ryoichi to work out an amnesty deal in exchange for access to the Unit's research data. According to his superiors, Dr. Naito was responsible for devising the strategy of Unit 731 officers, who, when interrogated, discussed everything except for "ta" and "ho"—code words for human subject experiments and biological warfare.

Dr. Naito Ryoichi was a surgeon and lieutenant colonel in the Japanese Imperial Army who had served as a bacteriologist in Unit 731 and had been Ishii's right-hand man. He had studied at the University of Pennsylvania before the war, and thus spoke English well. In 1939, Ishii sent him to the Rockefeller Institute for Medical Research in New York to obtain a yellow fever culture. They would not give it to him, and his subsequent attempts to obtain the bacteria using bribery also failed.

Lieutenant Colonel (Dr.) Murray Sanders arrived in Japan in September 1945. As he said:

> [I knew my] mission was biological warfare. I was to find what the Japanese had done, and when the [USS] *Sturgess* docked in Yokohama, there was Dr. Naito. He came straight toward me. He seemed to have had a photograph of me, and said that he was my interpreter."

Asked many years later if he knew that his "interpreter" had been a member of Unit 731, Sanders replied, "I didn't even know what 731 was."

Sanders found Dr. Naito to be "a very humble, shy person . . . very careful. He went home every night and came back the next morning . . . I found out later that he didn't go home, but went to the various Japanese headquarters." Naito provided sparse information about the BW research to Sanders. As an interpreter, he attended all interviews with officials, and steered the conversations to cover only what he wanted them to. After only ten weeks, Sanders was sent home when he contracted tuberculosis; his investigation was continued by Col. Arvo Thompson, a veterinarian.

The negotiations surrounding the BW data and amnesty turned into a game of high-risk, high-stakes poker. The United States was fascinated with the Japanese human experimental data, but the Japanese doctors wanted assurances that they would receive amnesty. The cat and mouse game continued until Naito was told that if they did not get cooperation, the United States would bring the Communists into the picture. This frightened the Japanese, and Naito "appeared the next morning with a manuscript which contained startling material. It was fundamentally dynamite. The manuscript said, in essence, that the Japanese were involved in biological warfare." Shortly after getting this information, the U.S. high command expressed their extreme interest, and Ishii felt safe enough to come out of hiding.

Although the local newspapers had declared Ishii dead and a mock funeral was held for him in his hometown, the doctor remained very much alive, and he finally surrendered to Allied authorities. Thompson interviewed Ishii for a month in early 1946, but Ishii gave few details. Talks continued and, on May 6, 1947, a top secret cable was sent from Tokyo to Washington stating:

> Experiments on humans were . . . described by three Japanese and con firmed tacitly by Ishii; field trials against Chinese took place . . . scope of program indicated by report . . . that 400 kilograms [880 pounds] of dried anthrax organisms destroyed in August 1945 . . . Reluctant statements by Ishii indicate he had superiors (possibly general staff) who . . . authorized the program. Ishii states that if guaranteed immunity from "war crimes" in documentary form for himself, superiors and subordinates, he can describe program in detail.

The same day, another top secret memorandum to U.S. authorities confirmed this information and their interest in it.

The U.S. government continued to pursue data on the BW experiments. Much information was obtained by granting the Japanese researchers immunity from war-crimes prosecution. On December 12, 1947, Edwin V. Hill, M.D., the chief of Basic Sciences at Camp Detrick, wrote that his objective was "to examine human pathological material which had been transferred to Japan from BW installations [in China]," and acknowledged the "wholehearted cooperation of Brig. Gen. Charles A. Willoughby, MacArthur's intelligence chief." Hill interviewed Ishii and other participants, who described, among other things, their anthrax, brucellosis, and botulism experiments, the number of people they infected, and the number that died.

Hill saw this information as a financial bargain:

> Specific protocols were obtained from individual investigators . . . [which] indicate the extent of experimentation with infectious diseases in human and plant species. Evidence gathered . . . has greatly supplemented and amplified previous aspects of this field. It represents data which have been obtained by Japanese scientists at the expenditure of many millions of dollars and years of work. Information has accrued with respect to human susceptibility to those diseases as indicated by specific infectious doses of bacteria.
>
> Such information could not be obtained in our own laboratories because of scruples attached to human experimentation. These data were

secured with a total outlay of Y [yen] 250,000 to date, a mere pittance by comparison with the actual cost of the studies. Furthermore, the pathological material which has been collected constitutes the only material evidence of the nature of these experiments. It is hoped that individuals who voluntarily contributed this information will be spared embarrassment because of it and that every effort will be taken to prevent this information from falling into other hands.

Another U.S. official, Dr. Edward Wetter, in a memo dated July 1, 1947, also affirmed that the value of the data overrode issues of justice:

This Japanese information is the only known source of data from scientifically controlled experiments showing the direct effect of BW agents on man. In the past it has been necessary to evaluate the effects of BW agents on man from data obtained through animal experimentation. Such evaluation is inconclusive and far less complete than results obtained from certain types of human experimentation . . . The value to U.S. of Japanese BW data is of such importance to national security as to far outweigh the value accruing from war crimes prosecution.

Although U.S. officials had first labeled reports of Japanese BW experimentation as a Soviet "smoke screen" to avoid discussing the whereabouts of Japanese POWs, and then dismissed them as mere "propaganda," they obviously were aware of the extensive human experiments. For example, during just one month in late 1947, Japanese scientists provided U.S. interrogators with more than 35 reports involving human experiments on 801 *maruta*, including 30 suicides. In fact, they apologized that they had autopsy records on only 1,000 of the *maruta* they sacrificed.

The U.S. government and the Japanese BW scientists finally completed a deal in 1948. The United States acquired information derived from Japanese BW experimentation "at a fraction of the original cost" for about $250,000. The data was sent to Camp Detrick in Maryland, which later became the U.S. Center of Biological and Chemical Warfare Development and Testing.

In 1985, Dr. Sanders sorrowfully (and disingenuously) admitted:

I feel terrible about it . . . If we had known they used human guinea pigs, I doubt we would have given immunity (but) we didn't have the foggiest notion . . . I would have been very happy to be part of the firing squad [for the Japanese involved] . . . The main reason for keeping silent was that we did not want to involve the Emperor . . . If at that point the Emperor was brought in, we would have had a lot of dead Americans and the war would have to be fought all over again.

The Americans were also worried that an open trial would give the Soviet Union vital information about biological warfare.

The International Military Tribunal for the Far East convened in Tokyo in 1946 and tried major Japanese leaders for two years. Initially, there were only 25 primary defendants. The court was made up of judges from most of the nations that Japan had brutalized. The Allies, headed by court president Sir William Webb of Australia and a U.S.-led team of lawyers, eventually prosecuted 5,570 Japanese for war crimes. No one directly involved with biological warfare was put on trial, although the U.S. Navy did prosecute 19 Japanese BW researchers in Micronesia.

On March 11, 1948, the Tribunal in Yokohama tried 30 people, 9 of whom were faculty at Japanese medical schools, on charges of vivisection, the wrongful removal of body parts, and cannibalism. None were BW scientists. Although the charge of cannibalism was dropped for lack of evidence, 23 Japanese were found guilty of the other charges: 5 were sentenced to death, 4 to life imprisonment, and 14 to jail. In September 1950, Gen. Douglas MacArthur reduced most of these sentences. No death sentence was carried out and, by 1958, all of them were free.

By the conclusion of the Allied war crimes trials in 1948, none of those who participated in the involuntary human experiments with biological warfare agents had been brought to justice. Indeed, some of those involved dominated Japan's National Institute of Health for the next 50 years—including seven directors and five vice directors. Given their backgrounds, it is not surprising that many of these researchers continued performing involuntary human experiments on prisoners, babies, soldiers, and psychiatric patients until the 1980s.

After intense negotiations, the Allies, led by the Americans, gave the prime instigator and the director of Japan's BW abominable human experimentation, Dr. Ishii Shiro, blanket immunity from prosecution. He lived in relative obscurity and inactivity until his death from laryngeal cancer in 1959, at age 69. Even those former colleagues who had high-level positions refused to hire him, not only because they wanted to distance themselves from him professionally, but also because his arrogant and domineering manner did not fit into the new post-war environment.

Commenting about the amnesty deal given the Japanese BW researchers, OSI Director Rosenbaum said, "I can't defend the decision not to prosecute them . . . They should have been prosecuted." Yet, while even more specific information about BW experiments on humans came out just after the war crimes trials concluded, a high-level decision was made to continue this amnesty.

The records forcibly acquired by the United States at the close of World War II were returned to Japan in February 1958. According to testimony by U.S. officials, only about 5 percent had been translated or copied. In a September 1986 statement at a U.S. House of Representatives Veterans' Affairs Subcommittee hearing, John H. Hatcher, Ph.D., chief of Army Records Management and the archivist of the Army, stated:

> It is possible that in one brief period we may have had some of those materials . . . [But after a] number of years, [they were] finally boxed up and sent back to Japan, because the problem of language was too difficult for us to overcome. It was written in many different dialects, many different alphabets, congu or conji, all of those things . . . In fact, they were so difficult that we did not even copy them. I think we boxed them up and sent them back to Tokyo.

That statement seems preposterous, especially because of the number of Japanese-Americans who had been held in numerous U.S. internment camps a few years before. Japan has now sealed the records.

According to Senator Diane Feinstein of California, who introduced a bill in 1999 to make documents concerning these events public:

> Although the Second World War ended over 50 years ago—and with it Japan's chemical and biological weapons experimentation programs—many of the records and documents regarding Japan's wartime activities remain classified and hidden in U.S. Government archives and repositories. Even worse, according to some scholars, some of these records are now being inadvertently destroyed.

When historian Sheldon Harris recontacted the public information officer who had previously granted him access to archived materials at Fort Detrick, he was told that, upon retiring from the military, the man had been ordered to "get rid of that stuff, meaning incriminating documents relating to Japanese medical war crimes."

A Penalty-Free Aftermath

Unlike the Germans, the Japanese are only now beginning to confront the horrors of the human experimentation that their physicians and scientists performed from about 1930 until 1945. Japan acknowledged the existence of Unit 731 only in the 1980s, after years of denial. In a terse reply to a parliamentary question, Japan's government confirmed that they had had a BW unit employing 1,285 military and 1,472 civilians, including Japanese Red Cross nurses. As of 2001, Japan has resisted both compensating the victims of its atrocities and making its records public.

In reality, tens of thousands of Japanese staffed the human experimentation facilities. For example, about 3,000 personnel worked at the Ping Fan complex at any one time, and an additional 300 men staffed each of the satellite facilities Ishii controlled. Physicians and scientists made up approximately 10 percent of the personnel in these complexes.

So as not to leave any doubt that his colleagues would be abandoning the precepts on which medicine is based, Dr. Ishii contrasted their work with that of other physicians in his speech at the opening of Ping Fan:

> Our God-given mission as doctors is to challenge all varieties of disease-causing microorganisms; to block all roads of intrusion into the human body; to annihilate all foreign matter resident in our bodies; and to devise the most expeditious treatment possible. However, the research work upon which we are now about to embark is the completely opposite of these principles, and may cause us some anguish as doctors.
>
> Nevertheless, I beseech you to pursue this research, based on the dual thrill of (1) as a scientist to exert efforts to probe for the truth in natural science and research into, and discovery of, the unknown world, and (2) as a military person, to successfully build a powerful military weapon against the enemy.

This marriage of scientific inquiry with military strategy may have helped many of those involved in human experimentation to absolve themselves of guilt. Toshimi Mizobuchi, a former training officer with Unit 731, was interviewed by Rabbi Abraham Cooper, associate dean of the Simon Wiesenthal Center for Holocaust Studies, in 1999. Toshimi described his feelings for the victims: "They were logs to me. Logs were not considered to be human. They were either spies or conspirators . . . They were already dead. So now they die a second time. We just executed a death sentence."

Most telling of all are the attitudes of participants at the time that these horrors were taking place. For example, when a group of 100 prisoners at Ping Fan tried to escape, they were sprayed with the pesticide chloropicrin and all were suffocated. According to witnesses, "Some of the doctors associated with the experimentation cried tears of regret when their valuable experimental materials were wasted."

Who were these men who joined Ishii in his gruesome experiments? As Sheldon Harris remarks in *Factories of Death*:

> Ishii's men, for the most part, joined him in Manchuria for an assortment of reasons. Some came out of a sense of adventure. Some were drafted by the military and could not refuse the order to report to Ping Fan. A few came to Ishii in order to assume technical positions of high importance. In 1938, seven faculty from Kyoto Imperial University were lured to Ping Fan by the promise that they would be employed as project directors or, if that were impossible, they would be given other important posts . . .
>
> Others, both civilian and military personnel, knowing what they would be expected to do once they were established in Ping Fan, or in any of the other laboratories under Ishii's jurisdiction, willingly enlisted in his cause because they could pursue research unhindered by either financial or ethical considerations. For them, ethics were not an issue.

According to author Robert Whymant, the Japanese hoped that the whole episode "would eventually fade away like an ill-remembered dream. Many Japanese regard their war as a state—like being drunk, which means that the worst excesses can be forgiven and forgotten the next morning. [There was an] official promotion of amnesia, which has enraged East Asian countries." Ishii Harumi, Ishii Shiro's eldest daughter, explained her father's behavior in this context:

> Were it not for the war and his chosen career, his genius might have flourished in a field other then medical science, possibly politics . . . What he did, or was alleged to have committed in the line of duty as a medical officer and soldier in the Imperial Japanese Army, shall be denounced by any moral standard. Even so, one must not forget that it all happened under extremely abnormal circumstances. It was war.

In the aftermath of the war, the Japanese medical community welcomed these researchers into their upper echelons. Many participants later became deans of Japan's medical schools, senior science professors, university presidents, and captains of industry. Professor Keiichi Tsuneishi, a Japanese expert on Unit 731, sums up the problem: "The way war criminals have been embraced by the medical community is indicative of a terrible moral sickness among doctors here."

Naoji Uezono, a member of Unit 731, had assumed that they would be tried as war criminals, adding, "The higher-ups did well out of the war—all the data from those experiments proved invaluable in promoting their careers." Both during and after the war, researchers published or presented more than

100 scientific papers about their work. In 1944, for example, Lt. Gen. Kitano Masaji published his wartime findings in prestigious journals. Along with Dr. Kasahara Yukio, Dr. Kitano described in one scientific article how, after injecting a prisoner with mouse-brain suspension of tick encephalitis, "this subject was sacrificed when fever was subsiding, about the 12th day."

After the war, the publications had to be a bit more circumspect. An October 1945 memo cautioned former Unit 731 members that wartime BW work should not be made public; researchers should call the prisons used for human subjects "central warehouses" and describe BW testing sites as "self-supporting farms." It also instructed personnel to say that some unit members spontaneously conducted BW research, but not under orders from their superiors. In his post-war descriptions of his wartime experiments, Kitano referred to his human subjects as "monkeys" or "Manchurian monkeys." The Japanese medical community, however, understood the references. The temperatures reported for Kitano's ill "monkeys" ranged up to 40.2°C. Not even the sickest monkey could endure such a high fever—although infected humans often do.

Dr. Shiro Kasahara, working with Dr. Kitano, produced hemorrhagic (Songo) fever from "blood or blood-free extracts of liver, spleen or kidney derived from individuals sacrificed at various times during the course of the disease." His subsequent medical publications, based on his human experiments at Ping Fan, helped him become vice-president emeritus of the Kitasato Hospital and Research Unit in Tokyo. When he was asked about his work at Unit 731, he gave a political response: "I feel very guilty about what I did . . . I *think* I did wrong." [original emphasis]

Dr. Yoshimura Hisato, who directed Unit 731's frostbite experiments, and his colleagues also made use of their data to further their post-war careers. Yoshimura held numerous prestigious posts, including a membership in the Antarctic Special Committee advising Japan's polar expeditions, professor emeritus at Hyogo Medical University, and chairperson of the Japanese Bio-meteorological Society. Without commenting on the nature of his war crimes, the English-language *Japan Journal of Physiology* published three reports in the early 1950s of freezing experiments that he conducted on more than 500 Mongols, Chinese, Siberian tribesmen, and others.

Acknowledged as one of the world's top authorities on human endurance to cold, Yoshimura could not hide his past forever. In 1982, he presented a review of his life's work—the comparative resistance of different races and age groups to extreme cold—to the prestigious Japan Physiological Society. He did not mention that he had performed this work on Unit 731's *maruta*, but a

Japanese newspaper reported his findings under the headline "Human Experimentation Blatantly Presented in Lecture." Student protests followed and Yoshimura was forced to resign his post as president of Kyoto Prefectural Medical College.

The BW researchers' chief post-war negotiator, Dr. Naito Ryoichi, had served as a surgeon and bacteriologist in Unit 731. Immediately after the war, he opened his own surgical practice, then joined with Dr. Kitano Masaji and Dr. Hideo Futagi, Unit 731's vivisection chief, to form the Japan Blood Bank in 1951. Awash in ex-Unit 731 members, the "Vampire Blood Bank" thrived by supplying the American army with blood during the Korean War.

The company grew to become *Midori Juji*, or Green Cross, an international pharmaceutical giant specializing in manufacturing interferon, plasma, and artificial blood. Green Cross bought Los Angeles-based Alpha Therapeutic Company, and Naito became company president in 1973 and chairman in 1978. In this capacity, he frequently traveled to the United States. Naito joined the New York Academy of Sciences and received an award from them in 1963. In April 1977, he received Japan's prestigious Order of the Rising Sun. Naito died in 1982. Green Cross was eventually acquired by Yoshitomi Pharmaceutical Industries, Ltd.

Not all of the unit members had successful post-war careers; the experience destroyed several. Ishida Gintaro, who served in Unit Ei 1644 in Nanking, was responsible for drawing pictures of prisoners infected with various pathogenic organisms. He spent the rest of his life selling fish. As he aged, he refused to receive medical treatment from doctors, believing that the Japanese medical establishment had been corrupted and that the public should be aware of the part they played in the atrocities.

Major General Kawashima Kiyoshi testified after the war:

> I committed a crime against humanity. I admit that testing the action of bacteriological weapons on living people by forcibly injecting them with serious infectious diseases, as was practiced by the detachment [Unit 731] with my participation, and also the wholesale slaughter of the experimentees with lethal bacteria are barbarous and criminal.

Just before he died, he talked with his granddaughter:

> I do not want to retract my memory of those days. That world filled with germs, drug reactions, and microscopes. The era in Nanjing is a shadow following me everywhere. Before WWII, I was a contemporary cartoonist with a certain reputation. Since the end of the war, I have never picked up my brush again. I have shaved my head like a monk and lived quietly. All this is an effort to flee from the shadow of Nanjing.

Yoshio Shinazuka was a laboratory technician at Harbin and helped produce plague-infected bacteria. He also assisted at autopsies on living Chinese subjects. He was 16 at the time, and later said:

> I had no idea I was a war criminal . . . I figured if a person can be shot with one bullet, what's wrong with using this person's body as an experiment for developing medical industries? Besides, I had been taught in school that the Emperor is the son of God and that we are different from other Asians.

The Chinese imprisoned Yoshio for five years, after which he became a Japanese civil servant and then entered a Buddhist monastery. In July 1998, the United States denied Yoshio Shinazuka entry, based on his war crimes, when he came to testify about the Unit 731 atrocities at a San Francisco exhibit.

Saburo Ienaga, a Japanese history professor who has tried to expose Japan's recent past, suggested, "It is possible that if the U.S. allows Shinazuka in and lets him speak, he will cause them problems, not because of what he did, but because of what he knows."

Epilogue

A number of Japanese who participated in the gruesome experiments have described their actions publicly. But, until November 2000, there was no such testimony in Japanese legal records. In 1997, families of the Chinese killed during these experiments filed a lawsuit against the Japanese government.

During the resulting trial, Yoshio Shinazuka testified in Tokyo District Court that he helped mass produce the bacteria that caused cholera, dysentery, and typhoid at a base near Harbin in the early 1940s. He also confirmed that Unit 731 participated in the 1939 Nomonhan BW incident and that the Unit dropped BW weapons in southern China in the 1940s. He said, "What I have done was something that nobody should have done as a human being. I cannot escape that responsibility."

Shortly thereafter, Shoichi Matsumoto, a former Unit 731 pilot, admitted spreading plague-infected fleas over Hangzhou in 1940 and Nanking in 1941. He also flew plague-infected rats to Singapore and Java. He said, "I committed all these war crimes because I was ordered to do so . . . I really think it's time for Japan to face this issue with humanitarian consideration."

Japanese textbooks have consistently avoided discussing Japanese atrocities—until the early 1980s, two of the Education Ministry's textbook reviewers were former members of Unit 731! Japanese activists have tried to inform

Japanese citizens about "the forgotten Holocaust" by mounting traveling exhibits.

After the intentional destruction of Japan's BW facilities at the end of the war, little remains as evidence of the horrors that occurred. The test center at Anda can no longer be identified. Two rooms in the ruins of Unit 731's headquarters now house a museum with only some germ warfare shells, laboratory equipment, and a few photographs of Japanese soldiers.

Many of the bioweapons that Ishii and his cohorts produced continue to be discovered in China. Scientists believe that the germs in these weapons are no longer active. However, China insists that Japan should pay for removing the 700,000 to 2 million deteriorating chemical bombs, most with mustard gas, that still lie in Manchurian warehouses and old munition dumps.

The use of biological warfare raises serious ethical questions. As with nuclear warfare, the massive and random destruction, the terror inflicted on civilian populations, and the lasting and ongoing damage it wreaks on people is unconscionable. The thousands of people exposed to BW agents by Japanese experimenters were not the only ones who suffered—the medical profession suffered as well. Military physicians, not the military hierarchy, initiated Japan's BW program, designed and implemented the barbaric human experiments, led the BW attacks, and helped cover up their crimes.

As Hal Gold said in *Unit 731: Testimony*: "Japanese military aggression made the human experimentation possible; the Japanese medical community was the silent inquisitor."

The History of Biological Warfare

Biological weapons are either living organisms that can reproduce, such as bacteria and viruses, or toxic materials produced by living organisms, such as toxins and physiologically active proteins or peptides. (Few biological weapons produce skin lesions; mycotoxin, which was used in Kampuchea around 1980, is the rare exception.) Since they must be either inhaled or ingested, biological warfare (BW) agents must be dispersed as 1µm to 10 µm particles or placed in food or water.

There are many potential BW agents among the thousands of naturally occurring bacteria and viruses. But only a limited number can actually be used in BW. The factors which determine their usefulness are:

1. Ease of production
2. Stability
3. Infectivity or toxicity

The bacteria that causes anthrax, *Bacillus anthracis*, is considered the best biological agent because in spore form it is stable for decades and it is easy to produce. Among viruses, Venezuelan equine encephalitis is one of the most lethal; among toxins, staphylococcal enterotoxin and botulinum toxin are excellent potential weapons.

Unlike chemical weapons (CW), which have immediate devastating effects, BW agents usually act more slowly and first produce symptoms similar to those of common illnesses. Since their full effects may not be seen for some time, this can lead to widespread epidemics before the problem, agent, or source is recognized. The terror produced by even the threat of using such weapons magnifies their effect on both military and civilian populations.

Military Use of Biological Warfare

Armies have used biological warfare for millennia. As early as the sixth century B.C., Assyrians poisoned enemy wells with rye ergot and Solon of Athens used hellebore (skunk cabbage) to poison the water supply during his siege of Krissa. In 400 B.C., Scythian archers dipped their arrows in blood and manure, attempting to make their enemies sick. The Greeks polluted their foes' drinking water with animal corpses in 300 B.C.; later, the Romans and Persians would adopt the same strategy.

At the battle of Tortona, Italy, in 1155, Barbarossa put human corpses in an enemy's water supply, successfully contaminating it. Catapulting diseased corpses into besieged cities was commonplace. In 1346–47, for example, Muslim Tatar De Mussis catapulted corpses infected with bubonic plague over the walls of Caffa in Crimea, causing an epidemic. The city surrendered and the defeated Christian Genoese sailors fled to Italy, possibly beginning the Black Death pandemic in Europe.

continued . . .

The History of Biological Warfare, continued

In 1422, during the siege of Karlstejn in the Holy Roman Empire, soldiers' corpses and 2,000 cartloads of excrement were hurled at the enemy. And, in 1485 near Naples, the Spanish supplied their French enemies with wine laced with leprosy patients' blood.

In the eighteenth century, BW was still unsophisticated but effective. In 1710, Russians catapulted plague-infected corpses into Reval, Estonia, which was held by the Swiss. In 1763, during the French and Indian War, British colonel Henry Bouquet gave smallpox-infected blankets to the Indians at Fort Pitt, Pennsylvania, triggering a devastating epidemic. While besieging Mantua, Italy, in 1797, Napoleon attempted to infect the inhabitants with swamp fever.

During the American Civil War, Dr. Luke Blackburn, who would later become Kentucky's governor, tried to infect Union troops by providing them with clothing exposed to smallpox and yellow fever. (At that time, no one knew that yellow fever can be transmitted only through mosquito bites.) It is not known if this plan was successful, even though friends and relatives claimed some Union officers died because of Dr. Blackburn's efforts. Confederates under General Johnson tried to contaminate water sources by leaving dead sheep and pigs in wells and ponds they passed while retreating in Mississippi in 1863. That same year, however, U.S. Army General Order No. 100 was issued, stating: "The use of poison in any manner, be it to poison wells, or food, or arms, is wholly excluded from modern warfare."

Bacteriological warfare became more sophisticated as microbiology developed; the causative organisms for many diseases were identified and many were grown in laboratories. During WWI, most biological attacks used anthrax and glanders and were directed at animals. The Germans launched BW attacks in Romania, Italy, France, Russia, and Mesopotamia. In the United States, the center for BW activity was in Maryland: A Johns Hopkins-trained surgeon, Dr. Anton Dilger, and his brother Carl produced bacteria that could be injected into military horses, mules, and cattle destined for the Allied Expeditionary Force in Europe. The United States military tested, but never used, a devastating biological toxin, "ricin," derived from castor beans. A 1918 report reads:

> These experiments show two important points: (1) easily prepared preparations of ricin can be made to adhere to shrapnel bullets, (2) there is no loss in toxicity of firing and even with the crudest method of coating the bullets, not a very considerable loss of the material itself . . . It is not unreasonable to suppose that every wound inflicted by a shrapnel bullet coated with ricin would produce a serious casualty . . . Many wounds which would otherwise be trivial would be fatal.

continued . . .

The History of Biological Warfare, continued

Biological Warfare Programs

Despite this research, in the mid-1920s, both the United States and the new League of Nations claimed that BW was impracticable, either because of inadequate delivery systems or because of enhanced public health and preventive medicine systems. BW was banned in the 1925 Geneva Protocol, which was signed by 28 nations (the U.S. Senate refused to ratify it). This was about the time that Dr. Ishii Shiro was on his two-year tour of foreign microbiological research facilities.

In 1931, as Japan's Prince Mikasa revealed in July 1994, his country's military laced fruit with cholera germs in an unsuccessful attempt to poison members of the League of Nations' Lytton Commission assigned to investigate Japan's seizure of Manchuria. As Japan began its human research experiments in BW and the Germans began testing offensive BW in the 1930s, the U.S. military was disparaging both the idea that it should be researched and the idea that it could be used. In an influential 1933 article in *The Military Surgeon*, Maj. Leon F. Fox wrote:

> Bacterial warfare is one of the recent scare-heads that we are being served by the pseudo-scientists who contribute to the flaming pages of the Sunday annexes syndicated over the Nation's press.

The U.S. military appeared to be nearly alone in this attitude. In 1929, the Soviet Union had opened a BW research facility north of the Caspian Sea and, by 1936, France had a large BW research program and Britain had established a group to investigate BW issues. By 1939, Sir Frederick Banting, who discovered insulin, had initiated Canada's BW research program with anthrax, botulinum toxin, plague, and psittacosis. Britain opened their BW laboratory in 1940.

During World War II, Germany had a relatively small BW program, working mainly with plague, cholera, typhus, and yellow fever. Japan had an extensive program, as described in this chapter. BW, however, proved lethal even for those working on or distributing the material. For example, during the 1940s, about 1,600 Japanese researchers and soldiers died from mishandling Unit 731's pathogens.

In 1941, when credible evidence arrived that the Japanese were using BW against Chinese troops, the U.S. government appointed a committee to study BW. By February 1942, the United States had established the War Research Service to coordinate defensive efforts against BW contamination of the nation's food and water supply. As the war progressed, the government established offensive BW research programs and supplied selected troops with defensive BW equipment. In June 1944, the U.S. government placed an order for one million four-pound SPD Mk I BW cluster bombs; they later canceled it when the war ended.

continued . . .

The History of Biological Warfare, continued

Biological Warfare Testing and Dissemination

In the 1950s, the United States continued its BW program, developing multiple delivery methods for BW agents. The most successful of these was the M114, a four-pound antipersonnel bomblet designed to be part of a cluster bomb. It contained 320 ml of *Brucella suis* (the bacteria causing brucellosis). The U.S. military also tested anthrax and yellow fever—and produced up to 500,000 mosquitoes a month to carry the yellow fever.

In several large-scale, open-air tests near heavily populated areas of the United States, the military used *Bacillus globigii, Serratia marcescens*, and inert particles to demonstrate that BW agents could be distributed using natural air currents, thus making them potent weapons of mass destruction. They also tested BW agents on human "volunteers," including civilian prisoners. During this period, the Soviet Union was also testing BW, and was producing and storing large amounts of BW agents.

By the 1960s, the U.S. military was testing vaccines against BW agents on human "volunteers." (In late 2000, the VA hospital system began testing former military personnel who may have taken part in BW testing without their knowledge.) These included immunizations against tularemia; anthrax; botulinum toxin; Rift Valley Fever; Q fever; and Eastern, Venezuelan, and Western equine encephalomyelitis.

The U.S. military had also developed the SD-2 Drone, a remote-controlled, recoverable aircraft with a 100 nautical mile range. This drone could travel at speeds up to 300 knots and carry more than 200 pounds of biological agents. They next developed the SD-5, which sped along at Mach 0.75, had a range of 650 nautical miles, and sprayed its 1,260 pounds of BW agents through a tail nozzle.

Estimates of Casualties Produced by Hypothetical Biological Attack*

Agent	Downwind Reach (Miles)	Dead	Incapacitated
Rift Valley Fever	0.6	400	35,000
Tick-borne Encephalitis	0.6	9,500	35,000
Typhus	>3	19,000	85,000
Brucellosis	>6	500	125,000
Q Fever	>12	150	125,000
Tularemia	>12	30,000	125,000
Anthrax	>12	95,000	125,000

*Release of 110 lbs. of agent from an aircraft along a 1¼ mile line upwind of a population center of 500,000. Adapted from: *Health Aspects of Chemical and Biological Weapons*, WHO, 1970.

continued . . .

The History of Biological Warfare, *continued*

The U.S. military also developed and mass-produced several BW bombs. In additional large-scale tests on unsuspecting civilians, they disseminated *Bacillus globigii*, a supposedly noninfectious agent with properties similar to anthrax, at public sites such as Washington, D.C.'s National [now Reagan National] Airport and Greyhound Bus Terminal and the New York City Subway system.

Finally, in November 1969, four months after the United Nations issued a report condemning the production and stockpiling of chemical and biological weapons, President Richard Nixon declared:

> I have decided that the United States of America will renounce the use of any form of deadly biological weapons that either kill or incapacitate. Our bacteriological programs in the future will be confined to research in biological defense, on techniques of immunization and on measures of controlling and preventing the spread of disease.

At the time, the United States had put the lethal BW agents for anthrax, tularemia, and botulinum toxin into delivery systems (in other words, they had been "weaponized"). The United States also had stockpiles of at least four incapacitating BW agents, as well as anti-crop agents. In February 1970, Nixon also banned BW toxins.

In the mid-1970s, there were reports that BW agents—mostly toxins—were being used in Southeast Asia and Afghanistan, primarily by the Soviet Union and Viet Nam. The Soviet Union had signed the Biological Weapons Convention in 1975 and specifically stated that "the Soviet Union does not possess any bacteriological agents and toxins, weapons, equipment or means of delivery." Yet, on April 3, 1979, an accidental airborne leak of anthrax spores occurred at a previously undetected biological weapons plant, the Soviet Institute of Microbiology and Virology in Sverdlovsk, Russia. Although only one BW weapon discharged and Soviet troops quickly attempted to decontaminate the facility and the city, 66 people who were downwind of the plant died of anthrax.

Only in 1992 did Russian President Boris Yeltsin admit that Russia had an offensive BW research program. It has since been discovered that they also tried to use recombinant DNA technology to produce lethal venoms in common bacteria.

Increasing Biological Warfare Risk

Over the past two decades, the risk of BW has actually increased. In the 1980s, authorities discovered that terrorist groups in the United States and Europe were manufacturing typhoid bacillus, ricin, botulinum toxin, and other BW agents for use on civilian populations. The reasons are obvious: ease of production and low costs. For example, NATO estimated that, in 2001, to produce 50 percent casualties in a square kilometer, it would cost about $9,000 for conventional

continued . . .

The History of Biological Warfare, continued

weapons, $4,000 for nuclear weapons, $3,000 for chemical agents and less than $5 for BW agents.

Biological weapons also have the benefit of not being detectable by ordinary means such as x-rays, dogs, and other devices, making them easy to transport. The delayed onset of symptoms ranging from a few hours to a few weeks; the ability of perpetrators to protect themselves against the agent with a vaccine; the difficulty in recognizing a BW attack; and the lack of a "signature" left at the scene all make it unlikely that the perpetrators would be caught.

In the 1990s, the Persian Gulf War produced evidence that Iraq had a large BW facility at al-Hakam. In 1995, Iraq admitted that this facility had prepared about 19,000 liters of botulinum toxin, 8,400 liters of anthrax, and 2,000 liters of aflatoxin and clostridium since 1988. They had "weaponized" some of this material and loaded it onto more than 200 missiles plus additional artillery shells, rockets, aircraft spray tanks, and bombs. Iraq is not alone in its offensive BW capability. Experts now believe that Iraq, North Korea, and Russia may have stockpiled the smallpox virus for BW use. Smallpox was eradicated from natural occurrence by intense worldwide public health efforts, so there is little immunity in any population.

In 1998, the world learned that Japan's Aum Shinrikyo cult, before its 1995 lethal nerve gas attack on a Tokyo subway, carried out at least nine BW attacks. Over a five-year period, they had tried to use BW agents against the Japanese legislature, the Imperial Palace, several sites in Tokyo, and U.S. Navy facilities. No deaths resulted, either because the agents were not sufficiently virulent or their delivery systems were faulty.

Civil defense agencies now take the threat of BW seriously and work to counteract terrorist groups that adopt Dr. Ishii's philosophy to employ the "silent enemy" of microbiology as a "silent ally."

In 2001, shortly after the World Trade Center tragedy, terrorists used the U.S. postal system to distribute deadly anthrax spores; thousands were exposed to the biological weapon and four died. At this writing, the identity of the perpetrators is unknown.

continued . . .

Common Biological Warfare Agents

Disease: Agent	Signs & Symptoms	Theoretical Toxicity*	Approx. onset (incubation) / Duration
Anthrax (Inhalation): *Bacillus anthracis*	Malaise, fatigue, myalgia, fever, and non-productive cough; followed by severe respiratory distress, chest pain, sweating, swelling, and shock.	One gram of spores could kill more than one-third of U.S. population. 50% exposed contract meningitis. 100% mortality rate without treatment; with treatment, >80%. 8,000–50,000 spores needed to infect. No person-to-person transmission.	1–6 days / 3–5 days.
Botulism: Botulinum Toxin, Type-A; *Clostridium botulinum*	Blurred vision, lid droop, difficulty swallowing and speaking, muscle weakness, respiratory distress, and death.	Few tenths of a microgram is lethal. 8 ounces could kill every living creature on the planet. No person-to-person transmission.	1–5 days (variable) / death in 1–3 days; lasts months if untreated.
Brucellosis: *Brucella suis, melitensis, abortus, canis* (human pathogenic types)	Localized inflammatory process, or acute febrile illness or chronic infection. Depression, headache, and irritability frequently occur.	10–100 organisms. No person-to-person transmission.	5–60 days (usually 1–2 months) / weeks to months.
Cholera: *Vibrio cholerae*	Abrupt onset of painless watery diarrhea (liters), vomiting without nausea, muscle cramps.	10–500 organisms. Person-to-person transmission is rare.	4 hours to 5 days (usually 2–3 days) / a week or more.
Glanders: *Pseudomonas mallei*	Ulcerating skin or mucosal lesions (skin contact); fever, chills, muscle and chest pain, fatigue, headache, photophobia, diarrhea, sepsis.	Thought to be relatively few organisms. Low rate of person-to-person transmission.	10–14 days (inhaled) / death in 7–10 days in septicemic form.
Plague: *Yersinia pestis*	Fever, headache, vomiting, chills plus: Pneumonia with blood-tinged sputum (pneumonic) or painful large skin blisters, altered mentation, abdominal pain (bubonic) or purpura, disseminated intravascular coagulation, abdominal pain, cyanosis/necrosis of fingers and toes (septicemic).	Disease caused by 1–10 organisms through the skin, or 100–500 inhaled. Up to 12% of those infected die. High rate of person-to-person transmission.	24 hours (inhaled); 1–8 days (skin); 2–6 days (septicemic) / 1–6 days in pneumonic form (usually fatal).
Q Fever: *Coxiella burnetii*	No common pattern. Most get fever, chills, sweating, weakness, weight loss, cough, and muscle aches.	1–10 organisms. Person-to-person transmission is rare.	2–10 days / 2 weeks or more.
Ricin: (derived from astor beans)	Fever, chest tightness, shortness of breath, nausea, muscle aches, hemorrhage from GI tract, necrosis of kidney, spleen, and liver.	3–5 µg/Kg kills half of the animals exposed to the toxin. No person-to-person transmission.	18–24 hours / days; if ingested, may cause death in 10–12 days.

continued . . .

Common Biological Warfare Agents, continued

Disease: Agent	Signs & Symptoms	Theoretical Toxicity*	Approx. onset (incubation) / Duration
Smallpox: *Orthopoxviridae varioloa*	Malaise, fever, rigors, vomiting, headache, backache, typical skin eruption.	Thought to be 10–100 organisms. High rate of person-to-person transmission.	7–17 days / 4 weeks.
Staph: Enterotoxin B derived from *Staphylococcus*	Fever, nausea, vomiting, diarrhea, headache, chills, muscle ache, non-productive cough, shortness of breath, chest pain, hypotension, shock.	0.03 µg/Kg incapacitates a person. No person-to-person transmission.	3–12 hours after ingestion / hours.
Trichothecene: Mycotoxins derived from *Fusarium*, *Myrotecium*, *Trichoderma*, *Cephalosprium*, *Verticimonosporium*, and *Stachybotrys* fungi	Loss of appetite, nausea and vomiting, weakness, dizziness, loss of coordination, shock, depressed immune system, diarrhea, sore mouth, bleeding gums, nosebleeds, cough, shortness of breath, blistered skin, diffuse bleeding.	Thought to be an intermediate amount of toxin. No person-to-person transmission.	2–4 hours / days to months.
Tularemia: *Francisella tularensis*	Fever, chills, headache, cough, myalgias, and pneumonia. Plus single ulcer and lymphadenopathy (ulceroglandular) or, more commonly, systemic symptoms and severe pneumonia, without local skin lesion or marked lymphadenopathy (typhoidal).	10–50 inhaled organisms. Without treatment, mortality rate 4% (ulceroglandular) to 35% (typhoidal).	2–10 days / weeks or more.
Typhoid: *Salmonella typhosa*	Chills, fever, cough, nose-bleed, weakness, abdominal swelling and tenderness, delirium, and rash.	1 lb. of culture in drinking water is as toxic as 11 lbs. of botulinum toxin or 10 tons of potassium cyanide.	10–12 days / duration varies.
Venezuelan Equine Encephalitis: *Alphavirus*	Chills, high fever, headache, malaise. Photophobia, sore throat, muscle aches, and vomiting are common. Encephalitis occurs in only 0.5% of adults and 4% of children. More incapacitating than lethal.	10–100 organisms. Low rate of person-to-person transmission.	2–6 days / days to weeks.
Viral Hemorrhagic Fevers: *Arenaviridae*, *Bunyaviridae*, *Filoviridae*, and *Flaviviridae* virus genuses	Fever, muscle aches, prostration—sometimes leading to shock and generalized bleeding. Depending on the virus, may cause liver or kidney failure or neurological damage.	1–10 organisms. Moderate rate of person-to-person transmission.	4–21 days / death in 7–16 days (depends on specific disease).

*If optimally distributed. Higher doses are generally used in BW weapons, since optimal dispersion generally cannot be achieved.

Adapted from: U.S. Army Medical Research Institute for Infectious Disease: *Medical Management of Biological Casualties Handbook*, 4th ed., 2001 [http://www.usamriid.army.mil/education/bluebook.html]; Sidell FR, Takafuji ET, Franz DR (eds.): *Medical Aspects of Chemical and Biological Warfare*. Washington, DC: Office of The Surgeon General, Walter Reed Medical Center, 1997; and other sources.

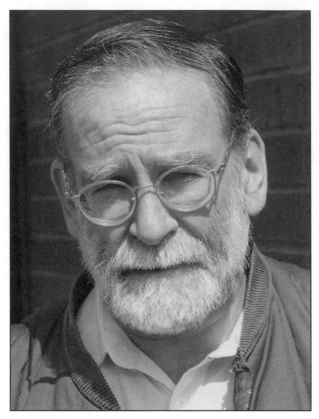

Dr. Harold Frederick Shipman, MBChB. (Courtesy of Cavendish Press, Manchester)

9

The Dr. Jekyll of Hyde

Harold Frederick Shipman, MBChB

Renate Overton, at age 45, was an outgoing divorcee who loved television soap operas and considered herself an expert in the characters and plots. A vital member of her community, she eagerly assisted any neighbor in need. Today, however, she wasn't feeling quite up to snuff, so Dr. Shipman had promised to stop by her house.

"So pleased you could come," she said as she let the doctor in the front door. "Won't you take a cup of tea?"

"No," he replied with a smile. "I'll just give you the injection you need and be on my way. I've lots more patients to see." He asked her to sit in an armchair in the living room and roll up her sleeve. Taking a syringe already prepared with the medication, he found the vein in her forearm and smoothly inserted the needle.

"That didn't hurt nearly as much as I thought it would," said Mrs. Overton. She smiled at the doctor as her eyes became heavy and her breathing slowed. Dr. Shipman stood over his victim, excited and pleased with himself.

Suddenly, Renate's daughter, Sharon, burst into the room. "What's going on?" she screamed, seeing her mother turning ashen. "She's taken a turn for the worse," said the doctor. "We had better ring an ambulance."

Mrs. Overton had lapsed into a coma, but she didn't die right away. She lingered in Tameside Hospital in a persistent vegetative state, while her daughter hovered over her and prayed for a miracle. Fourteen months later, she died without ever regaining consciousness. Dr. Shipman had killed his youngest victim.

~

Early Years

Harold Frederick Shipman was born January 14, 1946. He was a "celebration baby" born eight months after VE (Victory in Europe) Day. His parents, Harold and Vera, had married in 1937 and, after their first child, Pauline, was born in March 1938, Harold went off to war. Fred, later to become the infamous "Dr. Shipman," was born soon after he returned, followed four years later by his brother Clive.

His mother was extremely important in Fred's life—he wore a bow tie throughout his life because Vera thought it looked good. A small thin woman, she was said to have kept a spotless house and, although she provided her children with loving attention, she clearly expected that they would succeed in life. Vera had high hopes for Fred in particular. He attended High Pavement School, considered to be the best grammar (private) school in Nottingham. An average student, he was known for being serious, quiet, and polite. Although he rarely joined his classmates in their adolescent pranks, and was awkward around girls, he was stocky and tough. He excelled at rugby, and became the team's vice-captain in his senior year.

When Vera developed lung cancer during Fred's adolescence, it was a dreadful shock. Since his older sister was married and working and his younger brother was only 13 at the time, Fred was responsible for caring for his mother after school, and he watched her gradually wither away. She suffered greatly from her pain; her only relief was the doctor's daily visit, when he injected her with ever-increasing doses of morphine. This experience surely influenced Shipman's later obsessions with elderly women, morphine, and death. Certainly, it motivated him to be a physician. Vera died on June 21, 1963, when Fred was 17 years old. His classmates only discovered his mother had been ill and then died when he wore a black armband the day of her funeral.

Mr. Shipman carefully tended the children after his wife's death. To make a living, he held a succession of blue-collar jobs, finishing as a truck driver for local building firms. He died in 1985.

Although he demeaned anyone he thought inferior with the epithet "stupid," Fred failed to get the grades necessary to enter Leeds University Medical School on his first try. He retook his exams and entered the school in September 1965. Due to his family's financial situation, he qualified for an annual grant from the local government equivalent to about £3,280 (in 2002 pounds), which was enough to live on. At that time, the government paid the tuition and all fees for medical school, which consisted of five years at the university followed by at least one year as a "junior doctor" (intern) in a hospital.

Fred vowed he would have a new life as he went to Leeds to begin his career. Leeds had not been bombed during World War II, and the bustling city had retained its original charm. At the time Shipman was a student, both Leeds University School of Medicine, founded in 1831, and the University itself were rated as the most popular in Britain.

Shortly after he started medical school, Fred met Primrose Oxtoby on the bus they both took—she to her job as a window dresser, he to medical school. (In Britain, medical school begins after the equivalent of high school.) At least on the bus, Fred was something of a dandy, dressed for medical school in his sports jacket, tie, and flannel trousers. Seventeen-year-old Primrose was described as "nondescript, plain, . . . cheerful and friendly, but eminently forgettable."

Primrose was born in April 1949, to parents older than those of her classmates. She was a relatively lonely child; her sister, who was 13 years older, became a nurse and then an invalid with multiple sclerosis. Her father was a farm foreman; her mother, Edna, had a rigid philosophy of life that her daughter was expected to follow. Primrose's mother was something of a terror in the neighborhood, threatening neighbor children if they refused to play with her daughter. In the mid-1960s, Primrose became a bit rebellious. After high school, she attended a college class in art and design for a year, then started her job. She was still living at home in Wetherby, but her wages gave her a small feeling of independence.

A few weeks after meeting, Fred and Primrose became an item, solving the problem each had with loneliness and isolation from their peers. Near the end of Fred's first year in medical school, Primrose became pregnant, surprising everyone who knew her. Perhaps that is why Mrs. Oxtoby never liked her son-in-law. On November 5, 1966, with Primrose six months pregnant, the two married in the register office at Barkston Ash, about ten miles from where they lived. The Oxtobys and Fred's father were the only guests. On February 14, 1967, 21-year-old Fred and 17-year-old Primrose became parents for the first time when Sarah was born. They subsequently had three more children.

The Doctor

Medical school was difficult enough, but with a wife, a child, and very little income, it became extremely arduous. Nevertheless, after two years in the classroom and three years primarily in hospitals, Fred passed his final exams and graduated in 1970 with an MBChB degree (Bachelor of Medicine and Surgery, which is equivalent to M.D. and D.O. degrees.) Upon graduation, he was "provisionally registered" as a physician. He then left the university to become a "junior hospital registrar" (intern) at Pontefract General Infirmary, an outlying facility that, to attract house officers, made provisions for their families. With another baby on the way, this was important.

Fred spent his mandatory first year at Pontefract, where he served six months on surgery and six months on the internal medicine service. On August 5, 1971, Dr. Harold Frederick Shipman achieved "full registration with General Medical Council," becoming a fully licensed physician. He stayed at Pontefract for an additional two years and nine months, during which time he acquired a diploma in child health (DCH, September 1972) and another in obstetrics and gynecology (DRCOG, September 1973).

But Fred wanted to enter general practice and, on March 1, 1974, he joined a busy group practice at Abraham Ormerod Medical Centre in Todmorden. Todmorden, a pretty Yorkshire town, has been described as "a ribbon of dark Victorian millstone grit in a narrow defile where the River Calder cuts deep beneath high wild moors." He quickly established a good rapport with his patients, and, although he occasionally was aloof, his four partners noted that he was a very hard worker. After a month's probation, they made him a full member of the group.

When the Shipmans arrived in Todmorden, Primrose was already seriously overweight, but still presentable. She was also loudly abrasive or outgoing, depending on one's perspective. Fred threw himself into community activities, especially the arduous physical labor associated with restoring the old Rochdale Canal, a local landmark. The bearded and bespectacled Shipman was doing fine until he began to experience blackouts. His concerned partners referred him to a specialist, who diagnosed epilepsy. Because of his illness, Primrose had to drive him everywhere, including to his house calls. This circumstance may have saved one of Shipman's first intended victims.

Elaine Oswald, a 25-year-old government clerk, came into his office complaining of mild stomach pains. Although her symptoms were not severe, Shipman ordered her to go home and gave her Diconal® (a combination of cyclizine hydrochloride, an antiemetic, and dipipanone, a narcotic) for the pain that he said was possibly caused by kidney stones. He assured her that he would check on her later in the day. Oswald later said, "he told me to leave my front door unlocked, and said he would come straight up to the bedroom. In those days, you didn't question what the doctor said." True to his word, Dr. Shipman arrived early in the evening. "The last thing I remember," she said, "is him taking blood from one of my arms, then moving round the bed to inject something into my other arm."

Oswald awakened on the floor, bruised and bleeding from her mouth. Shipman was there, along with his wife and young son. Primrose had entered the house—and probably aborted the murder—when her son needed to use the bathroom. Dr. Shipman first said that Mrs. Oswald had overdosed. Later, when no one at the hospital believed his story, he claimed that she had suffered an allergic reaction to the medication. Christine McCafferty, a local Member of Parliament (MP), on hearing the story, later commented, "I have always thought it unlikely that he did not start his criminal activities in Todmorden." She added, "Now we think that Shipman was honing his skills here."

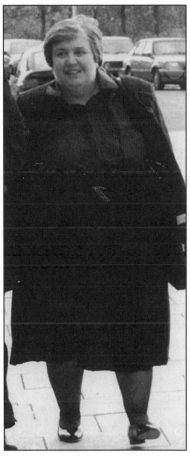

Primrose Shipman. (Courtesy of Cavendish Press, Manchester)

In reality, it was not epilepsy that caused Shipman's blackouts, but rather overdoses of pethidine (meperidine; Demerol®), a synthetic narcotic that he was injecting into himself at the rate of up to 700 mg a day (patients in pain generally receive about 100 mg). In July 1975, when a receptionist at Shipman's medical office raised concerns about his possible drug use, one of his partners began checking with patients for whom Shipman had supposedly prescribed the powerful drug; none had received it. In what would today be called an "intervention," the partners confronted Fred with the facts, which he readily admitted. He claimed to have become addicted when he was required to try the drug as part of his training (a ridiculous claim). He then asked his partners to ignore the problem—which may have involved a total of as much as 70,000 mg of pethidine. To their credit, they didn't, and insisted that he enter a hospital for treatment.

Shipman became furious and stormed out, saying that he would neither quit the practice nor enter a hospital. As he left, he threw his "night bag" (his doctor's bag for home visits) at them. An hour later, Primrose arrived and angrily announced that her husband would not resign, saying, "You'll have to force him out." It took the group six weeks to fire him for breaching practice rules and misusing drugs. During that time, he was on full salary.

Once things calmed down, the Home Office drug inspector, along with Shipman's partners, arranged for his admission to The Retreat, a famous psychiatric center in York. The facility, in 1975, was not prepared to handle drug addiction; of 320 admissions that year, only four patients were addicted to drugs. In November, West Yorkshire Police went to The Retreat to question Shipman about forging pethidine prescriptions. His career was in jeopardy.

The General Medical Council (GMC), which regulates physician behavior in Britain, decided, in a closed hearing, to allow him to continue treatment rather than taking action against him. He was forbidden to have controlled substances, such as narcotics, in his office. Unfortunately, the police, the medical authorities, and the British Government took no steps to enforce this prohibition or to prevent Shipman from prescribing, using, or amassing these drugs—a fact that came to light only after hundreds of his patients had died. He was forced to stop practicing medicine for a period that turned out to be one year and 294 days. One must wonder how many lives were saved by this hiatus.

Medical Practice in Hyde

In 1977, a "rehabilitated" Shipman arrived in the town of Hyde to replace a physician who was retiring from the seven-person Donneybrook practice. Hyde is a former milltown that has been absorbed into Greater Manchester. About seven miles from the center of Manchester itself, the town had a stable population of about 22,000. Ironically, in the mid-1960s, it had become infamous as the site where neo-Nazis Ian Brady and Myra Hindley sadistically killed five children in what became known as the "Moors Murders."

The Donneybrook group selected Shipman from among several applicants. When they interviewed him, Shipman readily admitted that he had been a pethidine addict, but assured them, "I am off it. I don't use it. You will have to trust me." They were impressed with the straightforward, well-qualified physician; they decided to give him a chance to prove himself. He would be with them for 15 years.

The Donneybrook practice was unique. Seven Hyde doctors had joined together in December 1967, in their own building, to share office space and equipment. When the town's other seven practitioners also decided to form their own group, the Clarendon practice, they built a double-sized building and split it down the middle to accommodate the two groups. The Donneybrook doctors, however, remained independent ("single-handed") practitioners. They formed an official group only after Shipman left.

Dr. Shipman quickly became popular with the patients. Unlike many other general practitioners, he spent a great deal of time talking with his patients; some described visits with him "like chatting with a favorite uncle." In addition to clinical questions, he would often chat about patients' personal lives. He was so popular that there was a yearlong wait to get on his "list," the panel of patients assigned to a doctor by Britain's National Health Service (NHS). Some colleagues described Shipman as a "workaholic," who would sometimes see other doctors' patients for them so that they could leave early. Dr. John Smith, a founding member of the Donneybrook group, later said, "As a doctor he was kind; there's lots of folks who stood by him when he was charged, just wouldn't believe it."

The non-physician staff at the practice were not as sanguine about Dr. Shipman. Apparently, he treated them as menial servants, abusing them with his biting sarcasm, especially the practice manager and the reception staff, who feared his temperamental outbursts. Vivian Langfield, the practice manager who later became a lay minister, recalled:

> [Shipman] was a bully who demanded that people look up to him and have regard to his position. If anyone queried anything to do with one of his patients he would say, "I am a good doctor. I have all the qualifications from Leeds Medical School. I have passed my exams," implying that you had better listen to him ... He didn't like people who were forceful, who stood up to him.

His physician colleagues, with whom he rarely socialized, described him as being "pushy" at their group meetings. He nearly always insisted that he was right—even when he clearly wasn't. Some people who knew him well later described Shipman as a "bully," a "control freak," and a "brilliant manipulator."

Despite his long hours at work and other activities, the Shipmans had two more children, David (March 20, 1979) and Sam (April 5, 1982). All the Shipman children have led exemplary lives. His oldest daughter, Sarah, later said that she was desperate to escape her father's grasp because he was so selfish and strict, although she has continued to support him.

Dr. Shipman became active in a number of medical activities outside the practice. As another local general practitioner (GP), Dr. Wally Ashworth, later commented, "He had a good personality for committee work: when we got some admin person in front of us, he would wipe the floor with them . . . He isn't a great brain, but he read up about things. In debate he could be aggressive, fiery, forthright." From 1980 to 1988, he became heavily involved in the local St. John Ambulance program, holding the positions of Divisional Surgeon, Area Surgeon, and Area Commissioner. As with his other positions, he quit abruptly and without apparent reason.

He also served on the Family Practitioner Committee, which later became known as the "Area Health Authority," and as secretary of the local Medical Committee. In the latter capacity, he checked that other doctors' offices were tidy and had appropriate facilities to accommodate patients. On at least one occasion, he was asked what two physicians should do about their partner whom they suspected of using controlled substances. Without disclosing his own drug-plagued background, Shipman counseled them to help him and, contrary to what had been arranged, failed to pass this information on to higher authorities. The two doctors did not find this out for some time, but they then reported the errant doctor themselves.

At Donneybrook, many of Shipman's elderly female patients who lived alone and were in apparently good health died suddenly. But Shipman was a sole practitioner, so his partners had little opportunity to notice a pattern. When he suddenly quit the group, his partners glimpsed his true nature. The informal papers establishing the group assumed that everyone would play fair, but Dr. Shipman used the contract's fine print and legal loopholes to take advantage of his associates.

In July 1992, he established his own practice, The Surgery, only 300 yards away from the Donneybrook building. Rather than leave his panel of 3,000 patients with the group, he took them with him, along with three receptionists and a district (visiting) nurse. He demanded that his former associates repurchase his £23,000 share in their building and he refused to pay his part of the group's tax bill from the prior year. While all this was technically legal, it was seen as both immoral and unprofessional. His duplicitous behavior, however, did not signal how bad things really were. His former partner, Dr. John Smith, later said, "He was shifty, arrogant, treacherous, but that does not make you suspect someone of being a mass murderer."

Dr. Shipman treated patients for six deadly years in his new clinic, called The Surgery, which was located in a row of shops along Market Street, known

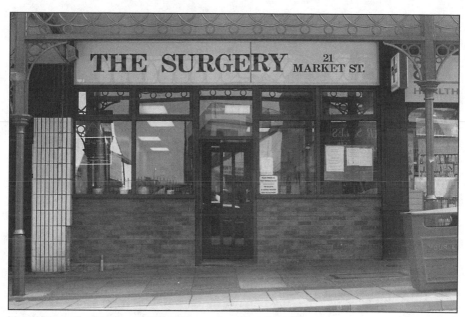

Dr. Shipman's clinic in Hyde. (Courtesy of Cavendish Press, Manchester)

locally as "Hyde Lane." After he left the Donneybrook group, Shipman became even more overbearing with his colleagues. Dr. Ian Napier later described Shipman's behavior at the local continuing medical education meetings:

> If I saw Fred there I avoided him, because he was embarrassing. As time went on he became more and more bristly, like a hedgehog. He'd interrupt the speaker—usually some eminent professor—and harangue him. Everyone would be embarrassed, thinking, "Oh, God, Fred, sit down and shut up." ... He was irascible, bad-tempered, yappy like a Jack Russell snapping at everyone's heels. He'd be trying to prove himself, and I imagine he thought we were all impressed by his knowledge.

Despite his mannerisms, the medical community considered Shipman to be a very good doctor. However, in 1985, the GMC received a complaint alleging that Shipman had provided inadequate medical care to a young man who had died from an undiagnosed illness. The complaint was referred to the Family Practice Committee and no action was taken. In 1989, Shipman was accused of prescribing the wrong dose of Epilim® (sodium valproate, an anticonvulsant) to a patient with epilepsy. He settled the medical negligence claim in February 2000, after his conviction for murder.

Generally, he spent inordinate amounts of time with his patients, made house calls, referred patients to specialists whenever necessary, and insisted that they receive the best medications, whether or not the drugs were on the approved formulary. As June Evans, a local councilwoman, said, "He never judged you, never criticized you. When you were in his surgery he treated you like the only patient he had." There was soon a wait of up to two years to become a patient at The Surgery.

Suspicions Mount

Eventually, several people noticed odd patterns, and began to think the unthinkable—that their kindly GP was killing his patients! One of these was the soft-spoken John Shaw, who, for 11 years until his retirement in 1999, ran a taxi service catering to Hyde's elderly women. He knew his customers well and helped them get around town and do their various errands. Shaw noticed that his clients were dying—and that nearly all were Dr. Shipman's patients. In 1996, when the numbers rose dramatically, he and his wife began to keep records of those elderly passengers associated with the doctor who died.

Although he confided in his wife, Shaw was afraid to go to the police, since he thought that no one would take him seriously—after all, he would be accusing one of the most popular men in town of an extraordinary crime. Shaw later recalled, "I kept losing my customers and it was always him who was the doctor. At first I thought he was unlucky or incompetent, then I realized it was something more sinister."

It was only after Kathleen Grundy's death was investigated as a murder that Shaw came forward. He gave his list, compiled over six years, of 20 customers who had died under Dr. Shipman's care to Detective Inspector (DI) Stan "The Hammer" Egerton. Egerton confirmed what Shaw had always believed: "Stan told me . . . They'd have assumed I had a grudge against Shipman. How could I, a taxi driver, question the work of such a popular and highly regarded doctor?"

Another group whose suspicions had been aroused were the operators of the Massey family funeral home, Frank Massey & Sons, who handled most of Dr. Shipman's deaths. In late 1996 or early 1997, they became aware that they were being called to an inordinately large number of deaths of Dr. Shipman's patients. They also noted that, unlike most deaths of elderly people, these were predominantly women, and about 90 percent of the decedents were found in their homes, alone and sitting in easy chairs fully dressed, often with a sleeve rolled up. (Most of those who die at home alone are found in bed, on the floor, in the bathroom, or near a telephone.) The accouterments that usually accompany chronic illness and presage death, such as medication bottles, hospital beds, walkers, and bandages, were absent for these deaths. Even stranger, on many occasions, Shipman was in attendance before or during the death—an extremely rare occurrence, even for a doctor who makes frequent house calls. In addition, there was never evidence that he had attempted any resuscitative measures.

Funeral Director Alan Massey, the firm's patriarch, confronted Shipman in his office with these concerns in late 1997. The doctor had already signed 47 death certificates that year, and Massey knew that the average British GP signs only about 8 annually. Massey recalled:

> [Dr. Shipman replied,] "There's no need to be concerned. It's all in the book, and anyone can look at the book." He gave me the deaths book which all doctors fill in, entering each death and the cause of death. It proved nothing: there was a medical term for the cause of death in each case, but it meant nothing to me, a layman.
>
> But I was reassured, mainly because he was so calm and matter-of-fact about it. He certainly didn't act like someone with something to hide, or someone who was nervous. I came away, after about fifteen minutes, feeling that perhaps we had been putting two and two together and making five.

Debbie Massey, Alan's daughter, remained unconvinced. She approached Dr. Susan Booth about her concerns at the Hyde chapel, where Dr. Booth had come to sign one of Dr. Shipman's cremation certificates. "Don't you think you're coming here a little bit too often?" she asked. That comment paralleled Dr. Booth's own misgivings about cremations of Dr. Shipman's patients. Shipman had pushed the families to cremate most of his victims' bodies, although this was not as difficult at it might have been elsewhere, since more than 70 percent of British dead are now routinely cremated. Still, it was unusual.

While a burial can occur with only one physician's signature on the necessary disposition forms, British rules require the signature of a second physician not in practice with the first for cremation. This is supposed to protect against using cremation to hide a crime. The second physician can sign the death certificate only after discussing the case with the primary doctor and, usually, viewing the body at the funeral home. But one can rarely determine or confirm the cause of death from such a superficial examination—and especially not if the patient was poisoned using narcotics. For this "rubber stamping" of the form, doctors are paid £41, which they call "ash-can money." Seeing this formality as a benefit, GPs have a saying: "The more you burn, the more you earn."

Because of the law, Shipman had to ask other physicians to sign the Authority to Cremate form. He normally asked members of Brooke Surgery to do this, which they did on a rotating basis. Professor Richard Baker performed the clinical audit for the National Health Service on Dr. Shipman's practice. He wrote:

> Since Shipman was able to ask several different practitioners to complete Form C [the confirmatory part of the cremation certificate], no single practitioner would automatically be exposed to an excess number of patient deaths. In these circumstances, if any practitioner did notice an excess, it could readily and credibly be ascribed to factors such as Shipman's large list [of patients] or his alleged preference to care for patients in their own homes in their final illnesses.

Dr. Susan Booth worked at Brooke Surgery, a group of doctors who had split from the Clarendon group and had an office across from Shipman's office. After Debbie Massey spoke to her, she and her partners discussed their concerns. By 1997, Dr. Linda Reynolds, a new Brooke partner, had noticed that Dr. Shipman seemed to be present at most of his patients' deaths. Dr. John Grenville, an early witness at the post-trial inquiry and an expert on general practice, commented:

> It is unusual for a patient to die in the presence of a GP or within a few hours of having seen the GP. The vast majority of such cases are where the patient is known to be terminally ill and the doctor has been visiting the patient at home on a regular basis at the end of the patient's life. It is extremely rare for no one else to be present … It is extremely uncommon for a deceased person to be sitting, head to one side, appearing peaceful and asleep. It is more usual to have a few moments of consciousness during which they will attempt to seek help and it is common to find a deceased patient lying on the floor near the chair on which they have been sitting but obviously have moved in the direction of the telephone or door.

Dr. Reynolds had mentioned her observations to her partners and, after Debbie Massey's conversation with Dr. Booth, the group decided to report their suspicions to the authorities, despite the caution urged by their Medical Defense Union (lawyers representing all British doctors). First, however, they did their own mini-survey. They found that their group, with 10,000 patients, had had only 15 deaths in the past year, while there had been three times as many deaths among Dr. Shipman's 3,000 patients. Both practices had patients who were essentially of the same age and social class.

On March 24, 1998, Dr. Reynolds called South Manchester's coroner, John Pollard (who had previously practiced criminal law), to discuss her suspicions. Although initially skeptical, he instructed the Greater Manchester police to conduct a quiet investigation. They assigned a detective to the case, and the local health authority checked the medical records of Dr. Shipman's patients who had died in the prior six months to see if the records matched the cause of death on their death certificates. They all correlated perfectly. But the authorities did not know that Dr. Shipman had altered (often sloppily) both the written and computer medical records. He probably did this first to be sure medical records and death certificates matched. Second, he wanted to be sure that no autopsy was performed. This could be done, for example, by citing the cause of death as a lethal disease.

Two weeks later, the officer assigned to the case told Dr. Reynolds that he could find no evidence of wrongdoing by Dr. Shipman. Although she reported that three more of Dr. Shipman's patients had died in the interim and were available for autopsy, the case was dropped.

The effort had not been entirely in vain. The next time Pollard received a phone call about a suspicious Shipman death, he took it much more seriously. Dr. Shipman's lethal career finally ended after relatives persuaded the police to investigate the bizarre circumstances surrounding the death of Kathleen Grundy.

The Victims

Unknown to the community, the kindly, hard-working, and slightly eccentric Dr. Harold Frederick Shipman was killing many of his patients. His victims were primarily elderly women. Kathleen Grundy was the best known of the group of 15 women for whose deaths Dr. Shipman was ultimately tried, and killing her would prove his downfall. Yet, despite the vital role these victims had played in their communities, journalists later noted that their identities as elderly women rendered them virtually invisible to almost everyone except their families and friends.

Laura Kathleen Wagstaff
Laura Kathleen Wagstaff, a kind widow, was killed on December 9, 1997. The 81-year-old's death may have been a mistake. Dr. Shipman drove to Dowson

Primary School, where Angela Wagstaff worked, and told her that her mother was dead. As it turned out, Shipman had gotten the relationship wrong—Wagstaff was actually Angela's mother-in-law. Her mother, Mrs. Royle, had delivered a bottle of gin to the doctor just that day as a Christmas present. Shipman listed Mrs. Wagstaff's death as being from a coronary thrombosis (heart attack).

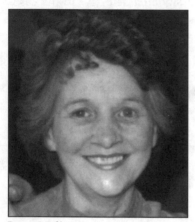

Joan Melia

Joan Melia, 73, was a trim, trendy, and smart-looking woman who, as her niece said, "was a natural counselor. If you went to her with a problem, you came away a lot lighter. She was such a kind person, very very loving, with a tremendous sense of humor."

When she died, the engagement ring that she never took off had disappeared. When her niece later called Dr. Shipman to discuss Melia's death, he was rude to her.

Joan Melia. (Courtesy of Cavendish Press, Manchester)

Ivy Lomas

Ivy Lomas, 63, was the only patient Shipman was convicted of murdering that died in his office. Shipman did not particularly like her, since she was opinionated and argumentative. As one lifelong acquaintance said, "Ivy could come across badly sometimes, a bit rough, but that was just her way." She spent much of her time caring for her son, who had psychiatric problems and had recently returned home after being in a residential facility.

On the day of her death, Mrs. Lomas walked into Dr. Shipman's office complaining of a minor pain in her arm. He took her into his treatment room and then came out, telling the receptionist that he was having trouble with the EKG machine. He then treated three other patients before returning to the room and "finding" her dead. He certified that she had died from coronary thrombosis and smoking.

Bianka Pomfret

Bianka Pomfret, 49, was one of Shipman's youngest victims. Unlike the others, who were all highly visible within their communities, Mrs. Pomfret suffered from manic-depression and had difficulty managing her daily activities. Even so, her neighbor described her as being "kind and gentle, especially with her children . . . She was a nice person, very quiet. You didn't know she was there." Dr. Shipman listed the causes of death as a blood clot in the heart, heart disease, smoking, and manic-depression.

Winifred "Winnie" Mellor

Winifred "Winnie" Mellor, 73, the mother of five children, was retired from running a chip shop. Full of energy and possessing a great sense of humor, she still played football with her grandsons. As her parish priest said, "Winnie Mellor was flying about . . . She was not sitting at home, looking into the fire. She gave her all to life and those around her." She read stories to elementary school children and gave communion to the bedridden. Dr. Shipman told her children that she suffered from angina and had refused hospitalization.

As he increasingly lost control, Shipman's killings accelerated. He began killing at least three to four patients a month; in February 1998, at least seven people succumbed to his lethal ministrations. According to prosecuting attorney Richard Henriques:

> [Dr. Shipman's patients] trusted him to care for them. Their relatives trusted him to tell the truth about the circumstances in which his patients died. The community trusted him to keep records and documentation with insight and knowledge . . . He did not care at all for these fifteen patients he killed. He did not tell the truth to their relatives—he duped them in order to save his own skin . . .
>
> [Shipman would] overbear, belittle and bamboozle [grieving relatives.] He took advantage of their lesser knowledge of medicine and procedures. As they grieved, this determined man employed every device to make sure no postmortem examination took place. The poisoner, of course, fears the pathologist. He fears ambulances and he fears hospitals.

Although its use is illegal for medical purposes in many countries, including the United States, Shipman probably injected his victims with diamorphine (heroin), which metabolizes rapidly to double-strength morphine and then to its glucuronide salts. The benefit to Shipman of using this drug was that it is very soluble—much more so than morphine; thus, a large amount of the drug can be administered in a small volume of liquid through a small-gauge needle. It is two to four times as potent as morphine when injected. According to Robert Forrest, Britain's leading forensic toxicologist, "[the victims] would die on the end of the needle, virtually. They would take a few breaths and be gone." However, diamorphine is also easily detected. That is why Shipman wanted to avoid autopsies and to cremate the corpses.

It is believed that Shipman told his elderly patients that he was giving them a flu shot, antibiotics, or vitamins. Since they died so quickly and quietly—some had friends in the other room at the time who didn't hear anything—he must have administered the medication intravenously.

He was able to stockpile the drug by over-prescribing it for terminally ill patients, getting the prescriptions from the pharmacies himself, and then giving his patients or their caregivers less than half, and sometimes none, of what he had obtained. In 1994, for example, he prescribed 1,000 mg of diamorphine for one patient who never received the drug. In at least five cases, he prescribed the drug for patients who were already dead and kept it for himself. He also collected any diamorphine that remained after his patients died, saying that he would dispose of it.

A visiting nurse, Marion Gilchrist, testified that she had questioned Shipman about entries in the drug records for a terminal patient because the amounts prescribed, administered, and remaining would not balance: "Dr. Shipman tried to explain why it was and I still couldn't understand. He said he had borrowed 100 mg of diamorphine from a friend and he had had to take 100 mg to return it." That explanation alone should have raised alarms, but it didn't.

Kathleen Grundy—The Turning Point

Kathleen Laura Grundy (née Platt) was an alert and fiercely independent 81-year-old widow. She was born in Hyde on July 2, 1916. When her husband, John, was mayor in 1962–63, she had served as mayoress of Hyde. John, a former schoolteacher, went on to become a lecturer at Manchester University. At the time of her death, she had been a widow for 30 years, and led a very active life in Hyde. Her home was a beautiful seventeenth-century cottage, located in Gee Cross, worth £200,000. She also owned a £90,000 cottage nearby and a £60,000 apartment in the Lake District. Mrs. Grundy was one of Dr. Shipman's many loyal patients, although she had few physical problems. She was an avid gardener and took long walks daily. She worked at the Age of Concern thrift shop twice a week, and served lunch three days a week at Werneth House, a local elder center.

Mrs. Grundy wrote compulsively about all her daily activities in her diary, a fact not known by many people. Later, police would use these records to

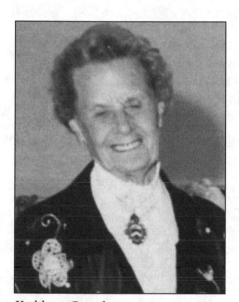

Kathleen Grundy. (Courtesy of Cavendish Press, Manchester)

further corroborate that Shipman had altered medical records to justify his patients' deaths. Two of his entries about Kathleen Grundy, for example, described office visits at times, as she had dutifully noted in her diary, that she had actually been shopping in another city or with her daughter.

On June 23, 1998, she told a friend that Dr. Shipman was coming to her house the next morning to take a blood sample and to have her sign some papers. When she failed to show up to help serve lunches at Werneth House, co-workers went to her home. Upon entering through an unlocked door, they found her fully clothed corpse curled up on the sofa.

Knowing that Dr. Shipman was her physician, they called him. He arrived ten minutes later and said that he had seen Mrs. Grundy just that morning "only for a talk." Shipman would later certify her death as resulting from "old age," a cause of death that no physician, even the sloppiest or least knowledgeable, ever lists on a death certificate. He declared her dead and advised Mrs. Grundy's friends to contact the law firm of Hamilton Ward for further instructions. When they did so, lawyers there said they were not Mrs. Grundy's agent, but that they had received her will, with an accompanying letter, that morning. The badly typewritten letter, dated June 22, 1998, and supposedly from Mrs. Grundy, began:

> Dear Sir, I enclose a copy of my will. I think it is clear my intention and wish Dr. Shipman to benefit by having my estate but if he dies or does not accept it, then the estate goes to my daughter.

It went on to say that Mrs. Grundy would stop by Ward's office in the next few days to verify the instructions. However, by the time Ward received them, she was already dead. He later testified that when he received the will, he thought it strange and put it on the corner of his desk. "When I got a phone call at lunchtime saying Mrs. Grundy had died, I became suspicious," he told the court.

Twelve days after Kathleen Grundy died, Brian Burgess from Hamilton Ward contacted Mrs. Grundy's only child, Angela Woodruff, to say that he had her mother's last will and testament. This was a surprise to Angela, who was a lawyer herself. She had always handled her mother's legal affairs and had a copy of what she thought was her mother's last will that she had prepared; this will left most of Grundy's estate to her family. The new will, in Ward's possession, read, in part:

> All my estate, money and house to my doctor. My family are not in need and I want to reward him for all the care he has given me and the people of Hyde. He is sensible enough to handle any problems this may give him. My doctor is Dr. HF Shipman.

Angela Woodruff was suspicious about the documents because the phrasing was unusual and the typing was sloppy. Her mother had been a secretary and had excellent typing skills—not to mention a passion for neatness. The will also stipulated that her body was to be cremated, but her mother had repeatedly told people that she wanted her body buried. Moreover, Mrs. Grundy had been active and alert until the day she died, and she and her family were on excellent terms.

The strange situation was compounded by another letter the lawyers received, dated four days after Mrs. Grundy's death, supposedly from an "S." or "J. Smith," that read, "I regret to inform you that Mrs. Kathleen Grundy of 79 Joel Lane died last week. I understand she lodged a will with you, as I am a friend who typed it out for her." No one by that name was ever located.

Woodruff decided to investigate the will and the circumstances of her mother's death. She visited the two "witnesses" for the strange will; it turned out that they were simply picked out of Dr. Shipman's waiting room when Mrs. Grundy had visited. Neither they, nor apparently Mrs. Grundy, knew what they were signing—they had believed it to be permission to participate in a survey on aging. Even so, as Woodruff later found out, the signatures on the will and the letter were actually forged copies, rather than the original signatures.

On July 24, 1998, Woodruff filed a complaint at the Leamington Spa police station in Warwickshire; they passed it on to the Greater Manchester police located in her mother's area. At first, the police thought that this was another case of a relative irate over being left out of a will, since Grundy's estate was valued at about £400,000 (about $660,000 at the time she died). But Woodruff and her family did not need the inheritance; they had inherited money from other relatives and both she and her husband, a physicist, had excellent jobs. When they combined the information that Woodruff had amassed with a re-evaluation of the prior investigation, the police decided that something was seriously amiss.

The Investigation and Arrest

When police revisited the Shipman case, they noticed something odd. The doctor was present at the deaths of many of his patients, and the majority of his patients died and were found within three hours of his having seen them. The typical pattern was:

1. Elderly woman.
2. Died unexpectedly.
3. Had received a home visit.
4. Decedent was dressed.
5. Sitting in chair.
6. Shipman lied about being called by decedent.
7. Shipman lied about calling ambulance.
8. Victim cremated.

To prosecute the case, the police knew that they had to acquire hard evidence. They started by examining the bodies of Shipman's victims. Kathleen Grundy was the first exhumation that the police in Greater Manchester had ever requested from the coroner, and they had to first develop a protocol for the procedure. The exhumation took place on Saturday, August 1, 1998, in a pouring rainstorm. Nighttime was selected so few people would notice. Nevertheless, staff at the adjacent Laurel Bank Nursing Home observed the unusual activity in the cemetery and notified the police. The newspapers, however, did not pick up the story until two weeks later.

UK Exhumation Services, called in to unearth Kathleen Grundy's body, would subsequently exhume all the bodies in the Shipman investigation. In addition to disinterring the body, they also followed routine forensic guidelines and took soil samples to be sure that chemicals in the ground around the casket had not contaminated the corpse. Kathleen Grundy's gravestone read: "Died Unexpectedly After a Lifetime of Helping Others." The exhumation of her body would ultimately help many more people—and end Dr. Shipman's killing spree.

One of the journalists who finally broke the story, Brian Whittle, wrote about the initial apathy by members of the press:

A query over the death of an elderly lady meant another "mercy killing" doctor, or possibly a case of medical negligence. There's a predictable newspaper scale of interest in death which tails off according to how remote from Britain the victims are (hundreds killed in an earthquake on the other side of the globe may rate only a couple of paragraphs) and how old the victims are: the murder of a child or a pretty young woman rates far more inches of newsprint than the death of an old woman.

Besides, there had been a spate of euthanasia stories, and although they merited a good debate on the feature pages of the broadsheets, they did nothing to boost circulation.

Kathleen Grundy's autopsy was performed at Tameside General Hospital later that day by Dr. John Rutherford, a local forensic pathologist. He told investigators that there was no immediately obvious physical cause of death. Mrs. Grundy's organs were in remarkably good shape for an 81-year-old woman and showed no signs of lethal disease. He sent tissue samples to North-West Forensic Science Laboratories at Chorley, Lancashire, for further analysis, although he could not provide any clues about what to look for.

To be sure that evidence was not destroyed on the day of the exhumation, police searched Shipman's office and home. When they approached the doctor as he was leaving work, he did not seem surprised. Rather, with a contemptuous smile, and after contacting lawyers at the Medical Defense Union, he helped police locate specific items they sought—such as his typewriter. As he handed it to police, Shipman made an unusual comment, "Mrs. Grundy borrows it from time to time." Investigators later discovered that it had been used to type the Grundy will and the letters sent to Hamilton Ward.

When officers searched Shipman's home, they were shocked at the grimy disarray: piles of papers and dirty clothes littered every room. One policeman later commented that the doctor had been growing penicillin on the stove; another said it was the sort of place where one wiped one's feet—upon leaving. Police found a lot of cheap jewelry, possibly "trophies" from his victims, and former patients' medical records.

Despite news reports that suggested Dr. Shipman might have killed many more women, The Surgery was still crammed with patients. He continued to exude a calm and confident air, but a few individuals found him distraught. He told his visiting nurse, Mrs. Gilchrist, that in the "thrillers" he read, "on the evidence they have, I would have me guilty." He also told her, "The only thing I did wrong was not having her [Kathleen Grundy] cremated. If I had had her cremated, I wouldn't be having all this trouble." He told a patient, Mrs. Lesley

Pulford, that he had not yet been arrested because toxicology tests took a long time to perform.

Many people in Hyde believed Shipman was guilty only of euthanizing suffering old ladies. The Surgery was flooded with flowers and cards and letters of support. Some were from relatives of those who would later be named as Dr. Shipman's victims. Other townspeople developed a type of black humor regarding the case and said, "Where there's a will, there's a way," or described imaginary films, such as *101 Cremations* and *Shipman's List*.

The investigation gathered momentum, and, on August 21, Detective Superintendent Bernard Postles requisitioned a large room at the Ashton-under-Lyne police station from which to manage the increasingly complex case. The preliminary investigation had identified at least 30 patients from The Surgery who had died in the past year. At the time of the trial, Postles, who was described as "smart, dapper and intelligent," had spent 27 of his 46 years as a police officer, 22 of them in the Criminal Investigation Division (CID). During the first months of the investigation, Postles and DI Stan Egerton would spend 12-hour days pouring over their data. Twenty-four detectives worked on the case, although more were added to carry out searches. This was one of the biggest cases any of them had ever worked.

Because there were so many potential victims, some of whose families refused to believe that they had been murdered, the detectives were divided into teams. Each team handled five or six dead patients. To prioritize their efforts, they scored each case to identify those that could most easily be prosecuted; cases with the highest number of points received the most attention. One point was awarded for each of the following circumstances:

- The body was buried rather than being cremated. Police initially did not believe that they could successfully prosecute those cases where the body was cremated.
- The patient's family expressed concern about the circumstances surrounding the death.
- The police had suspicions about the death due to such things as inconsistencies in the records or missing property.
- The written or computerized medical records had been altered.

A point was added for any case that scored four points, to emphasize its priority.

On September 2, Julie Evans, the toxicologist at North-West Forensic Science Laboratories, notified police that Mrs. Grundy's body contained sufficient diamorphine to have caused her death. Mrs. Grundy's death had become a murder case—and police now knew what poison to look for.

If Dr. Shipman's goal was to commit the perfect crime, then using diamorphine on his victims was his first error. While diamorphine itself degrades, its major metabolite—the glucuronide salt that forms within one to two hours in a cadaver with a warm liver (and functioning enzymes)—can be found in liver and other tissues. The drug can be detected as long as body tissue is present; it has even been found in thirteenth-century South American mummies.

To defend himself, Shipman later asserted that Mrs. Grundy had been a drug addict and that his medical records proved it. However, testimony at the trial by handwriting, medical, and computer experts would show that Shipman had altered his medical records to cover up the murders. For example, on December 10, 1997, when Bianka Pomfret's dead body was found propped up in a chair in her home, Dr. Shipman was in his office altering the records of her prior visits. In the 70 minutes before her body was discovered, the doctor made ten separate entries to document her supposed complaints of chest pain during the prior ten months.

At a time when many physicians shunned the new computer systems, Shipman tried to impress everyone with his knowledge of computers—which was rudimentary, at best. This ignorance would be his undoing. Although he had been a member of the advisory committee that instituted the 1996 update of Microdoc, the computerized recordkeeping system he used, Shipman ignored an important detail: the system stamped each entry with a permanent date and time that was unaffected by manually backdating the patient's record. This date-and-time stamp was accessible only by computer experts, and the police easily uncovered the incriminating data.

The toxicology results arrived on Wednesday. The police decided to arrest Dr. Shipman the following Monday, ostensibly so that he would have time to arrange for another physician to cover his practice. But no one informed either Shipman or his solicitor (non-litigating lawyer), Ann Ball, who had been assigned to him under the auspices of the Medical Defense Union.

On Monday morning, September 7, 1998, Shipman and Ann Ball arrived at the Ashton-under-Lyne police station to "help the police" with their investigation. But Shipman was skittish about going in; he persuaded Ball to go on a stroll through the nearby streets. When they finally entered, he was immediately arrested for Kathleen Grundy's murder, attempted theft by deception, and three counts of forgery. Shocked at his arrest, Shipman was also disgusted at being booked, photographed, and fingerprinted by a mere sergeant; he expected the chief constable to do it. Detective Chief Inspector Williams later joked, "He had been watching too many films."

The day of his arrest, Shipman's lawyer requested bail. Although friends pledged substantial sums in a drive that Primrose orchestrated, the judge refused to release him. Four days later, Joan Melia's body was exhumed for examination. She was the first of those who scored five points on the investigating team's scale. The next night, Winifred Mellor's body was dug up.

On September 28, at Hyde Municipal Cemetery, Bianka Pomfret's body was exhumed; as with the other exhumations, it took place in the middle of the night.

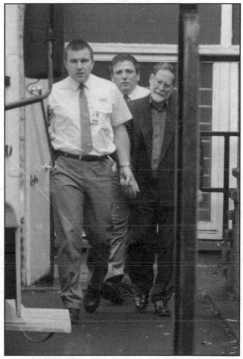

Shipman (right) at his arrest. (Courtesy of Cavendish Press, Manchester)

Although police were present to keep spectators at a distance, only one reporter and one photographer showed up. At later exhumations, when hordes of TV crews and reporters appeared, Stan Egerton would have his men turn some of the arc lights used to light the grave toward the crowd just as the coffin was removed from the ground, effectively blinding their cameras.

All the bodies, except that of Mrs. Grundy, were returned to their respective graves by the next afternoon—usually accompanied by a simple burial service. On December 9, the twelfth and final exhumation before the trial was completed, that of Elizabeth Mellor. This was the most individual exhumations ever undertaken in one case that did not involve war crimes. Although the names of possible murder victims kept piling up as the investigation continued, the police decided to stop at that point. As Coroner John Pollard remarked:

> The only word to sum up my feelings would be amazement. It was like Topsy, it just seemed to grow and grow. My main concern throughout was to see that justice was done, but to balance that against the cares and considerations of the family and friends. Exhumation is a disturbing experience

for everyone involved, including the police and, to some extent, myself as coroner, because I don't want to cause distress. But there is a need to prove if something has gone wrong.

On September 29, three weeks after Dr. Shipman's arrest, Britain's National Health Service finally held a hearing to stop him from practicing medicine. Shipman was officially charged with the murders of Joan Melia, Winifred Mellor, and Bianka Pomfret on October 5. When police told the doctor, he showed no emotion. But, when they told him that his backdated computer records had left an indelible trail, he collapsed on the floor, sobbing. His solicitor, Ann Ball, halted the interview because, as the doctor who had been summoned confirmed, he was "in a distressed and emotional state and unfit for interview."

He was interrogated the next day, and, on October 7, 1998, he was formally arraigned for the three additional murders in Tameside Magistrates' Court, as he stood sobbing and swaying from side to side. Over the next few days, Shipman quickly regained his confidence, arrogantly calling many of his police interrogators "stupid." The police soon stopped their interrogations, even after he was repeatedly brought back to court to be charged with more murders, because of Shipman's uncooperative response to each charge: "I treated them appropriately for their medical condition at the time."

Public Reaction

During the investigation and until Shipman's arrest, the press was free to write anything about the case. Newspaper headlines screamed out what seemed to be outrageous claims that Shipman had killed 50, or even 100 patients. Little did anyone imagine that the tabloids had grossly underestimated the body count. All this publicity prejudiced public opinion and complicated the jury selection for the trial. After the trial had begun and until he was convicted, the British press (but not the international press) was restricted to writing only about his court appearances.

From the time of Shipman's arrest until October 2000, the West Pennine Health Authority ran The Surgery using temporary physicians. They then appointed a permanent replacement, Dr. Amy Cumming. But the weekend before she was to begin, the Shipman children stripped the building of its furnishings, which belonged to Dr. Shipman. Dr. Cumming found it hard to serve patients, saying, "They did take everything and we only had a day to replace everything, which was a headache."

Nicci Gerrard, who covered Dr. Shipman's arrest and trial for Britain's *The Guardian Unlimited*, described the public reaction to the doctor and his actions:

> Shipman [is] Britain's worst serial killer by far—and perhaps the world's, too ...Yet he remains a weirdly unresonant figure, who baffles rather than horrifies us ... His face—clerkish and bespectacled, with a scratchy beard and aggrieved stare—doesn't send a frisson of terror through us ... He has not become one of our demons, not an icon of evil, and that's because he doesn't hold an evident meaning for us ...
>
> The majority of Harold Shipman's victims and assumed victims were elderly and they were female, which gave them a double invisibility. Everyone's assumption, when Shipman was first arrested, was that he was a mercy-killer, easing the sick patients out of a life they'd grown weary of . ..They weren't children, sweet innocents slaughtered, nor were they beautiful young women. They weren't the stuff of tragedy for us ...
>
> His murders were not Gothic and tormented, the stuff of horror stories and dark fairy tales, but mute and with a ghastly decorum. He didn't kidnap them, torture them, sexually abuse them, mutilate them or cut them up. He didn't boil them or bury them vertically in his garden or basement. He never listened to them scream. He simply killed them, one by one, down the years.

The Trial

Shipman was originally held in Strangeways Prison, officially known as Manchester Prison, on suicide watch. But, since many inmates and guards had relatives that Shipman could have killed, the authorities felt that it was not safe for him to stay there, so, in the fall of 1998, he was moved to Preston Prison. Later, he was moved again to Walton Prison in Liverpool. Sarah, his daughter, moved to a new home a mile from the prison so she could visit her father. His sons also visited him, often with Primrose.

Once in Walton, Shipman was given tranquilizers, which calmed him to the point that he took to prison life "like a natural," striding down the corridors "like he owns the place," according to the prison authorities. Before Shipman was later put into a cell alone, he shared a cell with Tony Fleming, a thief. While they were cellmates, the doctor saved Fleming's life when he tried to hang himself with Shipman's shoelaces. Annoyed at the interruption in his placid prison existence, Shipman commented, "Next time, use someone else's shoelaces."

His next cellmate was 34-year-old Peter Hall, who had bludgeoned his girlfriend and her sons, a 17-month-old and an 8-year-old, to death. He left a note for her ex-husband that read, "You are welcome to your family back." (Hall went to trial six months before Shipman and received three life sentences, since Britain has eliminated capital punishment.) Shipman counseled him on how to overcome his remorse; Hall hung himself in December 1999.

Shipman spent his time in prison answering letters, penning poetry, and writing reams of papers about his case. By the time his trial commenced, he had papers stacked ten feet high in his cell. Shipman also participated in social activities and played chess. He occasionally held office hours for prisoners and staff who wished to avail themselves of his medical services, but he was not permitted to prescribe any medications.

Preston was chosen as the site of the trial because Shipman's lawyers thought that the town was large enough and far enough from Hyde (35 miles) to impanel an impartial jury. Preston also has an impressive courthouse, known as "Old Bailey of the North" due to its similarity to the London original. Ironically, the town has its own disgraced physician: Dr. Thomas Monk, a nineteenth-century mayor who forged a will for one of his patients in an attempt to inherit his fortune. Monk went to prison, and his name was removed from a statue in the center of town.

Harold Frederick Shipman first appeared before Judge Thayne Forbes on October 5, 1999. Before the trial began, bookmaker William Hill offered 9:5 odds of the doctor being found guilty and 15:1 odds of him being acquitted. Shipman faced 16 charges: 15 for murder and 1 for forging Kathleen Grundy's will. The women he was accused of killing are: Elizabeth Adams, Muriel Grimshaw, Kathleen Grundy, Pamela Hillier, Jean Lilly, Ivy Lomas, Joan Melia, Winifred Mellor, Norah Nuttall, Bianka Pomfret, Marie Quinn, Irene Turner, Laura Kathleen Wagstaff, Maureen Ward, and Marie West.

Although the bodies of Alice Kitchen, Sally Ashworth, and Elizabeth Mellor had been exhumed, Shipman was not charged in these cases because the forensic evidence was lacking. Since the bodies had been buried for two years, there was not enough tissue (especially of the liver) to test for the breakdown products of diamorphine. According to the Department of Health report on Dr. Shipman:

> Toxicological tests were undertaken on samples of hair and thigh muscle of all nine patients, and on samples of liver in a small number of cases. The hair samples confirmed that all the patients could be regarded as

"morphine naïve," in other words they were not regular users of morphine. The thigh muscle and liver samples all revealed the presence of morphine in levels compatible with the administration of fatal doses, and in each case, the cause of death given by the Home Office Pathologist was morphine toxicity.

Prosecutors also decided they had sufficient evidence to charge Shipman with killing Marie West and Lizzie Adams, both of whose bodies had been cremated. This move established prosecutors' ability to charge Shipman with additional deaths as they were uncovered, even if they lacked strong forensic evidence.

Judge Queen's Counsel (QC) Forbes has a reputation for being scrupulously fair and meticulous. The reputation was well-earned, since not one conviction in his courtroom had ever been successfully appealed. Nicola Davies, QC, who specialized in medical cases, led Shipman's defense. Ann Ball had asked her to defend him in court, since she could not litigate cases. Both Davies and her junior partner, Ian Winter, seemed uncomfortable dealing with the working class witnesses, and appeared more at ease with the expert witnesses.

The prosecuting attorney was Richard Henriques, QC. Henriques had been named one of Britain's "fat cat" lawyers the year before, and reportedly earned £500,000 in fees annually. Educated at Oxford, he was the most senior and most respected trial lawyer in that part of Britain. He commented that he wished that every case he prosecuted had evidence as strong as there was in any one of the cases being brought against Shipman.

Thirty-eight seats in the courtroom were allocated to the press, including one, strangely enough, for a radio station, Rock FM. There were 7 men and 5 women on the jury, ranging in age from their mid-twenties to their late fifties. Sworn in on October 11, 1999, they had been painstakingly culled from a panel of 60 potential jurors who were all warned that the trial could take as long as five months.

Prosecutor Henriques led off with an eight-hour opening address, detailing the charges against Shipman and trying to explain why the kindly general practitioner had become a rampant serial killer. He said of the victims:

> None of them were prescribed morphine or diamorphine; all of them died most unexpectedly; all of them had seen Dr. Shipman on the day of their death. There is no question of euthanasia or what is sometimes called mercy killing. None of the deceased were terminally ill. The defendant

killed those 15 patients because he enjoyed doing so. He was exercising the ultimate power of controlling life and death, and repeated it so often that he must have found the drama of taking life to his taste.

More than 120 prosecution witnesses then were called to the court: elderly friends and middle-aged sons and daughters of the victims; police investigators; and various experts, including some from the United States, Germany, and Britain who described diamorphine's effects and the amount needed to kill a person. Dr. Shipman injected his victims with 30 mg of diamorphine (heroin), six times the normal 5 mg dose used to control pain. Professor Henry McQuay, from Oxford University, explained what happens when such an overdose is given:

> We would expect to see slowing of your breathing within two minutes. By five minutes your breathing would be very slow indeed, two to three breaths per minute … You would appear to be asleep. Your lips and fingers might well be blue and your toes might have a blue tinge to them. If your brain can't get any oxygen because your breathing has stopped, you would die.

Muriel Grimshaw's daughter testified twice, first about her mother's last days and then about how, after her husband's natural death of cancer in 1993, Dr. Shipman retrieved the leftover diamorphine. Although Shipman repeatedly denied stockpiling narcotics, police discovered drugs hidden in his home, still labeled with his patients' prescriptions. Hundreds of exhibits were introduced during the 25 days it took for the prosecution to present its case. The defense strategy would be completely different.

The defense began their task on November 25, 1999. QC Davies did not give an opening statement because, since it had to be based on available evidence, it would not have helped her client. Instead, she said, "I call Dr. Harold Frederick Shipman." It appeared that the doctor was not expecting this, as observers said he looked startled.

Appearing frail and nervous, Dr. Shipman would be the main witness on his behalf. Although Shipman claimed that prison was no greater strain than his medical internship, after 13 months in prison, he showed up in court thinner and grayer than when he entered prison. Observers said he looked "like a faded, homely chemistry teacher. From his appearance, he should have been wiping the froth from a half a pint of real ale off his beard in the snug of his local pub, rather than facing a murder trial."

Speaking quietly, he outlined his training and then proceeded, one by one, to describe the circumstances of each woman's death. His arrogance was clear to the jury; he interspersed technical language to demonstrate his superiority with street slang to "relate" to the jury. To portray himself as a merciful and humane physician, he described how, when Marie West and Marie Quinn died in his presence, he did not attempt to resuscitate them. He said that this was because he was "bothered by what we would end up with" if they survived, since "patients who survive often have a loss of personality and a loss of use of their body, and end up in a nursing home."

Despite all the evidence to the contrary, he still claimed to have tried to resuscitate Mrs. Kathleen Wagstaff for ten minutes after she collapsed. In reality, he never called for an ambulance or any other assistance. Slumping down in his seat, Shipman began crying while saying this. He then claimed that he had tried to resuscitate Ivy Lomas, who died in his office. However, he admitted that he did not request help from his office personnel—or even tell them she was dead—because he did not want "to disrupt the surgery [office]."

While Lomas's corpse lay in his treatment room, he calmly continued treating other patients. He later told police that "he considered her such a nuisance that he thought about having part of the seating area reserved for [her]," a statement that was repeated often at the trial. The doctor also admitted back-dating Pamela Hillier's medical records on the day she died, although he denied falsifying any information.

Numerous witnesses testified that Dr. Shipman barely glanced at their relatives before pronouncing them dead. When asked what criteria he used to pronounce these women dead, Shipman said he had felt for "brainstem activity" at the back of their necks. As an expert later testified at the post-trial inquiry: "This is nonsense. Brainstem activity does not produce any effect which can be felt by a hand on the back of the neck."

After Shipman's testimony for the defense, Prosecutor Henriques kept him on the witness stand another seven days, hammering at his inconsistencies and highlighting the eerily similar pattern in each death. Reporter Mikaela Sitford described Shipman as being "devoured" by Henrique's unrelenting examination, which intensified as it progressed. Henrique got Shipman to admit that he prescribed large, perhaps excessive, doses of narcotics, but the doctor claimed that the diamorphine found at his home was merely "an oversight." He could not explain how diamorphine got into the exhumed bodies, and restated (based on records he entered after her death) that Mrs. Grundy had been addicted to narcotics. He claimed to have sent blood samples to the hospital lab after visiting Mrs. Grundy, but said they must have disappeared.

Shipman's lawyers had no chance to mount a decent defense; his own testimony had convicted him. Shipman admitted that diamorphine killed his patients and he offered no suggestion how, other than through his administration, they could have died from the drug. The only other defense witness was a fingerprint expert who discussed the one print found on Mrs. Grundy's will. It belonged to Shipman, rather than to Mrs. Grundy or the two "witnesses."

When the trial was almost over, two bizarre incidents nearly caused a mistrial. The British Medical Association inexplicably e-mailed its members details about Shipman's drug addiction and convictions for stealing drugs and forging prescriptions in 1976. No one accepted responsibility, and the organization apologized. Justice Forbes ruled that since the jury had not found out about this incident, the trial would continue.

The second incident occurred when a "shock jock" on an FM rock station said on his prime time show, "We all know Shipman is as guilty as sin. Why don't we save the taxpayer a lot of money and end the trial now?" as his compatriot chanted "guilty, guilty, guilty" in the background. The judge was not pleased, but he concluded: "Fortunately for you, the jury has more sense than to listen to your sort of broadcast." He gave the broadcasters a warning rather than a contempt-of-court citation.

On December 13, the court recessed until January 5, 2000. When the trial resumed, Prosecutor Henriques addressed the jury with his summation. During this oration, Shipman doodled on a notepad, looking thoroughly dejected. His barrister then tried to sway the jury by portraying Shipman as a "caring if idiosyncratic" doctor who went out of his way to help his patients. She stressed, correctly, that the prosecution could find no real motive for the alleged murders, and she proclaimed the stockpile of diamorphine to be "a red herring." Davies described the toxicology evidence as being completely unreliable, due to both the decomposed state of the bodies and the tests that were used.

On January 10, Judge Forbes began his two-week summation of the case. He emphasized that each of the 16 charges needed to be considered separately, saying, "They do not stand or fall together." Finally, on January 24, the jury retired to consider their verdict. One week later, at 4:33 P.M. on Monday, January 31, 2000, the jury foreman announced to a hushed courtroom that they had arrived at a unanimous verdict for all counts. As Dr. Shipman stood emotionless, the foreman read out "guilty" 16 times—15 for murder and one for forgery.

Davies then requested that sentence be passed immediately. Judge Forbes complied, saying:

> You have finally been brought to justice by the verdict of this jury. I have no doubt whatsoever that these are true verdicts. The time has now come for me to pass sentence upon you for these wicked, wicked crimes.
>
> Each of your victims was your patient. You murdered each and every one of your victims by a calculated and cold-blooded perversion of your medical skills for your own evil and wicked purposes. For your own evil and wicked purposes you took advantage of them and grossly abused the trust that each of your victims placed in you. You were, after all, each victim's doctor. I have little doubt that each of your victims smiled and thanked you as she submitted to your deadly ministrations.
>
> None realized yours was not a healing touch, none knew in truth you had brought her death, death disguised as the caring attention of a good doctor. The sheer wickedness of what you have done defies description. It is shocking and beyond belief. You have not shown the slightest remorse or contrition for your evil deeds and you have subjected the family and friends of your victims to having to re-live the tragedy and grief you visited on them.

After imposing 15 life sentences and a four-year sentence for forgery, Justice Forbes broke with tradition by not sending his sentencing recommendation, in writing, to the Home Secretary. Instead, he said:

> In your case I am satisfied justice demands that I make my views known at the conclusion of this trial. I have formed the conclusion that the crimes you stand convicted of are so heinous that in your case "life" must mean life. My recommendation will be that you spend the remainder of your days in prison.

Dr. Shipman was then hurried out of the courtroom without a glance toward his family. The 57-day trial that Judge Forbes characterized as "deeply disturbing" and "historic" was finally over.

Why Did Dr. Shipman Kill?

Since Dr. Shipman has consistently denied killing anyone, despite incontrovertible evidence, we can only speculate on why he became history's most prolific serial killer. An unnamed physician who knew Shipman told the BBC:

> [Shipman] has got a huge defense mechanism against the incursion of reality. He probably found a way to disguise to himself what he has done.

The experience of killing was intensely personal and private to him and he is never going to give that up. We are never going to know the truth. All we can say is that he has been killing people for years.

In the case of Kathleen Grundy, the obvious motive seemed to have been greed, although his handling of the situation was so sloppy as to suggest that he wanted to be caught. In the case of other victims, objects—often of little value—were frequently missing from the victim's homes. Many of these items were later found in Shipman's home. He may have taken them as trophies, as do other serial killers.

Observers, including the prosecutor at his trial, have suggested that Dr. Shipman simply enjoyed killing and being present, with his enormous power over life and death, when his victims died. In that regard, he would be much like H. H. Holmes, the torture doctor. During his trial, Shipman gave some indication about his true feelings toward some of his more demanding patients when he called them "irritating."

Psychiatrist Ian Stephen told interviewers that Shipman "felt guilty that he had not been able to ease his mother's death with morphine when he was a teenager, so he set out to repeat her death and this time be in control of it." Psychologist Alan Wise thought that Shipman "was driven by the thrill of having the ultimate power over someone's life and death. He also had an obsessive-compulsive disorder. He developed this ritualistic act to kill and then felt compelled to repeat the act over and over."

A forensic psychiatrist who worked for the police suggested that Shipman's motivation might have been a form of necrophilia (having a bizarre sexual attraction for, and often performing sexual acts with, corpses). In Dr. Shipman's case, however, there is no evidence that there was physical sexual contact with his victims. Said Dr. Richard Badcock, "He was a necrophile—obsessed not with having sex with the dead, but with the act of inducing death and controlling the moment." This last is perhaps the best explanation for Shipman's motives, since necrophilia may result from transforming a fear of the dead (and death) into a desire for the dead—a "reaction formation" in psychiatric jargon.

Epilogue

The British Medical Profession

The post-Shipman fallout has been devastating to the British medical profession. By mid-2001, faced with other scandals within the health care community and granted emergency powers designed to protect patients, the General Medical Council was banning an average of one doctor a week from practicing medicine. One of the first casualties was Dr. Alan Banks, who advised the police during their first, aborted investigation of Dr. Shipman. Dr. Banks was suspended as an advisor to the health authority. Many others were not as fortunate; some physicians were removed from medical practice based on ridiculously little evidence. Innocent physicians were caught in the web of fear, and their patients were left without their longtime caregivers.

One example of the atmosphere of hysteria that overtook the medical community is Dr. Peter Lindsay, a GP from Pudsey in West Leeds. At 6:30 A.M. on January 24, 2001, police arrested the doctor at his home for the "very serious" charge of misusing lethal drugs on elderly patients. Although he had practiced medicine in the same town for 20 years, it took only an anonymous phone call (supposedly from another physician) and the accusation that some diamorphine was missing for police to arrest him.

Occurring as it did in the midst of the Shipman disaster, the inquiry immediately garnered local and national attention. Newspaper headlines such as "GP Quizzed Over Seven Deaths" ruined his reputation. Dr. Lindsay was stripped of his practice (the British National Health Service can do that simply by taking away a physician's patient list) and jailed on "suicide watch." Five months later, authorities "regretted" their mistake: the drugs were not missing, but rather being kept in the nursing homes and hospices or with district nurses that had to dispense them. There is no evidence that Dr. Lindsay ever acted improperly. The only impropriety that investigators found was that the doctor occasionally used *the wrong form* to record his drug use. Nevertheless, his career is ruined and his patients are without their physician. The authorities who acted so rashly have continued on without even a slap on the wrist.

These episodes are harming an already battered British medical system. Britain's physicians have been under nearly constant attack, as have those in the United States, for several years. This has led to a 15 percent drop, since 1997, in the number of applicants to the Britain's 24 medical schools. According to Dr. Ian Bogle, chairman of the British Medical Association, this was the first decrease in applicants in at least 40 years. Surveys of GPs have also shown that 60 percent of them are less likely than they were five years ago to recommend that young people enter the medical profession, and that they are increasingly likely to consider either quitting medicine or changing their career direction.

Nevertheless, the British government has established a complex bureaucratic system to "revalidate" British physicians and check the quality of their practices. The system, expected to cost between £7.85 million and £50 million by the time it is fully implemented in 2009, has been criticized from all quarters as being too cumbersome and time-consuming. Yet, even this new system is inadequate to address all the significant issues.

Professor Liam Donaldson, Britain's chief medical officer, tried to re-establish faith in the medical profession by saying, "Everything points to a doctor with the sinister and macabre motivation of a Harold Shipman as being a once-in-a-lifetime occurrence." A 2001 public poll showed that 89 percent of the British public still trusted their doctors to tell them the truth—up 2 percent from immediately after Shipman was convicted.

Dr. Shipman

Although many more alleged victims were identified after the trial, the chief prosecutor ruled out any more trials. He indicated that the massive publicity during the first trial would never again allow Shipman to have a fair trial in Britain. Eventually, people began speaking of the victims who were not among the 15 deaths for which Shipman was convicted as the "B" list. The police announced that Shipman would be charged with another 23 murders, although it is unlikely that he will ever go to trial. When this was announced, the press began calling Shipman "the British Mengele," comparing him to the notorious Nazi concentration camp doctor.

Until late April 2001, he refused to speak again with the police. At that point, he agreed to speak with detectives from West Yorkshire about 22 deaths that occurred when he worked in Todmorden in the mid-1970s, including three individuals who died on the same day. They interviewed him for a total of 30 hours at the local police station before taking him back to his permanent home at Frankland Prison in Durham, where he has the "soft job" of translating the Harry Potter books into Braille. Shipman has continued to refuse to speak with either the police or the coroner from the Manchester area who are responsible for investigating the deaths in Hyde.

Shipman's family still supports him and visits when possible. Primrose, whose only statement has been "no comment," lives alone in a bungalow in North Yorkshire. Since the NHS stripped the doctor of his pension, she has been forced to live on her savings. Sarah, the oldest child, works in public relations, while Christopher, the next oldest, is an engineer. The two youngest boys are studying engineering and agriculture.

The Public Investigation: How Many Victims?

In February 2000, the Secretary of State for Health arranged for a private inquiry into the Shipman matter, especially to address why the system failed to identify the abnormal number of deaths—and their cause. Only its final report was to be made public. In May 2000, under the authority of the Home Secretary, Coroner John Pollard began holding closed hearings on the 287 cases involving Dr. Shipman's patients. Each of the 27 inquests he completed took about one minute and fulfilled the legal niceties. He reached a verdict of unlawful killing in 25 cases and brought an "open verdict" in two more. He was quoted in the *Manchester Evening News* as saying, "The exact figure is the figure proved in court, but it is possible there are other deaths which have not been reported or come to light and that figure could be as many as 1,000."

The people of Hyde, especially the families of Dr. Shipman's dead patients, were not pleased with the government's off-hand, secret way of dealing with these issues. Richard Lissack, QC, the lawyer for many of the relatives, said that Shipman had "moved unchecked through families and streets and bit by bit murdered the heart of a community." The relatives successfully petitioned the government to hold full, open hearings into all of Dr. Shipman's possible murders. The British government then issued an order, under the Coroner's Act of 1988, to stop the coroner's inquests until the findings of new public hearings are completed and their report is issued.

In Britain, the Criminal Injuries Compensation Board, a government-funded organization, pays at least £10,000 to the close family (husband, wife, long-term partner, parent, or child) of a murder victim. If a widow dies and leaves several adult children, each receives £5,000. An additional £20,000 can be paid to individuals for excessive psychological damage. Since the perpetrator does not have to be convicted for the family to be compensated, more than 400 families can claim compensation in the Shipman case. Many have not yet heard that they can be compensated, so, as of mid-2001, the Board had paid only £700,000. According to solicitor Ann Alexander, "Compensation has never been an important issue for many of the relatives." However, the amount could eventually total nearly £5 million.

Public hearings, under Britain's 1912 Tribunal of Inquiry (Evidence) Act, into the deaths of 618 of Dr. Shipman's former patients began in mid-2001 in Manchester. The hearings will inevitably include some natural deaths among them. To be investigated are: the 451 deaths where some records exist, the deaths of the 15 women Shipman has already been convicted of killing, and at least 152 more deaths for which Shipman signed the death certificate. The families and friends of the decedents are viewing the proceedings via closed-circuit television from an annex of the Hyde library, only a two-minute walk from Shipman's former clinic. Security guards protect them from the media, and grief counselors are in constant attendance. Some survivors, even though they have repeatedly come to watch the proceedings, have not been able to step into the room; their grief is still too fresh.

The purpose of the inquiry, succinctly stated by counsel to the inquiry Caroline Swift, QC, is "wherever possible, worried relatives should receive an answer to the question, 'Did Shipman kill my parent, grandparent, aunt, uncle or friend?'" Dame Janet Smith, DBE, the High Court judge who chairs the investigation, voiced their concerns:

> That a doctor had been able to amass large quantities of diamorphine and to kill so many patients without detection. Why had the regulations which require a record to be made of the acquisition and supply of all controlled drugs, failed to prevent Shipman from obtaining diamorphine illicitly? Why had this not been noticed, especially in view of his convictions for drug abuse in 1976? Why had our systems of death certification with the availability of postmortem examination and coroner's inquest failed to detect and arrest the progress of this serial killer?

The inquiry will first attempt to determine exactly which patients were killed, and how. Investigating many of the deaths may be difficult. While the inquiry's investigation team initially examined 466 deaths, there are at least another 152 of Shipman's dead patients for which the only remaining evidence is an entry in the death registry. The medical records of those who died before 1991 were destroyed, according to standard procedures, before Dr. Shipman's murderous activities came to light. For many deaths prior to 1984, not even cremation certificates have survived. As Judge Smith said:

> [I] did not know whether it would be feasible for me to attempt to reach a decision on individual deaths. I wished to do so because I recognised the need for families to know the truth ... I have decided that I shall attempt to reach a decision in each individual case ... However, it will not be possible in every case for me to provide a definite answer, one way or the other.

Professor Richard Baker authored the clinical audit of Dr. Shipman's practice for Britain's National Health Service, which was published in January 2001. An epidemiologist, Dr. Baker works in the Clinical Governance and Research and Development Unit in the Department of General Practice and Primary Health Care, University of Leicester. Shipman issued 499 death certificates during 1978–1998. These were higher numbers than for any other practitioner in Hyde and Greater Manchester for almost every year during that period. In the understated language of statisticians, Dr. Baker noted, "The findings from the various components of the audit have dreadful implications, and give rise to grave concerns about the activities of Harold Shipman during his career as a general practitioner."

During this period, Baker found that, compared to Shipman's 499 deaths, the highest number of death certificates issued by any other practitioner was 210. Further, Shipman issued 297 (and possibly as many as 345) more death certificates than comparable colleagues during his entire medical career. His patients didn't die as often in the early 1990s, but, by 1995, they were dying at a brisk rate. In 1997, 39 of Shipman's patients died, while none of the other five GPs in Hyde reached double figures. Baker concluded that the death rates of general practitioners' patients should be included in Britain's monitoring system.

While Shipman had backdated some computerized records, the system to track these changes had not been in operation long enough to gather much data. The state of his written records was so atrocious that it was hard to say how many entries had been falsified. Shipman did admit in court, however, that he had backdated some medical records. He claimed he knew that the computerized system was tracking his changes.

Baker also found that during the 24 years Shipman spent as a GP, a significantly higher proportion of his older female patients died than compared to other GPs. The greatest number of excess deaths was for women aged 75 years or older; the second highest for women aged 65 to 74 years; and the third highest for men aged 75 years or older.

An extraordinary number of Shipman's patients died suddenly and at home. Baker discovered that there were 236 (and possibly as many as 277) more deaths at home among Shipman's patients than among his colleagues. According to Baker, this last figure may constitute the bulk of Shipman's murders. Statistics also showed that Shipman's patients had the unusual habit of dying on Monday, Tuesday, and Friday afternoons between 1 P.M. and 7 P.M. (presumably, when it would be more convenient for him).

A remarkable number of patients died when Shipman was either present or had recently seen them. Also, he certified the cause of death for an unusually large number of patients as "heart problems," "stroke," or "old age." The association between the cause of death listed was often not substantiated by the patients' medical records or the autopsy. Dr. Baker concluded that Dr.

Shipman had murdered patients throughout his career, not just in Hyde or during the latter years of his medical practice.

A separate, less-exact audit by a newspaper reporter in Todmorden revealed that for the time Shipman worked there (March 1, 1974, to September 30, 1975), there were 401 total deaths in the town. This was excessive compared to the 19 months before he arrived (348 deaths) and the 19 months after he left (372 deaths).

When investigators have determined what they believe to be a good estimate of the number of murders Dr. Shipman committed, the inquiry will move to "Phase Two," the in-depth examination of each of four elements of the case:

1. **Postmortem practices**
   Death and cremation certification. The roles of the informant, medical practitioners, medical referees, the registrar, and coroner. The custom and practice, generally and in Hyde. Should funeral directors have a role? The forms used. Should they be changed? What is considered good practice? The practices followed in the Shipman cases.
   Reporting and investigation of sudden deaths. The roles of the police, paramedics, and coroner. Good practice. The practices followed in the Shipman cases.
   The systems for monitoring or analyzing mortality rates. What did such systems reveal about Shipman?

2. **The first, aborted police investigation in March 1998**

3. **Controls on dangerous prescription medications**
   The procedures for prescribing, dispensing (to include provision on signed orders), collecting, delivering, storing, and disposing of controlled drugs and the monitoring of those procedures by the Home Office and the police. What did such monitoring reveal about Shipman?

4. **The monitoring system for British general practitioners**
   Whistle-blowing. The opportunity available to those in positions of responsibility (including medical colleagues, nurses, health visitors, practice staff, pharmacists, funeral directors, sheltered-housing staff, and staff of nursing and residential homes) to report concerns or suspicions about the conduct of a medical practitioner. Good practice. What reports of concern were made about Shipman and how were they dealt with? What further reports ought to have been made?

Disciplinary rules for general medical practitioners and the operation of the disciplinary processes operated within the NHS and by the General Medical Council. Powers of suspension. What happened in the case of Shipman?

The system for recording information about medical practitioners' qualifications and past history (including criminal convictions) and for communicating such information to those who may be considering appointing or employing them. What information is recorded arising from errors and complaints? What information was conveyed about Shipman?

The system for monitoring the performance of general medical practitioners, with particular reference to those in single-person practice, recordkeeping, and prescribing. The role of patients and their complaints in the monitoring of a GP's practice. The role of practice staff in reporting on the performance of a GP. The role of the former Regional Medical Officer. How was Shipman's work monitored and with what result? Accountability of GPs and Health Authorities.

During the inquiry, expert witnesses will testify in person, while lay witnesses will submit written testimony. All testimony will be made public and published, as will interim and final reports. Upon completion of the inquiry, the authorities will use the information gained to suggest how to change practices to better protect patients. The question of why Dr. Shipman killed hundreds of patients remains a matter of speculation, since he adamantly refuses to participate in this inquiry—or even to admit his guilt.

In mid-2001, Yorkshire TV produced a television dramatization of this case that has been condemned. Said a spokesman, "The memories of these awful events are still extremely painful for the close relatives of the victims and the people of Hyde. It is insulting to even contemplate making a TV drama at this time."

Perhaps the public has had a difficult time believing the extent of Dr. Shipman's evil deeds because, in the words of journalist Nicci Gerrard, he "offers us no glimpse into ourselves. He will not become a symbol of anything; his story spreads few ripples. His voice is dry, neutral. His face is blank. His eyes are polite and empty. His lips are closed. His heart is a mystery."

And Harold Frederick Shipman was a doctor.

Exhumations: Raising the Dead*

Exhumation, or *disinterment*, is the removal of an already-buried body from a grave or other burial site.

In recent times, authorities have permitted exhumations only for serious purposes and in "circumstances of extreme exigency." English secular law, for example, once strictly forbade disinterments. This was overcome by vesting exhumation authority in a religious officer, known as an "ordinary," who could authorize the exhumation under church law. Statutes now permit exhumations if they are in the public interest.

Normally, a court order is required before a body can be exhumed. In Britain, if the body is to be reinterred in the same churchyard gravesite from which it is exhumed, a church license (Bishop's Faculty) is also required. The British have, in the past, claimed to have less cause for exhumations than in the United States, since "it is very unusual [in Britain] for a victim of death from violence to escape a coroner's necropsy before burial." That, of course, was before Dr. Shipman. Objections to exhumations often come from family members, those who do not want further investigation of a case, and law enforcement officials who may be embarrassed by the results.

Disinterment is usually allowed if it is required to determine a cause of death, for historic/scientific purposes, to move a body to another burial site, or to establish a corpse's identity. Permission to exhume bodies has generally been denied if the request is made simply to gather information for a civil suit or to establish inheritance rights. In the past, however, corpses have often been disinterred for personal reasons.

Political and Religious Exhumations

At one time, the Catholic Church commonly tried the dead for heresy and other offenses. If convicted, their remains were exhumed and, if the offense would have warranted a death penalty, burned. Otherwise, the remains were usually reburied in unhallowed ground. For example, Pope Formosus' (d. 896) body was disinterred twice for his crimes. Pope Stephen VII, spurred by political motives, had the dead Pope's body exhumed and dragged through the streets. Then, after trying the corpse in what is popularly called the "Cadaver Synod," they cut off its fingers of consecration. The remains were again buried, but Pope Sergius III repeated the trial, disinterment, and punishment.

Although St. Ivo of Chartres stated in 1100 that the dead could neither be tried nor denied burial, the Church subsequently tried, exhumed, and "punished" several bodies, including Gherardo of Florence (d. 1250), who was tried for heresy in 1313, and John Wyclif (d. 1384), who was tried for heresy in 1425.

---

*Adapted from Iserson KV: *Death to Dust: What Happens To Dead Bodies?* 2nd ed. Tucson, AZ: Galen Press, Ltd., 2001.

continued . . .

Exhumations: Raising the Dead, continued

Not to be outdone, the Church of England convicted Thomas à Becket, the Archbishop of Canterbury and Chancellor to Henry II (d. 1170), of high treason around 1540. They exhumed his remains and publicly burned his bones.

There have also been exhumations for political retribution. For example, on January 30, 1661, the anniversary of the beheading of Charles I, the British House of Commons unanimously voted to exhume the bodies of Oliver Cromwell (d. 1658) and his two compatriots, Ireton (d. 1651) and Bradshaw (d. 1659). The remains were removed from their exalted resting places in Westminster Abbey and, "in their shrouds, [were] hanged by the neck until the going down of the sun." At sunset, their bodies were taken down; the heads were removed and placed on pikes outside Westminster for public exhibition, while the torsos were thrown into a pit under the gallows at Tyburn prison. Cromwell's skull remained rotting on a spike for about 18 years, until it was blown down in a storm and found by a passing soldier. In 1781, the soldier's daughter sold the skull to a private citizen for £118; it was later used as an exhibit in a peep show. It now resides at Sidney Sussex College in Cambridge, which Cromwell attended as a youth.

A tragic love story ended in a series of exhumations. Héloïse and Abelard, the famous unrequited lovers, were originally buried together. In 1630, however, an abbess decided that the burial of a monk and a nun in the same grave was indecent. (The couple had entered religious orders after they were forcibly separated during life.) She had the skeletons disinterred and reburied separately. During the French Revolution, their skeletons were disinterred again and purchased by a physician; later, the remains were given to the Museum of National Antiquities for display, where they joined the bones of the French writer Molière. Héloïse and Abelard's skeletons were eventually re-interred together in a special tomb. Molière's skeleton was reburied in the Parisian cemetery of Père-Lachaise.

Exhumations for Repatriation

Today a person's remains may be exhumed and transferred to another burial site for several reasons. Families or friends may often move a body so it can "rest" near those of other relatives. This is normally approved if all interested parties, such as next of kin and the owner of the cemetery (but not including the estate's executor), agree. When cemeteries are abandoned, the remains may be removed to another site.

On occasion, especially with deaths in foreign countries, bodies are buried temporarily with the clear intent of later moving them to their "final" resting spot. This usually causes no problems, as long as death was not from a serious easily transmitted disease such as diphtheria, typhus, or plague. In those cases, the body normally can be exhumed only if it is in an hermetically sealed container.

continued . . .

Exhumations: Raising the Dead, continued

One of the more unusual cases of "repatriating" the dead occurred in 1997. An aboriginal warrior, Yagan, was shot and killed in 1833 and his head was smoked. The head was on display at Liverpool City Museum until 1964, when it was haphazardly buried in the local cemetery among the remains of 22 babies. In 1997, the head was exhumed and returned to the Australian government. After its return, the Australians ceremoniously buried the head near the place where Yagan was shot.

Exhumations for Historical Purposes

Bodies have also been disinterred to enhance knowledge of medical history, to verify historical events, and to put bizarre theories to rest.

In 1972, the embalmed corpse of a 2,100-year-old "Chinese Princess" was found in the Hunan Province of China. She was exhumed and Chinese pathologists performed an autopsy. They found she had suffered from heart and gall-bladder disease, had been afflicted with three types of intestinal parasites and tuberculosis, had a poorly healed arm fracture, and had arthritis of her spine. Pathologists were also able to determine that she had borne children.

In 1508, St. Dunstan's remains were secretly exhumed more than 500 years after his death to retrieve part of his crown as a holy relic. The tomb of King Edward I of England was reopened in 1774 merely to document his burial clothes and accouterments (a robe of gold and silver tissue and another of crimson velvet, a scepter in each hand, and a jeweled crown).

Those exhumed are not always treated kindly. The body of King John (of Robin Hood fame) was accidentally exposed during repairs to the Worcestershire Cathedral in 1797. One worker took this opportunity to use a piece of the tyrant's body as fish bait—and he actually caught a fish using it. During the French Revolution, the body of King Henry IV was exhumed and torn to pieces by a mob. When the Bolsheviks took control of Russia in 1918, they entered the Kremlin to open the tombs and mock the bodies of the Czars. It is claimed that when they opened the tomb of Ivan Groznyi (the Terrible), his body was so well preserved and his visage so fierce that they quickly closed the tomb and left.

The tomb of the boy princes, Edward V and Richard, Duke of York (both killed by King Richard III), was opened in 1674 and again in 1932. The skeletal remains of the brothers, who had been first imprisoned and then murdered in the Tower of London, were examined both times for several reasons: to verify that the remains were indeed theirs, to determine a cause of death, and to try to determine who murdered them. The first exhumation was actually accidental, since Richard III had hidden their bodies. The second was done for scientific and historical reasons: The boys' identities and that of their killer were confirmed, but, since so much time had elapsed, no cause of death could be verified.

continued . . .

Exhumations: Raising the Dead, continued

To test an old conspiracy theory, forensic scientists exhumed the body of Zachary Taylor, twelfth President of the United States, in the early 1990s. Using modern scientific methods, they analyzed the remains to check for poisons; none were found. Permission to exhume and re-autopsy the bodies of John F. Kennedy and presidential assassin John Wilkes Booth has, however, been repeatedly denied.

Similarly, the body of Dr. Carl Weiss, the alleged assassin of Senator Huey Long of Louisiana, was exhumed to look for missing bullets (none were found). To test one of the many conspiracy theories, Lee Harvey Oswald, President John F. Kennedy's assassin, was exhumed to be sure that he, and not a Soviet agent, was buried in his grave. It contained his remains. In 1985, the purported remains of war criminal Dr. Josef Mengele, the German mass murderer at the Auschwitz death camp, were exhumed from a small cemetery near Sao Paulo, Brazil. All types of analysis available, including video superimposition of facial photographs, were used to ascertain the corpse's identity; it was he.

Forensic Exhumations

Forensic pathologists rarely undertake exhumations. In part, this is due to the high cost of disinterment-reinterment: to open and close the grave; replace or repair a vault, grave liner, or casket; and pay for the pathologist may total $4,000 or more. The frequency of exhumations depends on various factors, including an area's political climate, dominant religions, funding, legal system, and autopsy rate.

Forensic pathologists exhume bodies to:

1. Investigate the cause or manner of death.
2. Collect evidence (such as bullets or hair fragments).
3. Determine the cause of an accident or the presence of disease.
4. Gather evidence to assess malpractice.
5. Compare the body with another person thought to be deceased.
6. Identify war and accident victims who were hastily buried without identification.
7. Settle accidental death or liability claims.
8. Search for lost (often valuable) objects.

Exhumed bodies are not pretty. According to Dr. Jesse Carr, former Chief of Pathology at San Francisco General Hospital:

> An exhumed embalmed body is a repugnant, moldy, foul-looking object. It's not the image of one who has been loved. You might use the quotation "John Brown's body lies a-moldering in the grave"; that really sums it up. The body itself may be intact, as far as contours and so on; but the silk lining of the casket is all stained with body fluids, the wood is rotting, and the body is covered with mold.

continued . . .

Exhumations: Raising the Dead, continued

To counteract the odor, pathologists put benzoin on their masks, spray fragrant aerosols, or freeze the remains before the examination. Before gloves came into routine use in the mid-1900s, pathologists often put soap under their fingernails before starting an autopsy on decomposed or exhumed bodies to prevent the smell from lingering on their hands.

Aside from bones, the connective and adipose (fat) tissues and some tissues in the internal organs (interstitial and perivascular) are preserved the longest. Sufficient heart and lung material for adequate examination may remain after several years. Adipocere (a fatty change in tissue due to water immersion) helps preserve some tissues. As analytical methods have improved, exhumation to perform toxicological tests has become more important. One group, for example, found parathion (a potent insecticide sometimes used as a poison) in an exhumed body 17 years after burial.

While pathologists now autopsy exhumed corpses in the morgue, these autopsies were once routinely conducted at the graveside. By necessity, this practice was also used in disinterments carried out during the post-World War II war-crimes investigations. Disinterment and autopsy may take place behind screens, although some have been done in full view at the graveside—and the resulting distress has occasionally resulted in court-imposed damages awarded to the family. The next of kin or their representatives are commonly invited to be present for the disinterment.

In a disinterment for medicolegal reasons, photographs are taken as soon as the casket is opened. After the remains are removed and transferred to an autopsy table, the body is weighed, measured, and, in many cases, x-rayed. Fingerprints and hair samples are obtained whenever possible. Mold is cleaned off to reveal scars, tattoos, birthmarks, or other identifying information. Dental structures and abnormalities are carefully recorded for use in identification, and dental x-rays may be taken. Pathologists perform as much of a forensic autopsy as possible, including tests for toxins. After the examination, the body is reburied.

The most sensational disinterments have been done to investigate homicides, suspected homicides, and deaths resulting from other criminal activity. When bodies are exhumed by accident, such as happens at archaeological digs, paleontological sites, and construction sites, or by natural events, such as floods, forensic pathologists and anthropologists must determine whether the body was a routine burial or is evidence of criminal activity.

Criminal cases may warrant disinterment if new evidence appears after a victim has been buried without recognition of foul play, such as in the Shipman cases. In one instance, a 9-year-old girl died in a fire and, because of new evidence, she was exhumed 10 years later. The new autopsy revealed that she had died from a stab wound to the neck. (Attempting to hide a murder with a fire is

continued . . .

Exhumations: Raising the Dead, continued

relatively common, and forensic pathologists rarely miss this.) In another case, the initial autopsy determined that a man had died as a result of being run over by a car. A second autopsy after exhumation revealed three bullets in his brain, the actual cause of his demise.

Suspicion of foul play may lead to exhumation, especially if no autopsy was originally performed, the results are questioned, or new tests have been developed. In a bizarre case, authorities exhumed the body of an 89-year-old woman when they suspected that Mark Villella, a funeral director in Orange City, Florida, had murdered his wife. They found his wife's body stuffed under the elderly woman in her casket. Villella stabbed his wife when she told him she wanted a divorce, and then took her body to the funeral home and stored it in the cooler. Four days later, he placed her body underneath the elderly woman for burial.

Pathologists have also used exhumation to determine the extent of therapeutic catastrophes. In 1964 and 1965, up to 24 Belgians with prostate cancer were inadvertently given pills containing large doses of digitoxin (a long-acting heart medication and potential poison), instead of estradiol, a hormone. They died and were buried before anyone suspected there was a problem. A forensic team disinterred the bodies from 17 to 40 months after death and determined the true cause of their deaths—accidental poisoning.

Political and wartime mass murders have been reasons to exhume bodies. Some of the most notorious are the Russian massacre of Polish soldiers in the Katyn Forest during World War II, the German massacre of Italian civilians in Rome's Ardentine caves, the deaths of prisoners in German concentration camps, and the thousands of civilians who "disappeared" under the former Argentine dictatorship. Recent mass exhumations have occurred in Kosovo, Croatia, Mexico, Russia, and Rwanda. Disinterment techniques also reconstructed the events of General Custer's last battle at Little Bighorn.

Exhumations for Other Reasons

Occasionally, bodies have been exhumed for very personal reasons. One family had their son's body exhumed to retrieve a wallet buried with him. It contained $64 and some credit cards. The exhumation cost $2,149!

Also, in 1960, an English man disinterred his mother who had been buried earlier that morning. He took the body to an empty house where he attempted to revive her by feeding her a mixture of plasma, sugar, lime juice, and milk. He then used electric shocks, connecting her foot to the house's electric source until it short-circuited. Abraham Lincoln, for example, in an expression of unassuaged grief, reportedly had the body of his favorite child, Willy, disinterred twice so he could gaze upon the boy's face.

continued . . .

Exhumations: Raising the Dead, continued

A romantic, albeit macabre, exhumation took place at Highgate Cemetery in London. The well-known nineteenth-century poet and painter, Dante Gabriel Rossetti, buried the only manuscript of several poems with the body of his wife, Elizabeth Eleanor Siddal. Seven years later, in 1869, he decided to retrieve the poems. One autumn night, by the light of a great bonfire, the lady's body was disinterred. Onlookers reported that the corpse's very long flaming-red hair covered the manuscript and some strands were removed with the book. Rossetti wrote to his brother, "All in the coffin was found quite perfect; but the book, though not in any way destroyed, is soaked through and through and had to be still further saturated with disinfectants." After the manuscript was dried and disinfected, it was returned to its author.

With the ability to do DNA analysis, increasing numbers of researchers and lawyers are seeking to exhume bodies for identification and to test paternity claims. Some of those exhumed for DNA testing include: French singer Yves Montand (he wasn't the father); Anna Anderson Manahan, who claimed to be Russian Princess Anastasia (she wasn't); Jesse James's remains in Missouri (it's him); and Butch Cassidy and the Sundance Kid in Bolivia (they only found a German miner's remains). Requests to test dictators Juan Peron's and Benito Mussolini's remains for paternity are pending.

10

Serial Killers: Psychology & Behavior

How could there be so much evil in the world? Knowing humanity, I wonder
why there is not more of it.

— Woody Allen, *Hannah and Her Sisters*

How many serial killers and murders are there?

Like the bogeyman, serial killers continue to haunt us. In 1983, LAPD
homicide investigator Pierce Brooks estimated that as many as 12,000 people
were murdered by serial killers every year. However, many experts believe that
number is too high. In 1988, for example, Holmes & De Burger estimated that
of the approximately 5,000 unsolved murders each year (a number that has
remained fairly constant), between 25 and 65 percent, or 1,250–3,250, are
serial murders.

Based on investigators' interviews with serial killers, it appears that, on
average, each one kills 10 to 12 people over a several-year period. As Dr.
Shipman demonstrated, some will greatly exceed this number. Most experts
estimate that there are about 35 serial killers operating at any one time in the
United States. Most will never be apprehended.

Serial killings may be on the rise. Robert Ressler, who was instrumental in
the formation of the FBI's Behavioral Science Unit, said, "I think it's at epidemic proportion. The type of crime we're seeing today did not really occur
with any known frequency prior to the fifties. An individual taking 10, 12, 15,
25, 35 lives is a relatively new phenomenon in the crime picture of the U.S."

Holmes & Holmes, in *Profiling Violent Crimes: An Investigative Tool* (1996), stated:

> [It] would be an error to assume that we are all potential victims of serial killers, or that there is a serial killer around every corner. However, from our own experiences with police departments across the United States, we believe that current estimates concerning numbers of victims may be too high, but estimates of numbers of killers may actually be too low ...
>
> It is our estimate that there are at least 100 serial murderers currently active in the United States. Estimates of the numbers of victims have been questioned by many experts ...
>
> It should be kept in mind that some serial killers may kill no more than one victim a year, or none at all during particular periods of time (perhaps because they are prevented from doing so by illness or incarceration). But there is no doubt that a substantial number of the victims who fall prey to serial predators, including killers, each year are not recognized as serialists' victims because of lack of communication among law enforcement agencies, law enforcement turf issues, and some law enforcement personnel's simple refusal to identify or accept some cases as instances of serial murder.

Even the number of deaths that can be attributed to those serial killers who are apprehended is in doubt. While some take their secrets to the grave, others seek the limelight once they have been caught. As Douglas & Olshaker wrote:

> We're all conditioned by the media ... Serial criminals are like that too. Many of them are proud of their "accomplishments," and once they're incarcerated, they want to be known as the biggest, the baddest, and the best. The late and unlamented Ted Bundy used to get off on academics writing to him saying they wanted to study the sophisticated criminal mind. Henry Lee Lucas claimed credit for at least seventy murders he did not commit.

How did experts develop a definition of a "serial killer"?

Most work on psychopaths (and related diagnostic labels) has centered on males, since experts believe that less than 10 percent of psychopaths are women. Italian psychiatrist Cesare Lombrosos launched scientific criminology in the late nineteenth century after examining thousands of prisoners and soldiers. In a description that now seems both quaint and simplistic, he identified five types of criminals, based on unique facial traits that police could use to identify potential criminals:

1. The born criminal
2. The insane criminal
3. The criminal by passion
4. The habitual criminal
5. The occasional criminal

In his 1941 book, *The Mask of Sanity*, Hervey Cleckley expanded on Lombrosos's work and described the clinical characteristics of psychopaths. Among these are a lack of empathy or anxiety, and being hot-headed, manipulative, irresponsible, self-centered, and shallow. Psychopaths are likely to commit more types of crimes than other offenders, are more violent, are more likely to repeat crimes, and are less likely to respond to treatment.

Psychological descriptions of multiple murderers have long been confusing, overlapping, and nonspecific. These individuals have been called psychopaths, sociopaths, and sufferers from an "Antisocial (U.S. definition) or Dissocial (Europe) Personality Disorder." The criteria for such personality disorders emphasize persistent violation of society's rules, a callous disregard for others, repeated violation of other people's rights, and an inability to experience guilt or to profit from experience—especially punishment. These disorders are usually diagnosed in late childhood or adolescence based on the individual's behavior, such as repeatedly breaking the law, lying for personal benefit, impulsiveness or failure to plan ahead, repeated fights or assaults, recklessly disregarding others' safety, failure to keep a job or honor financial obligations, and being indifferent to or rationalizing behavior that hurts others. (These actions must not have occurred during acute schizophrenic or manic episodes.)

In 1952, "sociopathic personality" replaced "psychopath" in official psychiatric jargon. In 1968, the official *DSM-II* term became "personality disorder, antisocial type," with those affected being unsocialized, impulsive, without guilt, selfish, callous, and failing to learn from experience. R. D. Hare and his associates later developed a 22-item Psychopathology Checklist for rating potential psychopaths. Their criteria included a lack of remorse or empathy, shallow emotions, manipulativeness, lying, egocentricity, glibness, low frustration tolerance, episodic relationships, parasitic lifestyle, the persistent violation of social norms, need for stimulation, and criminal versatility.

The checklist used these elements grouped around a narcissistic personality and antisocial behavior. Otto Kernberg, in *Borderline Conditions and Pathological Narcissism* (1975), describes the antisocial personality as being based on "malignant narcissism," or amorality and self-absorption with a sadistic component. Despite the professional jargon, the common term for such individuals remains "psychopath."

Various pseudoscientific terms have also been attached to serial killers. These include "dacomaniac," those with a mania for killing; "homicidomaniac," those with an insane compulsion to kill; "phonomaniac," an insane individual with homicidal tendencies; and "murderholic," an individual addicted to killing.

Why does someone become a serial killer?

No one really knows.

It can be almost impossible to determine the root cause for the behavior of many of these killers. In 1898, the Journal of the American Medical Association claimed that "only about 20 to 25 percent of criminals are born criminals. Three-fourths of the crime in our land is caused by neglected education." Things haven't changed much in the last hundred years; we are still asking the same question: Are serial killers born that way, or does their behavior stem from their environment?

Multiple killers have usually had some experience at a very young age that teaches them that they are rewarded with pleasure for their socially unacceptable behavior. Unfortunately for researchers, many of these individuals have repressed the memory of the experience. In addition, multiple killers do not view their behavior as deviant or abnormal, but they do realize that it must be hidden to prevent society's retribution.

While still children, these killers recognized that manipulating others gave them a sense of power that they lacked in other areas of their lives. They established preferred behaviors in the same way all people do, by receiving personal rewards—"reinforcement"—when they performed certain acts. In their case, these rewards are for what most people view as aberrant acts, and may include a sense of power, vindication, and even joy. As with all learned behaviors, if they do not get this type of reinforcement, they stop doing it.

Psychologist Lonnie Athens, in *The Creation of Dangerous Violent Criminals*, suggests that people become violent in four stages, all brought on by external factors: brutalization and subjugation (as powerless children), belligerency, violent coaching (by parents and acquaintances), and criminal activity. Other explanations for such behavior include childhood abuse, chemical imbalances, brain injuries, exposure to traumatic events, and perceived societal injustices.

But the environment may not be the only factor. Some studies suggest that children can inherit a sociopathic predisposition. One Danish study of twins who had been raised apart since birth found that biological relatives of psychopaths were four to five times more likely to be sociopathic than the average person.

Further insight into such individuals' minds comes from their own (rare) statements. Unlike most medical killers, Arthur Warren Waite was surprisingly candid about his motivation. Waite, a dentist, murdered his in-laws in 1916. He planned to kill the rest of his family using arsenic, ground glass, influenza germs, a nasal spray of tuberculosis organisms, and chloroform. Waite explained:

> I have always been for myself, and never cared for others. If I wanted money, I got it. I am a coward, and whenever I have been in a hole, I took the easiest way out. My life consisted of lying, cheating, stealing, and killing. My personality was that of a gentleman, and I went in for music, art, and poetry—as far as I thought it was required by my vocation.

Douglas cautioned, however, that "while an abusive or dysfunctional background can explain why you might become a dysfunctional, unhappy, or otherwise psychologically messed-up adult, it doesn't explain away, or let you off the hook for, perpetrating acts of violence against other human beings." Many people with backgrounds identical to mass killers have become normal, well-adjusted members of their community. It also raises anew forensic psychologist Dr. Stanton Samenow's question, "How [can] you expect to *rehabilitate* an individual who has never been *habilitated* in the first place." [original italics] That these individuals may not be candidates for rehabilitation comes through clearly in a quotation from Dr. Mudgett/Holmes, whose confession was published and serialized by William Randolph Hearst in 1896:

> Like a man-eating tiger of the tropical jungle, whose appetite for blood has once been aroused, I roamed about the world seeking whom I could destroy . . . I committed this and other crimes for the pleasure of killing my fellow beings, to hear their cries for mercy and pleas to be allowed even sufficient time to pray and prepare for death.

Dr. Holmes' words seem eerily similar to comments made by modern serial killers.

Are there early warning signs or predisposing factors to identify potential serial killers?

For more than a century, researchers, psychologists, and police investigators have tried to identify childhood characteristics that could be used to determine who might become a serial killer. They have had only limited success. The problem is that it is difficult to assess identifying traits in adolescents, since most adolescents are angry, moody, and defiant. Experts believe that children and adolescents who exhibit a persistent pattern of antisocial behavior should be monitored, however, since about half of these children become adult psychopaths. Eighty-two percent of sociopaths report day-dreaming so much as a child that it became a problem for them, 71 percent report chronic lying, 80 percent report running away from home, and 83 percent had severe temper tantrums.

Of course, not all such children become criminals, although they may become sociopaths. John McHoskey and his colleagues demonstrated the prevalence of sociopathy in children using a testing instrument they developed based on the sixteenth-century writings of Niccoló Machiavelli. Called the "Kiddie-MACH," it tests the strategies that people use to gain and maintain interpersonal power.

Profilers, psychologists, and others who study serial killers have noted the prevalence of three childhood behaviors that together have come to be called (somewhat simplistically) the "homicidal triad": bedwetting (enuresis) beyond an appropriate age, fire starting (pyromania), and cruelty to animals or smaller children. Although such information is often difficult to ascertain, some estimate that 60 percent of multiple murderers wet their beds past adolescence. As FBI profiler John Douglas, one of the first to note this pattern, was quick to point out:

> Not every boy who displays these traits is going to grow up to be a killer, but the combination of the three was so prominent in our study subjects [well-known multiple murderers] that we began recommending that a pattern (rather than isolated incidents) of any two of them should raise a warning flag for parents and teachers.

The strongest predictor of deviant behavior is the presence of extreme stress at a child's home or in their immediate environment. In this respect, all of society contributes to producing mass killers. Family members contribute by being poor role models, through physical or sexual abuse, or by interceding to protect their child from deserved consequences, by neglect, by failing to provide a nurturing environment, or by using money as a substitute for parenting. Because of such dysfunctional backgrounds, mass killers lack self-confidence and a feeling of self-worth.

Fathers are often implicated in their children's psychopathology. Seventy-two percent of serial killers report that they lack attachment to, and have no positive view of, their fathers. John Wayne Gacy's father, for example, was a violent alcoholic who beat John's mother, shot his dog, and berated him by calling John a sissy, a queer, and a failure. Albert DeSalvo's father broke his mother's fingers as young Al watched helplessly. Mothers have also been implicated. As Steven Egger notes in *The Killers Among Us*: "Serial murderers are frequently found to have unusual or unnatural relationships with their mothers . . . Perhaps we find comfort in this cliché—the mother is a ready-made excuse, particularly in our contemporary era of obsessive parenting."

Nancy H. Allen listed factors that can be used to assess the likelihood that a person will become a serial killer. These are listed on page 6 in the *Introduction*.

Do serial killers share any common characteristics?

While all serial killers are sociopaths, not all sociopaths are serial killers.

Essentially, sociopaths lack those traits that help people get along with each other in a society. One of these traits is the ability to love—serial killers develop no lasting relationships except those from which they directly benefit. Sociopaths identify with aggressive role models, and are fascinated by violence, injury, and torture. They are capable only of sadomasochistic relationships based on power. Most are highly impulsive individuals who repeatedly demonstrate aggressive behavior and who constantly search for new stimulants (thrill seekers).

As Ronald Markman, a forensic psychiatrist, wrote, "They lack the internal prohibitions, or conscience, that keep most of us from giving full expression to our most primitive, and sometimes violent impulses." As Holmes & De Burger noted, Ted Bundy exemplified the classic sociopathic aspects of the serial killer: he was unable to love and had a sadistic nature combined with anti-social personality traits such as an evasive personality, strong feelings of insecurity, general anger, and a tendency to run from problems. Not all sociopaths, however, are killers; many become successful in business or other professions. Perhaps you know some?

Between 3 and 5 percent of men are sociopaths; considerably less than 1 percent of women are sociopaths. Serial killers tend to be white males, 25 to 34 years old, lower to middle class, intelligent or at least "street smart," charming and charismatic, and police "groupies" or interested in police work. As illustrated in many of the stories in this book, as they progress in their killings, they experience a degeneration of their personality, take less time to plan their crimes, have less time between killings, and increase the level of violence. Often, they collect newspaper clippings or mementos that document their exploits, so that they can repeatedly use them to relive their fantasies during their "cooling-off periods."

Even though they may not appear so to others, serial killers perceive themselves to be society's rejects. Those who work with them agree. Former FBI profiler Robert Ressler, for example, characterized most serial killers as "complete losers and completely inadequate people in society." John Douglas classified them as "underachieving, underemployed loners." He went on to note, "there is a phenomenon with some of these guys we refer to as the 'dangerous forties.' When they get to that age and take stock, if it doesn't look as though life is going quite the way they planned it, they can pop." Talk about a midlife crisis!

Most serial killers will not speak in detail about their crimes or motivation. John Douglas, the FBI's legendary profiler, however, could sometimes get them to talk by asking them to speculate about what "the killer" might have been thinking—that is, to speak about themselves in the third person. Ronald Holmes persuaded one serial killer to let him tape an interview on the condition of anonymity. Holmes published part of the interview in his book, *Profiling Violent Crimes: An Investigative Tool.* As that killer said:

> This need for self-magnification is always, I believe, a mandatory prerequisite to any episode of violence. Just prior to his every decision to victimize, a serial killer always first experiences a sudden and precipitous psychological fall, an extreme low, which he can neither tolerate nor deal with in any rational fashion. Throughout his day-to-day existence, all of his meaning is derived from the fact that he thinks himself profoundly special, unique, and perfect over all other human beings on the face of the earth...The acting out of his cherished fantasies, he knows, will elevate him from his intolerable and infuriating psychological low; they will make things "all right" and cause him to feel good about himself; they will "prove," without any shadow of doubt, that he is really somebody...
>
> The specific methods of violence he chooses to act out, then, are perceived as "good" and "righteous," perfectly appropriate for the present, as

they have already been tried and tested in the imagination for their ability to restore his feelings of supremacy ...The consequences of this outlook are that the struggles, the pain, and the outcries of a serial killer's victim inspire nothing in the way of pity; his victim is a worthless object, wholly depersonalized, and is therefore ineligible for such a human expression as pity ... His victim's misery is the elixir that thrills him beyond all measure, for it is his tangible assurance that all is proceeding according to his well-ordered plan; it is his visible "evidence" that he is the magnificent, all-powerful creature he always knew himself to be.

In the final analysis, all serial killers, including those in this book, have one thing in common: they kill many people for their own gratification.

How do serial killers' fantasies progress to violence?

Serial killers' lives revolve around fantasy. Insecure and helpless when they cannot control a situation, they cope by manipulating violent images in their minds. There they conjure up the perfect victim and imagine what they will do to him or her. Initially, this may be an innocent pastime, but, as with any other addiction, these fantasies grow until they are uncontrollable. Eventually, the individual becomes obsessed with the fantasies and feels compelled to carry them out. The resulting violence only feeds their imagination, leading to thoughts and actions that are progressively more violent. According to FBI testimony before Congress:

> [The] fantasy has become a situation in which the killer is always in control, always powerful. This fantasy has gone so far as to become another reality for the killer, equivalent to, and as viable as, the real world. Indeed, the fantasy world is so real to the killer, that he believes he can move between fantasy and reality, that there is no distinguishable difference.

As the serial killer's fantasies develop, the killings and torture may become more elaborate. Ted Bundy called this a "learning curve": the more murders one commits, the more skilled he or she becomes. Compelled to continue, serial killers can stop only if they are caught or successfully undergo psychotherapy. Holmes & De Burger note, however, that the success rate of psychotherapy has essentially been nil.

A serial killer described the progression of these violent fantasies (speaking in the third person) to Ronald Holmes for his book, *Profiling Violent Crimes*:

The entire sum of his initial violent activity takes place only in his imagination, and usually minus the presence of any outwardly directed feelings of hatred. At first, he is perhaps only intrigued by the mind-pictures he allows into his imagination. Then, gradually these begin to provide him with a sense of pleasure and self-gratification, this arising from the heady sense of control and power and accomplishment he feels as he places himself in the role of the aggressor within his make-believe arena of violence . . . At this early stage, he almost certainly gives no serious thought to the possibility of carrying out violence over to actual living victims.

As he continues dwelling on such images, however, he becomes like the budding heroin addict who finds he requires a more powerful jolt, a more powerful means of self-gratification . . . Gradually, he grows more and more dissatisfied with the limited collection of mind-pictures that his imagination has worn out to excess, so he begins to search out newer and more sophisticated imagery to play out in his mind. This imagery—which he obtains from books, magazines, movies, or any other sources depicting new examples and new methods of violence—is introduced and tried out upon his still-imaginary victims, thus further reinforcing mental violence as his primary means of self-fulfillment.

The next step in the progression is that violence upon imaginary victims . . . begins to lose its gratifying effects upon the future serial killer. Thus, he switches gears anew and starts practicing his mental violence on real, living people—people he sees or knows from his school, neighborhood, or his workplace . . . probably convinced that, despite the fact that he might actually enjoy inflicting real violence . . . he still would never consider doing such a thing to them, or to any other living human being, outside the space of is own imagination . . . But even this new practice soon loses its novelty and gratifying effects . . . His deterring inhibitions gradually begin to dissolve in the face of his need for a more effective stimulus. For the first time, he begins seriously considering the thought of real violence against live human beings.

Finally, then, the decisive moment of choice arrives, and the inevitable occurs. He has practiced violence in his mind for so long and has derived such intense feelings of personal fulfillment from this imagery that his appetite for this, when it arises, is virtually insatiable. Imagery, however, no longer cuts the mustard . . . His brutal fantasies must be acted out, that only this real violence will give him the measure of relief that his compulsion craves.

What do serial killers think about their victims?

Serial killers visualize victims as objects they can dominate. Even if they know their victims well, as did Drs. Shipman and Palmer, at some point they no longer see them as human beings they care about. To be certain that they can both objectify and control their victims, they choose weak, unimportant (to them) people who approximate their fantasy ideal. As Ted Bundy remarked, "What's one less person on the face of the earth anyway?" Ronald Holmes's serial killer also had some insights in this area:

> In the case of most serial killers, the physical and personal characteristics of those on their respective list of victims only infrequently coincide with the desired traits of their imagined "ideal" . . . There are two basic, interrelated reasons for this disparity. The first centers on the extreme caution exercised by a serial killer in his predatory search for a victim; the second, upon the nature of the compulsion that drives him to violence . . . A serial killer is among the most alert and cautious of all human beings, this arising from his foremost concern to carry out his activities at the very lowest minimum of risk to himself.

The domination serial killers seek is an extension of the typical societal relationship between men and women, which the killers pathologically enhance in their fantasies. Serial killers cannot recognize the difference between small, social forms of dominance, such as leading a dance, and more aggressive forms, such as rape. The fantasy world of a serial killer is so violent that he responds fiercely to nearly every situation in real life. Ted Bundy, for example, said that he wanted total control over his victims, "possessing them physically as one would possess a potted plant, a painting, or a Porsche. Owning, as it were, this individual."

The serial killer's need to dominate and demonstrate his power over helpless victims often includes dismembering their bodies. Cutting apart the corpses proves that, in fact, his victims were nothing—and now are no more than little pieces of scrap. Central to his idea of possession is the need to dehumanize the victim. Medical training teaches physicians to distance themselves from their patients, this may help physician-killers to dehumanize their victims. As one of Dr. Shipman's colleagues, Dr. Ian Napier, said, "Being a doctor is a very numbing experience; it requires detachment. You couldn't be a good doctor if you cared too much . . . I don't think Fred Shipman saw his victims as human beings. He was completely desensitized." Ronald Holmes's serial killer, quoted in *Profiling Violent Crimes*, addressed this subject:

> Well before he ever crosses paths with his next victim, he has already stripped that person of all human meaning and worth; he has unilaterally decreed, in absentia, that the person is deserving of no human consideration whatsoever . . . This, then, is a serial killer's personal perception of all

his future victims; each one is nothing more than a mere object, depersonalized in advance, with each existing only for himself and only to be
seized and used as he sees fit . . . After years of nurturing and reinforcing
his compulsion for violence within his imagination, each serial killer comes
to a place where he finds it absolutely necessary to act out his brutal
mind-images.

Ted Bundy admitted that he often kept his female victims for hours or
days in a coma or dead before disposing of them. He told FBI agent Bill
Hagmaier, "murder isn't just a crime of lust or violence. It becomes possession.
They are part of you . . . You feel the last bit of breath leaving their bodies . . .
You're looking into their eyes . . . A person in that situation is God!"

These killers may also take body parts as "trophies" or, in some cases, may
cannibalize their victims. Jeffrey Dahmer ate some of his victims, symbolizing
complete possession and total annihilation. Similarly, California serial killer
Edmund Kemper sliced off part of one girl's leg and put it into his macaroni
casserole. Very often, rather than taking something with intrinsic worth, they
take worthless souvenirs. Dr. Shipman had many small pieces of costume
jewelry, presumably from his victims, including a box of rings that fit no one
in his household. As with any souvenirs, these are reminders of the fulfilled
fantasy that allow the killer to relive the thrill of the event and, in some cases,
prevent police from identifying the victim. Both trophies and souvenirs often
have an aphrodisiac effect on these killers.

How do serial killers justify their actions?

Given their weak personalities, perhaps it is not surprising that serial killers
rarely take responsibility for their heinous acts. If they admit their crimes,
serial killers often try to excuse their acts by blaming their mother, a spouse,
their childhood, or a nebulous conspiracy. Henry Lee Lucas blamed his
upbringing, Jeffrey Dahmer claimed that he was born "with a part missing,"
and Ted Bundy blamed his actions on the influence of pornography. Herbert
Mullin, who killed 13 people in Santa Cruz, California, claimed that "voices"
told him it was time to "sing the die song."

Bobby Joe Long, who killed at least 10 women in Florida in the early
1980s, claimed that a head injury from a motorcycle accident made him
hypersexual and, eventually, a serial killer. One of the most psychopathic
killers, John Wayne Gacy, was executed by lethal injection on May 10, 1994, for
sodomizing and killing at least 33 young men. Gacy first claimed that another
personality actually committed the crimes. He never showed remorse for his

crimes, and subsequently said that his victims deserved to die—he was simply fulfilling destiny.

As mentioned earlier, serial killers rarely talk about their crimes. When they do, it is often difficult to distinguish fact from fantasy. The poisoner-blackmailer Dr. Neill Cream and the torturer-embezzler Dr. H. H. Holmes so embellished their confessions that one is uncertain whether they were confessing, bragging, or simply confabulating. Drs. Palmer, Shipman, and Petiot followed the more common route and simply refused either to admit their guilt or to discuss their situation.

What is "profiling"?

Whoever fights monsters should see to it that in the process he does not become a monster. And when you look long into an abyss, the abyss also looks into you.
— Friedrich Nietzsche

The FBI's Behavioral Science Unit developed the art of profiling to determine a criminal's social and psychological makeup. The ultimate purpose is to develop clues to help identify a criminal and to give police possible strategies to use when interviewing suspects. Police in many jurisdictions now use profiling, also known as "investigative criminal profiling," to determine specific characteristics to look for in suspects, recognize a crime pattern that may help them locate suspects, and ask the right questions when they interview suspects. Police most commonly use profiling when it appears that one offender is repeating major crimes, such as homicide, rape, and arson.

Profilers focus on the criminal's behavior during crimes, the *modus operandi*, which provides clues to their personality and motivation. The perpetrator's psychological needs motivate him to kill specific victims in a specific manner. The distinct and unchanging elements of the crime, which John Douglas terms the "signature," often reveal more about a criminal than the method used. As shorthand for profiling, Douglas uses the equation:

Why? + How? = Who?

Profiling is gradually being transformed from an art to a science as it becomes integrated with the other forensic sciences. Profilers often begin with whatever behavioral clues they can find at a crime scene. For example, they carefully look at the state of the body: What did the killer do with and to the corpse? Did he "overkill" the victim, attacking the corpse long after death or inflicting injuries far worse than were necessary to kill? If so, investigators assume that the killer was expressing severe anger, and possibly knew his victim. If he wrapped up the body, positioned it in a specific way, or covered the face, the killer may feel remorse, and may have known the victim before the crime. If the killer leaves the body in plain sight or casually dumps it at a convenient site, it may suggest contempt for the victim.

The importance of profiling derives from the serial killer's anonymity; police only know a serial killer's identity once they capture him. Called UNSUBs, or Unknown Subjects, by profilers, serial killers are difficult to identify because they hide behind carefully constructed facades of normalcy. While they do not know how to feel sympathy for others, they learn how to simulate it through observation. They are smooth talkers—glibness is part of their persona. These psychopaths know society's rights and wrongs, and outwardly act and speak as if they, too, hold these values. When they are finally caught, they may assume a mask of insanity, and use every possible psychiatric ploy to avoid responsibility for their acts. Robert Louis Stevenson translated this duality into the title character in *Dr. Jeckyll and Mr. Hyde*.

Profilers also try to determine a serial killer's age. John Douglas says that "when we're trying to determine the age of the UNSUB in a violent crime, we usually start at 25 and add or subtract years based on the degree of sophistication." Profilers also know that these men are commonly fascinated with the police and with authority in general. Many join the military or impersonate law enforcement officials, since carrying badges and driving police-type vehicles makes them feel important. This behavior is an extension of the serial killer's pathological need for dominance, and a way to bring their fantasy into reality.

Police do not expect to talk to a serial killer until they apprehend him. As the saying goes, "Killers don't call, and callers don't kill." People who call police usually have a profit motive, such as kidnappers. Serial killers rarely call law enforcement personnel, although they may send other messages. When they do, profilers can use psycholinguistic analysis of their words or symbols to further characterize the individual's personality, level of sophistication, motivation, and threat level.

Profiling, of course, has its limitations, but it remains a powerful tool. When asked about the most infamous serial killer in history, Jack the Ripper, John Douglas said "It would be difficult to come up with the Ripper's specific identity at this late date, but even after a century we can very legitimately profile the UNSUB and say with reasonable assurance the type of individual he was."

What types of serial killers are there?

Investigators classify serial killers according to several factors, including where the crime is committed, how organized they are, and their apparent motive. Such information aids profilers as they try to determine the killer's identity, and how to capture him.

Crime Scene

One common method that police use to classify serial killers is the nature of their crime scenes. This relates to their method of operation, or *modus operandi* (MO), meaning their pre- and post-killing behavior. This helps police gain insights into their motivation and personality. The FBI's standard categorization for violent crime scenes is: organized, disorganized, or mixed.

Organized crime scenes indicate a deliberate, preplanned killing with significant preparation, a methodical approach, and advance knowledge of the victim and the crime scene. These individuals are similar to Holmes & De Burger's "act-focused" killers, who murder quickly and efficiently after meticulously planning their attacks. They may stalk their victim for weeks, bring their own weapon, and make elaborate plans for the disposition of the body. Drs. Holmes, Petiot, and Shipman had organized crime scenes.

The *disorganized* and *mixed* crime scenes demonstrate a lack of planning—the killer picks victims almost at random, uses weapons of opportunity, and is extremely violent. There is either no plan at all or the plan goes awry, such as in Dr. Cream's killings. These murderers kill for the idea of killing. They are similar to what Holmes & De Burger refer to as "process-focused" killers, who use excessive violence and often dismember or abuse the dead victim.

Mobility

Police and profilers also classify serial killers by their *degree of mobility*, or the geographic area from which they obtain their victims. Many serial killers live in the same area for a long period, killing their victims in adjacent neighborhoods and disposing of the bodies nearby. This is the pattern for most physician-serial killers: Because their killings often appear to be natural deaths, there is no reason to hide or to dispose of the bodies. In addition, most have a professional practice to maintain, and so are restricted to the same locale. Other serial killers, however, travel frequently or, even, continuously in an effort to confuse and thwart the police. Extremely mobile serial killers may be the hardest to catch, since they go from one police jurisdiction to the next and decades may pass without anyone noticing a pattern.

Motive

Police also classify serial killers by the *motive*, or the *reason they killed*. Killers have both intent and motive. Intent refers to making a choice to commit the crime. In the case of serial killers, there is no question about whether their actions are deliberate—they mean to kill. More important for identifying the serial killer and, perhaps, predicting who may become such a monster in the future, is the question of motive. Why do serial killers perform their heinous acts? According to Douglas & Olshaker, "the key to that is in the victimology. Who has he chosen as his victims, and why? Are they victims of opportunity, or was a careful and deliberate choice made? . . . Why did he do it? The who? follows directly from there." In their book *Serial Murder*, Holmes & De Burger describe four types of serial killers based on motive:

- **Visionary:** This type kills in response to voices or visions that they receive from an evil force or from God.

- **Mission-oriented:** This type selects some specific group (such as prostitutes in Dr. Cream's case and their "enemies" in the cases of the two Japanese physicians in *The Minor Players*) who they want to eliminate.

- **Hedonists:** This type obtains sexual gratification from violence and killing; they are also called lust or thrill killers. Others in the hedonistic group kill for personal gain. Individuals with a sexual motivation usually suffer from *paraphilias*, disorders of sexual aim or direction. Drs. Petiot and Holmes represent this group.

- **Power/Control-oriented:** Power/control killers also get sexual gratification from having the power of life and death over their victims. This group includes many in this book; Dr. Shipman certainly falls into this category.

The table on the next page attempts to relate crime scene characteristics with these four types of serial killers.

The Crime Classification Manual divides homicidal motives into four categories to help identify the killers: *criminal enterprise, personal causes, group cause*, and *sexual motivation*. The names of the categories are descriptive enough so that a further explanation really isn't necessary. The physicians in this book who killed for *criminal enterprise* are Drs. Weil, Hyde, Hazzard, and Palmer. Those killing for *personal causes* include Drs. Ruxton, Kappler, Suzuki, Takahashi, Green, Crippen, and Webster. Those with a *group cause*, such as political, religious, or socioeconomic extremists, are the World War II Japanese physicians and Stalin. Because their crimes involve multiple participants, these

Crime Scene Analysis of Suspected Serial Murder Cases

Crime Scene Characteristics	Type of Serial Killer			
	Power/ Control	Hedonist	Visionary	Mission
Controlled crime scene	Yes	Yes	No	Yes
Overkill	No	Variable	Yes	No
Chaotic crime scene	No	No	Yes	No
Evidence of torture	Yes	Yes	No	No
Body moved	Yes	Yes	No	No
Specific victim	Yes	Yes	No	Yes
Weapon at scene	No	No	Yes	No
Relational victim	No	No	No	No
Victim known	No	No	Yes	No
Aberrant sex	Yes	Yes	No	No
Weapon of torture	Yes	Yes	No	No
Strangles the victim	Yes	Yes	No	No
Penile penetration	Yes	Yes	Variable	Yes
Object penetration	No	Yes	Yes	No
Necrophilia	Yes	Variable	Yes	No
Usual gender	Male	Male	Male	Male

Adapted from: Holmes, RM, Holmes ST: *Profiling Violent Crimes: An Investigative Tool*, 2nd ed. Thousand Oaks, CA: Sage Publications, 1996, p. 81.

extremists seek a convenient, secluded spot at which to safely commit their crimes. The Japanese military physicians used secret bases in occupied Manchuria; Stalin used his prisons. Sexually motivated killers include Drs. Cream, Holmes, and Petiot.

Sexual homicides, the category for most serial killers, are also usually sadistic crimes, in which the killer derives the greatest satisfaction from the victim's response to torture. Drs. Holmes and Petiot are in this category. In these instances, the level of violence always exceeds that which is necessary to force the victims to comply with the sexual act. The victim's pain, fear, and discomfort arouse the perpetrator sexually. The torture methods used are often custom-made. These killers focus their violence on the erogenous parts of the victims' bodies and have already prepared elaborate methods to dispose of the bodies.

In attempting to determine the motive for the killings, investigators are taking the first step toward identifying the killer. This is an integral part of profiling.

Bibliography

Introduction: Physicians as Multiple Murderers

Danto BL, Bruhns J, Kutscher AH (eds.): *The Human Side of Homicide.* New York: Columbia Univ. Press, 1982.

Douglas J, Olshaker M: *The Anatomy of Motive: The FBI's Legendary Mindhunter Explores the Key to Understanding and Catching Violent Criminals.* New York: Pocket Books, 1999.

Douglas J, Burgess AW, Burgess AG, Ressler RK: *Crime Classification Manual: A Standard System for Investigating and Classifying Violent Crimes.* San Francisco: Jossey-Bass, 1997.

Eckert WG: Physician crimes and criminals. the historical and forensic aspects. *Amer J Forensic Med Path.* 1982;3(3):221–30.

Furneaux R: *The Medical Murderer.* New York: Abelard-Schuman, 1957.

Hall A: *Crimes and Punishment: A Pictorial Encyclopedia of Aberrant Behavior.* Vol. 3. Paulton, England: BPC Pub., 1973, pp. 9–30.

Hickey EW: *Serial Murderers and Their Victims.* 2nd ed. Washington, D.C.: Wadsworth, 1997.

Holmes RM, De Burger J: *Serial Murder.* Beverly Hills, CA: Sage, 1988.

Holmes RM, Holmes ST: *Profiling Violent Crimes: An Investigative Tool.* 2nd ed. Thousand Oaks, CA: Sage, 1996.

Jones F: *Beyond Suspicion: True Stories of Unexpected Killers.* Toronto: Key Porter, 1992.

Scott SL: *What Makes Serial Killers Tick?* (film) Dark Horse Entertainment, 2000.

Simon RI: *Bad Men Do What Good Men Dream: A Forensic Psychiatrist Illuminates the Darker Side of Human Behavior.* Washington, D.C.: American Psychiatric Press, 1996.

Chapter 1: William Palmer, M.D.

Anon.: *Illustrated Life and Career of William Palmer of Rugeley.* London: Ward & Lock, 1856.

Anon.: *The Illustrated and Unabridged Edition of* The Times *Report of the Trial of William Palmer.* London: Ward & Lock, 1856.

Bunaby E: "The Fatal Gambles of William Palmer." In: Goodman J (ed.): *Medical Murders: Classic True-Crime Stories.* London: BCA, 1991, pp. 67–77.

Davison A: Murder and medicine. *Report of Proceedings of the Scottish Society of the History of Medicine.* 1969–70:15–27.

Glaister J: The trial of William Palmer. *Saint Bartholomew's Hosp J.* 1956;60:273–81.

Graves R: *They Hanged My Saintly Billy.* London: Cassell & Co., 1957.

Haines M: *Doctors Who Kill.* Toronto: The Sun, 1993, pp. 9–12.

Knott GH (ed.): *The Trial of William Palmer (for Murder by Poisoning).* 3rd ed. (rev. by Watson ER) London: William Hodge, 1952.

Linnett MJ: William Palmer. *Saint Bartholomew's Hosp J.* 1956;60:268–72.

Ward J: *Crimebusting Breakthroughs in Forensic Science.* London: Blandford, 1998, pp. 47–60.

Chapter 2: Thomas Neill Cream, M.D., C.M.

Altick RD: *Victorian Studies in Scarlet.* New York: W.W. Norton, 1970, pp. 259–67.

Bensley EH: McGill University's most infamous medical graduate. *Canadian Med Assoc J.* 1973;109:1024–27.

Boswell C, Thompson L: *Practitioners of Murder.* New York: Collier Books, 1962.

Haines, *Doctors Who Kill,* pp. 43–47.

Jesse FT: *Murder and Its Motives*. London: Harrap, 1952.

McLaren A: *A Prescription for Murder: The Victorian Serial Killings of Dr. Thomas Neill Cream*. Chicago: Univ. of Chicago Press, 1993.

Miller O: *Twenty Mortal Murders: Bizarre Murder Cases from Canada's Past*. Toronto: MacMillan of Canada, 1978.

Shore WT (ed.): *Trial of Thomas Neill Cream*. London: William Hodge, 1923.

Chapter 3: Herman Webster Mudgett, M.D., alias Dr. H. H. Holmes

Ashbury H: *The Gem of the Prairie: An Informal History of the Chicago Underworld*. New York: Knopf, 1940.

Boswell, Thompson, *Practitioners of Murder*, pp. 83–103.

Franke D: *The Torture Doctor*. New York: Hawthorn Books, 1975.

Geyer FP: *The Homes-Pitezel Case: A History of the Greatest Crime of the Century and of the Search for the Missing Pitezel Children*. (No city given): Publishers' Union, 1896.

Miller, *Twenty Mortal Murders*, pp. 142–56.

Schechter H: *Depraved: The Shocking True Story of America's First Serial Killer*. New York: Pocket Books, 1994.

U.S. Five: *The Devil's Rood: A Group Novel about America's First Serial Killer* (fictionalized account). Berkeley, CA: Creative Arts Book Company, 1999.

Chapter 4: Linda Burfield Hazzard, D.O.

Gevitz N: *The D.O.'s: Osteopathic Medicine in America*. Baltimore: The Johns Hopkins Univ. Press, 1982.

Hazzard LB: *Diet in Disease and Systemic Cleansing*. Wanganui, N.Z.: H. I. Jones & Son, 1917.

Hazzard LB: *Fasting for the Cure of Disease*. Seattle: Hazzard Pub. Co., 1908, 1910.

Hazzard LB: *Scientific Fasting: the Ancient and Modern Key to Health*. (5th ed. of *Fasting for the Cure of Disease*). New York: Grant Pub., 1927.

Olsen G: *Starvation Heights: The True Story of an American Doctor and the Murder of a British Heiress*. New York: Warner Books, 1997.

Chapter 5: The Russian Doctors' Plots

Birstein VJ: *The Perversion of Knowledge: The True Story of Soviet Science*. Cambridge, MA: Westview Press, 2001.

Conquest R: *The Great Terror: A Reassessment*. New York: Oxford Univ. Press, 1990.

Orlov A: *The Secret History of Stalin's Crimes*. New York: Random House, 1953.

Rancour-Laferriere D: *The Mind of Stalin: A Psychoanalytical Study*. Ann Arbor, MI: Ardis, 1988.

Rapoport L: *Stalin's War against the Jews: The Doctors' Plot and the Soviet Solution*. New York: The Free Press, 1990.

Rapoport Y: *The Doctors' Plot of 1953*. Cambridge, MA: Harvard Univ. Press, 1991.

Rappaport H: *Joseph Stalin: A Biographical Companion*. Santa Barbara, CA: ABC-CLIO, 1999.

Talbott S (trans., ed.): *Khrushchev Remembers*. Boston: Little Brown, 1979.

Tushnet L: Murder by disease. *Ann Med Hist*. 1939:121–27.

"Vicious Spies and Killers under the Mask of Academic Physicians." *Pravda*. January 13, 1953, p. 1. Wolfe PR (trans.)

Volkogonov D: *Stalin: Triumph and Tragedy*. Shukman H, ed., trans. London: Weidenfeld & Nicolson, 1991 [English]. Orig. pub. as *Triyumf I Tragediya: politicheskii portret I. V. Stalina*. Moscow: Novosti, 1989.

Chapter 6: Marcel André Félix Petiot, M.D.

Grombach JV: *The Great Liquidator*. Garden City, NY: Doubleday, 1980.

Haines, *Doctors Who Kill*, pp. 117–26.

Heppenstall R: *Bluebeard & After: Three Decades of Murder in France*. London: Owen, 1972.

Maeder T: *The Unspeakable Crimes of Dr. Petiot*. Boston: Atlantic Monthly Press, 1980.

Massu (Commissaire) GV: *L'enquête Petiot: La Plus Grande Affaire Criminelle du Siècle*. Paris: Libraire Arthème Fayard, 1959.

Seth R: *Petiot: Victim of Chance*. London: Hutchinson, 1963.

Sobran J: "Murder Most Patriotic." Griffin Internet Syndicate, 1999.

Chapter 7: The Minor Players

Ablow KR: *The Strange Case of Dr. Kappler: The Doctor Who Became a Killer*. New York: Free Press, 1994.

Anon.: "Deadly Doctors." In: Hall, *Crimes and Punishment*, pp. 9–30.

Anon.: *The Trial of Professor John White Webster*. New York: Chas. Scribner's Sons, 1928.

Anon.: *Trial of John W. Webster for the Murder of Dr. George Parkman*. Jersey City, NJ: F. D. Linn & Co., 1879.

Blundell RH, Wilson GH: *Trial of Buck Ruxton*. Edinburgh: Hodge, 1936.

Borowitz A: "The Janitor's Story." *A Gallery of Sinister Perspectives: Ten Crimes and A Scandal*. Kent, Ohio: Kent State Univ. Press, 1982.

Carlson ET: "The Unfortunate Dr. Parkman." *Amer J Psychiat*. 123:Dec. 6, 1966.

Carus WS: *Bioterrorism and Biocrimes: The Illicit Use of Biological Agents Since 1900*. Washington, D.C.: Center for Counterproliferation Research, National Defense Univ., August 1998 (Rev. February 2001).

Goodman J (ed.): *Medical Murders: Classic True-Crime Stories*. London: BCA, 1991, pp. 5–24.

"Grand Jury Testimony." *Kansas City Star*. April 24, 1910, p. A4.

Irving HB: *A Book of Remarkable Criminals*. New York: Hyperion, 1975.

Musick J: "Debora Green Back in Court." *New York Times*. May 25, 2000.

Rizzo T: "Green Asks To Withdraw Pleas of No Contest to Killing Children." *Kansas City Star*. January 6, 2000.

Rabson 3M: Doctors delinquent: the trials of two physicians charged with murder. *JAMA*. 1971;216(1):121.

Rule A: *Bitter Harvest : A Woman's Fury, a Mother's Sacrifice*. New York: Simon & Schuster, 1998.

Smith EH: *Famous Poison Mysteries*. New York: Dial Press, 1927.

The Complete Newgate Calendar, Vol. IV.

Ward, *Crimebusting Breakthroughs*, pp. 165–175.

Young F: *The Trial of H. H. Crippen*. London: Notable British Trials Series, 1920.

Chapter 8: Japan's Inhuman Experiments

Blumenthal R: "Japan Rebuffs Requests for Information about Its Germ-Warfare Atrocities." *New York Times*. March 4, 1999, p. A12.

Gold H: *Unit 731: Testimony*. Singapore: Yenbooks, 1996.

Harris SH: *Factories of Death: Japanese Biological Warfare, 1932–45, and the American Cover-Up*. New York: Rutledge, 1994.

Kristof ND: "Japan Confronting Gruesome War Atrocity." *New York Times*. March 17, 1995.

Materials on the Trial of Former Servicemen of the Japanese Army Charged with Manufacturing and Employing Bacteriological Weapons. Moscow: Foreign Languages Pub. House, 1950.

Sidell FR, Takafuji ET, Franz DR (eds.): *Medical Aspects of Chemical and Biological Warfare*. Washington, D.C.: Office of the Surgeon General, Walter Reed Army Medical Center, 1997.

Thompson A, Lt. Col., V.C.: *Report on Japanese Biological Warfare (BW) Activities*. U.S. Army. May 31, 1946. Declassified September 10, 1970.

Thomas P: "War Crimes List Bars 16 Japanese from U.S." *The Washington Post*. December 4, 1996, p. A1.

Tyler PE: "In Chinese Village, Germ Warfare is Remembered Nightmare." *New York Times*. April 2, 1997.

U.S. Senate: *Congressional Record*. (10 November 1999), pp. S14533-S14571. (Bill S.1902).

Whymant R: Butchers of Harbin. *Connecticut Med*. 1983;47(3):163–65.

Williams P, Wallace D: *Unit 731: The Japanese Army's Secret of Secrets*. London: Hodder & Stoughton, 1989.

Zilinskas RA (ed.): *The Microbiologist and Biological Defense Research: Ethics, Politics, and International Security*. New York: New York Academy of Sciences, 1992.

Chapter 9: Harold Frederick Shipman, MBChB

Baker R: *Harold Shipman's Clinical Practice 1974–1998: A Clinical Audit Commissioned by the Chief Medical Officer*. London: British Dept. of Health, 2000.

Carter H: "Doctor 'duped families to save his skin.'" *The Guardian*. January 6, 2000.

Gerrard N: "The True Evil of this Killer Doctor." *The Guardian Unlimited*. January 7, 2000.

Iserson KV: *Death to Dust: What Happens to Dead Bodies?* 2nd ed. Tucson, AZ: Galen Press, Ltd., 2001.

Sitford M, Panter S: *Addicted to Murder: The True Story of Dr. Harold Shipman*. London: Virgin Pub., 2000.

Whittle B, Ritchie J: *Prescription for Murder: The True Story of Mass Murderer Dr. Harold Frederick Shipman*. London: Warner, 2000.

Chapter 10: Serial Killers: Psychology & Behavior

Danto et al., *Human Side of Homicide*, 1982.

Douglas, Olshaker, *Anatomy of Motive*, 1999.

Douglas et al., *Crime Classification Manual*, 1997.

Hickey, *Serial Murderers*, 1997.

Holmes, De Burger, *Profiling Violent Crimes*, 1996.

Scott, *What Makes Serial Killers Tick?*, (film), 2000.

Simon, *Bad Men Do What Good Men Dream*, 1996.

Index

Permissions

About the Author

Kenneth V. Iserson, M.D., MBA, FACEP, is a Professor of Emergency Medicine and Director of the Arizona Bioethics Program at the University of Arizona Health Sciences Center, Tucson, Arizona. He practices emergency medicine and is the medical director of southern Arizona's major search and rescue operation. While Dr. Iserson has written about death, after-death counseling (*Grave Words: Notifying Survivors About Unexpected Deaths*), and the multitude of dispositions for corpses (*Death to Dust: What Happens to Dead Bodies? 2nd ed.*) nothing that he has done in his 30-year medical career has made him eligible to be a subject of this book. He promises that his energies will remain with writing and practicing medicine and bioethics—and that he will not let his talents drive him over to "the dark side."

Galen

Galen of Pergamum (A.D. 130-201), the Greek physician whose writings guided medicine for more than a millennium after his death, inspired the name, Galen Press. As the father of modern anatomy and physiology, Galen wrote more than 100 treatises while attempting to change medicine from an art form into a science. As a practicing physician, Galen first ministered to gladiators and then to Roman Emperor Marcus Aurelius. Far more than Hippocrates, Galen's work influenced Western physicians and was the "truth" until the late Middle Ages, when physicians and scientists challenged his teachings. Galen Press, publishing non-clinical, health-related books, will follow Galen's advice that "the chief merit of language is clearness . . . nothing detracts so much from this as unfamiliar terms."

Also by Galen Press, Ltd.

After-Death Planning Guide
Kenneth V. Iserson, M.D.

Civil War Medicine: Challenges and Triumphs
Alfred Jay Bollet, M.D.

Death to Dust: What Happens to Dead Bodies? 2nd ed.
Kenneth V. Iserson, M.D.

Death Investigation: The Basics
Brad Randall, M.D.

Ethics in Emergency Medicine, 2nd ed.
Edited by Kenneth V. Iserson, M.D., Arthur B. Sanders, M.D.,
and Deborah Mathieu, Ph.D.

Get Into Medical School! A Guide for the Perplexed
Kenneth V. Iserson, M.D.

Getting Into A Residency Companion Disk for Windows™

Grave Words: Notifying Survivors about Sudden, Unexpected Deaths
Kenneth V. Iserson, M.D.

House Calls, Rounds, and Healings: A Poetry Casebook
David Schiedermayer, M.D.

Iserson's Getting Into A Residency: A Guide for Medical Students, 5th ed.
Kenneth V. Iserson, M.D.

Non-Standard Medical Electives in the U.S. & Canada, 2nd ed.
Kenneth V. Iserson, M.D.

Résumés and Personal Statements for Health Professionals, 2nd ed.
James W. Tysinger, Ph.D.

The Cost-Effective Use of Leeches and Other Musings of A Medical School Survivor
Jeffrey A. Drayer, M.D.

The International Medical Graduate's Guide to U.S. Medicine
Louis B. Ball

For more information, please contact:

Customer Service, Galen Press, Ltd.
P.O. Box 64400, Tucson, AZ 85728-4400 USA
http://www.galenpress.com
Tel: (520) 577-8363   Fax: (520) 529-6459

Pocket Protocols
for Notifying Survivors about Sudden, Unexpected Deaths
Pocket-sized booklet containing the protocols from *Grave Words*

ISBN: 1-883620-05-8 $ 6.95 (Bulk discounts available)

Slides for Grave Words

- Slide Sets of the Protocols & other tables from Grave Words
- Build your own Death Notification and Death & Dying Course using the specialized slide sets

Slide Set	Number of Slides
A. Main Protocol for Death Notification	65
B. General Set: Sudden Death/Nurse Interactions/ Grief/Communication/Survivors' Questions	50
C. Chaplains/Religions	42
D. Emergency Medicine/Trauma	35
E. Phrases: Helping and Hurtful	23
F. Telephone Notification Protocol	20
G. Students' Deaths	17
H. Emergency Medical Services	16
I. Telling Friends	16
J. Children: Telling & Grieving	13
K. Obstetrics	14
L. Disaster Survivors' Protocol	10
M. Organ Donation	10

Prices:

Item 1: Complete set of 330 slides: $ 395.00

Item 2: Main Protocol + Any three other sets: $ 345.00

Item 3: Main Protocol + Any two other sets: $ 295.00

Item 4: Main Protocol + Any one other set: $ 250.00

Item 5: Individual set: $3.00/slide

Items 1-4: Includes one copy each of *Grave Words & Pocket Protocols*.
Add shipping of $15 for each item.

To order, and for more information, please contact Galen Press, LTD., at:
P.O. Box 64400 Tucson, AZ 85728-4400 USA
Internet: www.galenpress.com
Tel: (520) 577-8363 Fax: (520) 529-6459

Previews: We keep our prices low by not offering previews. See our 30-Day Guarantee.

Thirty Day Money Back Guarantee: You may return your purchase *within thirty days* for a refund of the purchase price. (Shipping costs not refundable.)

Note: Prices subject to change.

Order Form

Yes! . . . Please send me:

_____ copies of **Demon Doctors: Physicians as Serial Killers,**
   @ $28.95 each $ _____

_____ copies of **Civil War Medicine: Challenges and Triumphs,**
   @ $44.95 each $ _____

_____ copies of **Death to Dust: What Happens to**
   Dead Bodies? @ $48.95 each $ _____

_____ copies of **Getting Into A Residency: A Guide For**
   Medical Students, 5th ed. @ $36.95 each $ _____

_____ copies of **The Companion Disk** @ $12.00 $ _____

_____ copies of **Grave Words: Notifying Survivors about**
   Sudden, Unexpected Deaths @ $38.95 each $ _____

_____ copies of **Pocket Protocols** @ $6.95 each $ _____

_____ copies of **Ethics In Emergency Medicine, 2nd ed.**
   @ $39.95 each $ _____

_____ copies of **Résumés and Personal Statements for Health**
   Professionals, 2nd ed. @ $18.95 each $ _____

_____ copies of **Death Investigation: The Basics** @ $24.95 each $ _____

_____ copies of **Get Into Medical School! A Guide for the**
   Perplexed @ $34.95 each $ _____

_____ copies of **The International Medical Graduates' Guide**
   to U.S. Medicine @ $31.95 each $ _____

_____ copies of **House Calls, Rounds, and Healings:**
   A Poetry Casebook @ $12.95 each $ _____

_____ copies of **The Cost-Effective Use of Leeches and Other**
   Musings of a Medical School Survivor @ $14.95 each $ _____

AZ Residents – Add 7.6% sales tax $ _____

Shipping: $3.50 for 1st Book, $1.00 / each additional $ _____

Priority Mail: **ADD** $3.00 for 1st Book, $2.00 / each additional $ _____

TOTAL ENCLOSED (U.S. Funds Only) $ _____

❑ Check   ❑ VISA   ❑ MasterCard

SHIP TO: Name _____

  Address _____

  _____

  City/State/Zip _____

  Phone **(required)** _____

CREDIT CARD Number: _____

Expiration date: _____   Signature: _____

Send completed form and payment to:

Galen Press, Ltd.   Tel (520) 577-8363
PO Box 64400-D2   Fax (520) 529-6459
Tucson, AZ 85728-4400 USA   Orders: 1-800-442-5369 (US/Canada)

Visit our Home Page at www.galenpress.com
Also available through your local bookstore.
Prices Subject to Change

Pocket Protocols
for Notifying Survivors about Sudden, Unexpected Deaths
Pocket-sized booklet containing the protocols from *Grave Words*

ISBN: 1-883620-05-8 $ 6.95 (Bulk discounts available)

Slides for Grave Words

- Slide Sets of the Protocols & other tables from Grave Words
- Build your own Death Notification and Death & Dying Course using the specialized slide sets

Slide Set	Number of Slides
A. Main Protocol for Death Notification	65
B. General Set: Sudden Death/Nurse Interactions/ Grief/Communication/Survivors' Questions	50
C. Chaplains/Religions	42
D. Emergency Medicine/Trauma	35
E. Phrases: Helping and Hurtful	23
F. Telephone Notification Protocol	20
G. Students' Deaths	17
H. Emergency Medical Services	16
I. Telling Friends	16
J. Children: Telling & Grieving	13
K. Obstetrics	14
L. Disaster Survivors' Protocol	10
M. Organ Donation	10

Prices:
Item 1: Complete set of 330 slides: $ 395.00
Item 2: Main Protocol + Any three other sets: $ 345.00
Item 3: Main Protocol + Any two other sets: $ 295.00
Item 4: Main Protocol + Any one other set: $ 250.00
Item 5: Individual set: $3.00/slide

Items 1-4: Includes one copy each of **Grave Words & Pocket Protocols.**
Add shipping of $15 for each item.

To order, and for more information, please contact Galen Press, Ltd., at:
P.O. Box 64400   Tucson, AZ 85728-4400 USA
Internet: www.galenpress.com
Tel: (520) 577-8363   Fax: (520) 529-6459

Previews: We keep our prices low by not offering previews. See our 30-Day Guarantee.

Thirty Day Money Back Guarantee: You may return your purchase *within thirty days* for a refund of the purchase price. (Shipping costs not refundable.)

Note: Prices subject to change.

Order Form

Yes! . . . Please send me:

_____ copies of **Demon Doctors: Physicians as Serial Killers,**
    @ $28.95 each $ _____

_____ copies of **Civil War Medicine: Challenges and Triumphs,**
    @ $44.95 each $ _____

_____ copies of **Death to Dust: What Happens to
Dead Bodies?** @ $48.95 each $ _____

_____ copies of **Getting Into A Residency: A Guide For
Medical Students, 5th ed.** @ $36.95 each $ _____

_____ copies of **The Companion Disk** @ $12.00 $ _____

_____ copies of **Grave Words: Notifying Survivors about
Sudden, Unexpected Deaths** @ $38.95 each $ _____

_____ copies of **Pocket Protocols** @ $6.95 each $ _____

_____ copies of **Ethics In Emergency Medicine, 2nd ed.**
@ $39.95 each $ _____

_____ copies of **Résumés and Personal Statements for Health
Professionals, 2nd ed.** @ $18.95 each $ _____

_____ copies of **Death Investigation: The Basics** @ $24.95 each $ _____

_____ copies of **Get Into Medical School! A Guide for the
Perplexed** @ $34.95 each $ _____

_____ copies of **The International Medical Graduates' Guide
to U.S. Medicine** @ $31.95 each $ _____

_____ copies of **House Calls, Rounds, and Healings:
A Poetry Casebook** @ $12.95 each $ _____

_____ copies of **The Cost-Effective Use of Leeches and Other
Musings of a Medical School Survivor** @ $14.95 each $ _____

AZ Residents – Add 7.6% sales tax $ _____

Shipping: $3.50 for 1st Book, $1.00 / each additional $ _____

Priority Mail: **ADD** $3.00 for 1st Book, $2.00 / each additional $ _____

TOTAL ENCLOSED (U.S. Funds Only) $ _____

❐ Check   ❐ VISA   ❐ MasterCard

SHIP TO: Name _____

  Address _____

  _____

  City/State/Zip _____

  Phone **(required)** _____

CREDIT CARD Number: _____

Expiration date: _____ Signature: _____

Send completed form and payment to:

Galen Press, Ltd.   Tel (520) 577-8363
PO Box 64400-D2   Fax (520) 529-6459
Tucson, AZ 85728-4400 USA   Orders: 1-800-442-5369 (US/Canada)

Visit our Home Page at www.galenpress.com
Also available through your local bookstore.
Prices Subject to Change

Pocket Protocols
for Notifying Survivors about Sudden, Unexpected Deaths
Pocket-sized booklet containing the protocols from *Grave Words*

ISBN: 1-883620-05-8 $ 6.95 (Bulk discounts available)

Slides for Grave Words

- Slide Sets of the Protocols & other tables from Grave Words
- Build your own Death Notification and Death & Dying Course using the specialized slide sets

Slide Set	Number of Slides
A. Main Protocol for Death Notification	65
B. General Set: Sudden Death/Nurse Interactions/ Grief/Communication/Survivors' Questions	50
C. Chaplains/Religions	42
D. Emergency Medicine/Trauma	35
E. Phrases: Helping and Hurtful	23
F. Telephone Notification Protocol	20
G. Students' Deaths	17
H. Emergency Medical Services	16
I. Telling Friends	16
J. Children: Telling & Grieving	13
K. Obstetrics	14
L. Disaster Survivors' Protocol	10
M. Organ Donation	10

Prices: **Item 1:** Complete set of 330 slides: $ 395.00
Item 2: Main Protocol + Any three other sets: $ 345.00
Item 3: Main Protocol + Any two other sets: $ 295.00
Item 4: Main Protocol + Any one other set: $ 250.00
Item 5: Individual set: $3.00/slide

Items 1-4: Includes one copy each of **Grave Words & Pocket Protocols**.
Add shipping of $15 for each item.

To order, and for more information, please contact Galen Press, LTD., at:
P.O. Box 64400 Tucson, AZ 85728-4400 USA
Internet: www.galenpress.com
Tel: (520) 577-8363 Fax: (520) 529-6459

Previews: We keep our prices low by not offering previews. See our 30-Day Guarantee.

Thirty Day Money Back Guarantee: You may return your purchase *within thirty days* for a refund of the purchase price. (Shipping costs not refundable.)

Note: Prices subject to change.

Order Form

Yes! . . . Please send me:

_____ copies of **Demon Doctors: Physicians as Serial Killers,** @ $28.95 each $ _____

_____ copies of **Civil War Medicine: Challenges and Triumphs,** @ $44.95 each $ _____

_____ copies of **Death to Dust: What Happens to Dead Bodies?** @ $48.95 each $ _____

_____ copies of **Getting Into A Residency: A Guide For Medical Students, 5th ed.** @ $36.95 each $ _____

_____ copies of **The Companion Disk** @ $12.00 $ _____

_____ copies of **Grave Words: Notifying Survivors about Sudden, Unexpected Deaths** @ $38.95 each $ _____

_____ copies of **Pocket Protocols** @ $6.95 each $ _____

_____ copies of **Ethics In Emergency Medicine, 2nd ed.** @ $39.95 each $ _____

_____ copies of **Résumés and Personal Statements for Health Professionals, 2nd ed.** @ $18.95 each $ _____

_____ copies of **Death Investigation: The Basics** @ $24.95 each $ _____

_____ copies of **Get Into Medical School! A Guide for the Perplexed** @ $34.95 each $ _____

_____ copies of **The International Medical Graduates' Guide to U.S. Medicine** @ $31.95 each $ _____

_____ copies of **House Calls, Rounds, and Healings: A Poetry Casebook** @ $12.95 each $ _____

_____ copies of **The Cost-Effective Use of Leeches and Other Musings of a Medical School Survivor** @ $14.95 each $ _____

AZ Residents – Add 7.6% sales tax $ _____

Shipping: $3.50 for 1st Book, $1.00 / each additional $ _____

Priority Mail: **ADD** $3.00 for 1st Book, $2.00 / each additional $ _____

TOTAL ENCLOSED (U.S. Funds Only) $ _____

❏ Check   ❏ VISA   ❏ MasterCard

SHIP TO: Name _____

Address _____

_____

City/State/Zip _____

Phone **(required)** _____

CREDIT CARD Number: _____

Expiration date: _____   Signature: _____

Send completed form and payment to:

Galen Press, Ltd.   Tel (520) 577-8363
PO Box 64400-D2   Fax (520) 529-6459
Tucson, AZ 85728-4400 USA   Orders: 1-800-442-5369 (US/Canada)

Visit our Home Page at www.galenpress.com
Also available through your local bookstore.
Prices Subject to Change